Advances and Refinements in Asian Aesthetic Surgery

Editor

LEE L.Q. PU

CLINICS IN PLASTIC SURGERY

www.plasticsurgery.theclinics.com

January 2023 • Volume 50 • Number 1

ELSEVIER

1600 John F. Kennedy Boulevard ● Suite 1800 ● Philadelphia, Pennsylvania, 19103-2899

http://www.theclinics.com

CLINICS IN PLASTIC SURGERY Volume 50, Number 1
January 2023 ISSN 0094-1298, ISBN-13: 978-0-323-92021-6

Editor: Stacy Eastman
Developmental Editor: Jessica Nicole B. Cañaberal

Clinics in Plastic Surgery (ISSN 0094-1298) is published quarterly by Elsevier Inc., 360 Park Avenue South, New York, NY 10010-1710. Months of issue are January, April, July, and October. Business and Editorial Offices: 1600 John F. Kennedy Blvd., Suite 1800, Philadelphia, PA 19103-2899. Periodicals postage paid at New York, NY and additional mailing offices. Subscription prices are $559.00 per year for US individuals, $1024.00 per year for US institutions, $100.00 per year for US students and residents, $625.00 per year for Canadian individuals, $1218.00 per year for Canadian institutions, $696.00 per year for international individuals, $1218.00 per year for international institutions, $100.00 per year for Canadian Students and $305.00 per year for international students/residents. To receive student/resident rate, orders must be accompanied by name of affiliated institution, date of term, and the *signature* of program/residency coordinator on institution letterhead. Orders will be billed at individual rate until proof of status is received. Foreign air speed delivery is included in all *Clinics* subscription prices. All prices are subject to change without notice. **POSTMASTER:** Send address changes to *Clinics in Plastic Surgery*, Elsevier Health Sciences Division, Subscription Customer Service, 3251 Riverport Lane, Maryland Heights, MO 63043. **Customer Service: 1-800-654-2452 (US and Canada). From outside of the United States and Canada, call 314-447-8871. Fax: 314-447-8029. E-mail: JournalsCustomerService-usa@elsevier.com (for print support); JournalsOnlineSupport-usa@elsevier.com (for online support).**

Reprints. For copies of 100 or more of articles in this publication, please contact the Commercial Reprints Department, Elsevier Inc., 360 Park Avenue South, New York, New York 10010-1710. Tel.: +1-212-633-3874; Fax: +1-212-633-3820; E-mail: reprints@elsevier.com.

Clinics in Plastic Surgery is covered in *Current Contents, EMBASE/Excerpta Medica, Science Citation Index, MEDLINE/ PubMed (Index Medicus), ASCA,* and *ISI/BIOMED.*

Contributors

EDITOR

LEE L.Q. PU, MD, PhD, FACS, FICS
Professor of Surgery, Division of Plastic
Surgery, Department of Surgery, University of
California, Davis Medical Center, University of
California, Davis, Sacramento, California, USA

AUTHORS

ZIN MAR AUNG, MD, PhD
Department of Plastic and Reconstructive
Surgery, Shanghai Ninth People's Hospital,
School of Medicine, Shanghai Jiao Tong
University, Shanghai, China

WEIGANG CAO, MD, PhD
Department of Plastic and Reconstructive
Surgery, Shanghai Ninth People's Hospital,
Shanghai Jiao Tong University School of
Medicine, Huangpu District, Shanghai, China

GANG CHAI, MD, PhD
Department of Plastic and Reconstructive
Surgery, Shanghai Ninth People's Hospital,
School of Medicine, Shanghai Jiao Tong
University, Shanghai, China

CHENG-JEN CHANG, MD, PhD, FACS, FICS
Department of Plastic and Reconstructive
Surgery, Chang Gung Memorial Hospital,
Chang Gung University, Department of Plastic
Surgery, Taipei Medical University Hospital,
Department of Surgery, School of Medicine,
College of Medicine, Graduate Institute of
Biomedical Optomechatronics, College of
Biomedical Engineering, Taipei Medical
University, Taipei, Taiwan

JIE CHEN, BSN
Department of Plastic and Reconstructive
Surgery, Peking Union Medical College
Hospital, Peking Union Medical College and
Chinese Academy of Medical Sciences,
Beijing, China

XIAOJUN CHEN, MD, PhD
Department of Plastic and Reconstructive
Surgery, Shanghai Ninth People's
Hospital, School of Medicine, Shanghai
Jiao Tong University, Shanghai,
China

YU-RAY CHEN, MD
Professor, Department of Plastic and
Reconstructive Surgery, The Craniofacial
Center, Chang Gung Memorial Hospital,
Taoyuan, Taiwan

CHIH-KANG CHOU, MD, MS
Charming Institute of Aesthetic and
Regenerative Surgery (CIARS), Qianjin District,
Kaohsiung City, Taiwan

HAIYAN CUI, MD
Professor, Department of Plastic and
Cosmetic Surgery, Tongji Hospital, Tongji
University School of Medicine, Shanghai,
China

CHUANCHANG DAI, MD, PhD
Department of Plastic and Reconstructive
Surgery, Shanghai Ninth People's Hospital,
Shanghai Jiao Tong University School of
Medicine, Shanghai, China

LI DONG, MD
Department of Plastic Surgery, Peking
University Third Hospital, Haidian District,
Beijing, China

RUIJIA DONG, MD
Department of Plastic and Reconstructive Surgery, Beijing Tsinghua Changgung Hospital, School of Clinical Medicine, Tsinghua University, Beijing, China

DOMINIK DUSCHER, MD, PhD
The Face and Longevity Center Munich, Munich, Germany; Department of Plastic, Reconstructive, Hand and Burn Surgery, BG-Trauma Center, Eberhard Karls University Tübingen, Tübingen, Germany

MIN GONG
Beijing Yimei Medical Cosmetology Plastic Clinic, Beijing, China

WENQING HAN, MD, PhD
Department of Plastic and Reconstructive Surgery, Shanghai Ninth People's Hospital, School of Medicine, Shanghai Jiao Tong University, Shanghai, China

WILSON W.S. HO, MBCHB, FRCSED
Medical Director, The Specialists: Lasers, Aesthetic and Plastic Surgery, Private, Central, Hong Kong

JIUZUO HUANG, MD
Department of Plastic and Reconstructive Surgery, Peking Union Medical College Hospital, Peking Union Medical College and Chinese Academy of Medical Sciences, Beijing, China

SHU-HUNG HUANG, MD, PhD
Division of Plastic Surgery, Department of Surgery, Hyperbaric Oxygen Therapy Room, Kaohsiung Medical University Hospital, Department of Surgery, School of Medicine, Graduate Institute of Medicine, College of Medicine, Kaohsiung Medical University, Kaohsiung City, Taiwan

ZHAO JIANFANG, MD, PhD
Department of Plastic Surgery, Peking University Third Hospital, Haidian District, Beijing, China; Department of Plastic and Burn Surgery, Peking University First Hospital, Xicheng District, Beijing, China

CHIA CHI KAO, MD
KAO Plastic Surgery Institute, Santa Monica, California, USA

BYEONG SEOP KIM, MD
Department of Plastic and Reconstructive Surgery, Shanghai Ninth People's Hospital, School of Medicine, Shanghai Jiao Tong University, Shanghai, China

FACHENG LI, MD, PhD
Plastic Surgery Hospital, Chinese Academy of Medical Sciences and Peking Union Medical College, Beijing, China

SHENGLI LI, MD, PhD
President of Chinese Society of Rhinoplasty, Professor of Plastic Surgery, Department of Plastic and Reconstructive Surgery, Shanghai Ninth People's Hospital, Shanghai Jiao Tong University School of Medicine, Shanghai, China

YUNZHU LI, MD
Department of Plastic and Reconstructive Surgery, Peking Union Medical College Hospital, Peking Union Medical College and Chinese Academy of Medical Sciences, Beijing, China

JENG-YEE LIN, MD, PhD
Freya Aesthetic Institute, Taipei, Taiwan

LI LIN, MD, PhD
Department of Plastic and Reconstructive Surgery, Shanghai Ninth People's Hospital, School of Medicine, Shanghai Jiao Tong University, Shanghai, China

TSAI-MING LIN, MD, PhD
Charming Institute of Aesthetic and Regenerative Surgery (CIARS), Qianjin District, Kaohsiung City, Taiwan

YUN-NAN LIN, MD
Division of Plastic Surgery, Department of Surgery, Kaohsiung Medical University Hospital, Kaohsiung City, Taiwan

KAI LIU, MD, PhD
Department of Plastic and Reconstructive Surgery, Shanghai Ninth People's Hospital, School of Medicine, Shanghai Jiao Tong University, Shanghai, China

XIAO LONG, MD
Department of Plastic and Reconstructive Surgery, Peking Union Medical College Hospital, Peking Union Medical College and Chinese Academy of Medical Sciences, Beijing, China

JIE LUAN, MD
Department of Breast Plastic Surgery, Plastic Surgery Hospital of Chinese Academy of Medical Sciences

MING NI
Beijing Yimei Medical Cosmetology Plastic Clinic, Beijing, China

LEE L.Q. PU, MD, PhD, FACS, FICS
Professor of Surgery, Division of Plastic Surgery, Department of Surgery, University of California, Davis Medical Center, University of California, Davis, Sacramento, California, USA

LINGLING SHENG, MD, PhD
Department of Plastic and Reconstructive Surgery, Shanghai Ninth People's Hospital, Shanghai Jiao Tong University School of Medicine, Huangpu District, Shanghai, China

MENGZHE SUN, MD, PhD
Department of Plastic and Reconstructive Surgery, Shanghai Ninth People's Hospital, School of Medicine, Shanghai Jiao Tong University, Shanghai, China

HIDENOBU TAKAHASHI, MD
Department of Surgery, Kaohsiung Medical University Hospital, Kaohsiung City, Taiwan

CHUNMEI WANG, MD, PhD
Department of Plastic and Aesthetic Surgery, Institute of Dermatology, Southern Medical University, Guangzhou, China

DONG WANG
Beijing Yimei Medical Cosmetology Plastic Clinic, Beijing, China

GUOBAO WANG, PhD
Department of Plastic and Cosmetic Surgery, Tongji Hospital, Tongji University School of Medicine, Shanghai, China

XIAOJUN WANG, MD
Department of Plastic and Reconstructive Surgery, Peking Union Medical College Hospital, Peking Union Medical College and Chinese Academy of Medical Sciences, Dongcheng District, Beijing, China

YUNENG WANG, MD
Plastic Surgery Hospital, Chinese Academy of Medical Sciences and Peking Union Medical College, Beijing, China

JIAO WEI, MD, PhD
Department of Plastic and Reconstructive Surgery, Shanghai Ninth People's Hospital, Shanghai Jiao Tong University School of Medicine, Shanghai, China

CHIN-HO WONG, MBBS (Singapore), MRCS(Ed), MMED (Surg), FAMS (Plast Surg)
W Aesthetic Plastic Surgery, Singapore, Mount Elizabeth Novena Specialist Center, Singapore, Singapore

YI-CHIA WU, MD, PhD
Division of Plastic Surgery, Department of Surgery, Kaohsiung Medical University Hospital, Department of Surgery, School of Medicine, College of Medicine, Kaohsiung Medical University, Kaohsiung City, Taiwan

YIDING XIAO, MD
Department of Plastic and Reconstructive Surgery, Peking Union Medical College Hospital, Peking Union Medical College and Chinese Academy of Medical Sciences, Beijing, China

HAISONG XU, MD, PhD
Department of Plastic and Reconstructive Surgery, Shanghai Ninth People's Hospital, School of Medicine, Shanghai Jiao Tong University, Shanghai, China

ALAN YAN, MD
Department of Plastic and Reconstructive Surgery, The Craniofacial Center, Chang Gung Memorial Hospital, Taoyuan, Taiwan

AN YANG, MD
Department of Plastic Surgery, Peking University Third Hospital, Haidian District, Beijing, China

CHANG-CHIEN YANG, MD
Board Certified Plastic Surgeon, Director of Artwood Plastic Surgery Clinic, Taipei, Taiwan

CHAO YANG
Beijing Yimei Medical Cosmetology Plastic Clinic, Beijing, China

DAPING YANG, MD
First Beijing BCC Plastic Surgery Hospital, Beijing, China

XIANXIAN YANG, MD, PhD
Department of Plastic and Reconstructive Surgery, Shanghai Ninth People's Hospital, School of Medicine, Shanghai Jiao Tong University, Shanghai, China

BO YIN, MD
Plastic Surgery Hospital, Chinese Academy of Medical Sciences and Peking Union Medical College, Beijing, China

HAIYANG YU, MD
Litchi Cosmetic Medical Clinic, Hangzhou, China

HAILIN ZHANG, MD
Department of Plastic and Reconstructive Surgery, Peking Union Medical College Hospital, Peking Union Medical College and Chinese Academy of Medical Sciences, Beijing, China

ZIWEI ZHANG, MD, PhD
Department of Plastic and Reconstructive Surgery, Shanghai Ninth People's Hospital, School of Medicine, Shanghai Jiao Tong University, Shanghai, China

YANCHUN ZHOU, BA
Department of Nursing, Shanghai Ninth People's Hospital, School of Medicine, Shanghai Jiao Tong University, Shanghai, China

DEJUN ZHU, MD
Nike Cosmetic Medical Clinic, Zhongshan City, China

Contents

 Video content accompanies this article at http://www.plasticsurgery.theclinics.com.

The highest level of esthetic treatment serves not only as a procedure but also as an artistic creation under the limitations of medicine. Based on oriental esthetic and anatomic features, the authors have proposed the " Future Codes" design in Chinese calligraphy describing the art of facial rejuvenation in Asians to help doctors perform well. The concept encompasses a systematic overall design for the art of facial rejuvenation in Asians, associated with beautiful meanings and is easy to learn and perform safely, including the 5 principles of minimally invasive facial rejuvenation: adding, subtracting, tightening, brightening and flexing.

Asians are of different ethnic origins. Nevertheless, they share the common facial structural deficiencies and consequences of the aging process that create the opportunity for esthetic intervention. As a result, Injectables are widely used in young Asians to achieve an oval facial shape with increased facial height and projection. In mature Asians with lifelong structural deficiencies, the beauty treatment plan is more complex than removal of signs of aging. Therefore, apart from injectables, other treatment modalities for tissue repositioning, neocollagenesis and skin quality improvement are also required to obtain the optimal result.

 Video content accompanies this article at http://www.plasticsurgery.theclinics.com.

Autologous fat grafting and facial liposuction are widely used to reshape facial contours. But up to now, there is no surgical design idea for Asian women. The article aimed to provide a facial esthetic design to guide the combined operation of facial liposuction and fat grafting for Asians, that is, the "three-line and nine-point" design method. In retrospective reviews, the surgical results of clinical practice were satisfactory, and a more attractive facial appearance was obtained. Our technique can easily be learnt and can be mastered by the most well-qualified plastic surgeons for satisfactory outcomes.

 Video content accompanies this article at http://www.plasticsurgery.theclinics.com.

Minimally invasive facial rejuvenation techniques are gaining attention because of their advantages such as less trauma, quick recovery, high safety, obvious results, and repeatable operation. In this article, the principle, the operation method, advantages, and disadvantages of the new fast recovery suspension technique modified by the authors are described in detail, and the clinical cases are listed to further illustrate the efficacy of the modified operation. The authors also compared this procedure with other common facial rejuvenation techniques. It is hoped that our article can provide a reference for clinicians to better use facial rejuvenation technology.

Radiofrequency (RF)-assisted liposuction treatment is a minimally invasive skin-tightening technique for the patient population with skin laxity. The authors recommend facial liposuction combined with the RF procedure for the treatment of skin laxity. Minimal-invasive liposuction creates working channels for RF treatment and sufficiently exposes the subdermal fibrous septal network tissue so that the RF energy can directly act on the collagen of the fibrous septal network for thermal shrinkage, leading to better surgical results. In this article, the authors describe their preferred technique and experience for face rejuvenation and contouring.

 Video content accompanies this article at http://www.plasticsurgery.theclinics.com.

Asian anatomy and concepts of beauty differ from whites. Traditional SMAS face-lifts are developed based on a white patient population and not ideal to achieve the aesthetic goals of Asian patients. The characteristics of the ideal facial rejuvenation techniques for Asians comprise hidden incisions to avoid hypertrophic scarring and cultural stigma. The authors' approach addresses the Asian face in all dimensions using minimally invasive modalities combined with skin regenerative methods. This surgical technique is called the "Ponytail Lift." It simulates the vertical lift of the face when having the hair pulled up in a high ponytail.

The complications associated with polyacrylamide hydrogel injection including tissue infection, nodular formation, and migration along tissue planes have been well-documented. Complete removal of injected material is seldom possible. Patients who underwent removal of injected material were significantly more likely to express interest in facelift. We provide an open surgical technique with facelift incision to deal with the removal of polyacrylamide hydrogel and complication due to volume deflation and tissue descent.

 Video content accompanies this article at http://www.plasticsurgery.theclinics.com.

In this article, authors mainly introduce new digital technology in facial bone contouring surgery. In our experience, these new technologies are crucial in ensuring the satisfaction of surgical accuracy. Our previous studies have shown surgeons can use precise pre-operative design to reduce operative time, reduce bleeding during surgery. Additionally, augmented reality can enhance the perspective perception of surgeons combining virtuality and reality. What's more, robot-assisted surgical technology also has a strong application prospect in facial contouring surgery. In the future, the combination of soft tissue contouring surgery will make the facial bone contouring surgery safer and more effective.

An esthetic smile is an integral feature of beauty. Improvement of the smile can be achieved by a combination of orthognathic surgery, orthodontics, and cosmetic dentistry. Preoperative evaluation serves to address a patient's surgical goals; it allows a surgeon to perform a detailed facial analysis and identify patients who are contraindicated for surgery. LeFort I and bilateral sagittal split osteotomy are performed to minimize the risk of complications. Injuries to the inferior alveolar nerve are the most common complication after orthognathic surgery, in which 90% of patients experience transient sensory disturbance of the lower lip in the postoperative period.

 Video content accompanies this article at http://www.plasticsurgery.theclinics.com.

A primary concern in facial aesthetics is the rejuvenation of periorbital areas through soft tissue recontouring, skin texture improvement, and harmoniousness with souring anatomic tissues. Currently, the ease of harvesting, abundance in volume, and lack of immune rejection make autologous fat transplantation a disruptive strategy in aesthetic medicine. The evolution and improvements made by myriad surgeons have contributed to the popularity of periorbital rejuvenation and have highlighted its indispensability in Asian patients. Lin and colleagues have advocated the technique of microautologous fat transplantation since 2007 for facial recontouring and rejuvenation. This article illustrates more in-depth technical details and innovative concepts for the improvement of the periorbita.

 Video content accompanies this article at http://www.plasticsurgery.theclinics.com.

Asian upper blepharoplasty is one of the most popular cosmetic procedures for Asians, but less optimal result is still common. The authors' comprehensive approach to Asian upper blepharoplasty includes (1) to determine both the height and length of the upper skin crease; (2) to create more ideal anatomy of the upper eyelid; (3) to reconstruct the desirable anatomic structure of the upper eyelid skin crease; and (4) to add a medial epicanthoplasty if needed to enhance cosmetic results.

Revision of Asian upper blepharoplasty can be extremely challenging to surgeons when encountering cases with multiple complications and very limited tissue sources. In this article, the author is going to guide the newcomers or revision Asian upper blepharoplasty by showing the theory of double-fold formation to help them to make a workable surgical plan when dealing with revision Asian upper blepharoplasty cases. The pathogenesis of complications of upper blepharoplasty can be classified systematically and the solution to each individual complication is also illustrated. Typical clinical cases of revision Asian upper blepharoplasty are then sampled as integrated practice.

 Video content accompanies this article at http://www.plasticsurgery.theclinics.com.

The lower eyelid is one of the commonest areas Asian patients present for rejuvenation. The spectrum of patients presenting for treatment ranges from the young to the more mature. Young patients present with "premature" aging due to an anatomical predisposition. These are patients we figuratively call those who "do not age well." Even patients with strong skeletal support manifest aging, in a predictable and progressive manner. Such patients eventually benefit from quality esthetic surgery of the lower eyelid and mid cheek.

To explore a pyriform aperture augmentation method that is suitable for Asian patients with mid-face concavity, we designed a novel prosthesis to perform pyriform aperture augmentation. Three different rhinoplasty schemes are designed according to the degree of mid-face concavity: (1) simple implantation around the pyriform aperture, (2) implantation around the pyriform aperture and augmentation rhinoplasty is performed concurrently, and (3) implantation around pyriform aperture combined with nasal extension technique. Comprehensive rhinoplasty with pyriform aperture augmentation can substantially improve the aesthetic relationship between nasal and facial areas. This technique is suitable for comprehensive rhinoplasty of Asian patients with mid-face concavity.

The demands of the revision rhinoplasty in Asian populations are increasing nowadays. Rhinoplasty-related complications frequently occurred in clinical practice, for example, implants deviation, extrusion, infection, nasal contraction deformities, and skin necrosis after primary or multiple surgeries. To obtain a successful revision rhinoplasty in Asian, early detection, prompt management, and appropriate treatment of complications are essential for minimizing postoperative adverse consequences. In revision rhinoplasty for Asian patients, autologous tissues play an important role as new support grafts for nasal structure reconstruction.

 Video content accompanies this article at http://www.plasticsurgery.theclinics.com.

Breast augmentation with implants is becoming a more widely accepted and popular procedure in Asia. The axillary approach remains the preferred incision for Asian women. Endoscope technique is the best option for transaxillary breast augmentation. It greatly increases control over the process, avoids various drawbacks, reduces the incidence of complications, and improves the stability of clinical effects of transaxillary implant breast augmentation. Freestyle endoscopic technique may greatly improve the flexibility and efficiency of the endoscope operation through the axillary approach. This article introduces the freestyle endoscopic-assisted transaxillary breast augmentation with high position dual-plane technique.

Advantages of standard endoscopic surgery include diminished incidence of scarring, numbness, bleeding, and edema, making endoscopic surgery preferable to the conventional suprapubic approach. Endoscopic-assisted abdominoplasty can also treat diastasis recti deformity with minimal excess skin. For enhanced results, a learning curve is expected to achieve optimal technical expertise.

Refined buttock augmentation with fat grafting in Chinese women during the past decade is introduced. The ideal buttock contouring outcome and figure silhouette come from the proper individualized plan and meticulous maneuvers through fat grafting to the buttocks combined with liposuction procedures on the surrounding areas of the buttocks as well as on the other body parts. The fat grafts are collected, filtered, and condensed by gravitation in a sterilized canister during liposuction. It is recommended that fat grafts were only transplanted into the subcutaneous layers and with no injection into the musculatures of the buttocks. High patients' satisfaction was obtained with no major complications and fewer minor complications.

 Video content accompanies this article at http://www.plasticsurgery.theclinics.com.

Female genital cosmetic surgery consists of multiple procedures, usually including labiaplasty, clitoral prepuce reduction, labia majora augmentation, and vaginoplasty. The reasons for women to undergo these surgeries can be categorized as functional and aesthetic ones. In this study, we introduced the modified vaginoplasty with acellular dermal matrix (ADM) and briefly reviewed our experience in the combination of multiple procedures to achieve the optimal effect.

With the increasing demand of breast augmentation with fat grafting in the past decade, the techniques of fat grafting have been continuously improved or refined and the science behind has been extensively investigated. Therefore, the safety and efficacy of fat grafting to breasts have met the standard for primary breast augmentation. The key to a successful outcome and reducing fat necrosis is meticulous fat harvesting, graft processing, and injection. In this article, authors propose our preferred techniques of rimary breast augmentation with fat grafting and an algorithmic approach for the management of fat necrosis based on the most scientific studies.

CLINICS IN PLASTIC SURGERY

SERIES OF RELATED INTEREST

Facial Plastic Surgery Clinics
https://www.facialplastic.theclinics.com/
Otolaryngologic Clinics
https://www.oto.theclinics.com/

THE CLINICS ARE AVAILABLE ONLINE!
Access your subscription at:
www.theclinics.com

Preface

Advances and Refinements in Asian Aesthetic Surgery

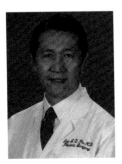

Lee L.Q. Pu, MD, PhD, FACS, FICS
Editor

As the Editor of the first-ever comprehensive textbook on Asian aesthetic surgery, entitled *"Aesthetic Plastic Surgery in Asians: Principles and Techniques,"* and as the Associate Editor of the *Aesthetic Plastic Surgery*, the official journal of the International Society of Aesthetic Plastic Surgery (ISAPS), I have witnessed the fast development of Asian aesthetic surgery from its infancy to the current state. It is one of the fastest growing subspecialties in aesthetic plastic surgery. The unique features of anatomy in Asian patients along with their cultural background and sense of beauty and different expectations after aesthetic surgery may stand alone and deserve attention in our specialty worldwide. For the last two decades, the scope of Asian aesthetic surgery has expanded from double eyelid surgery and nasal dorsal augmentation to facial rejuvenation, breast enhancement, body contouring including gluteal augmentation, and even gynecologic cosmetic procedures. Worldwide aesthetic plastic surgeons are eager to learn the common aesthetic surgical techniques for their Asian patients. Furthermore, they also want to learn more advanced or refined techniques in Asian aesthetic surgery.

Because there is an urgent need to publish updated techniques in Asian aesthetic surgery, I have accepted another invitation from the publisher of *Clinics in Plastic Surgery* to publish a special issue that focuses on advances and refinements in Asian aesthetic surgery. With my strong connection with the entire membership of the World Association for Plastic Surgeons of Chinese Descent (WAPSCD), I had decided to put

such an issue together by inviting many excellent aesthetic plastic surgeons together from Mainland China, Taiwan, Hong Kong, Singapore, and the United States. Therefore, this special issue itself not only covers traditional topics of Asian aesthetic surgery, such as double eyelid procedure and nasal dorsal augmentation, but also includes many new contents, such as minimally invasive procedures for facial rejuvenation, periorbital rejuvenation, aesthetic facial skeleton contouring procedures, aesthetic breast surgery, abdominoplasty, gluteal augmentation, and vaginal rejuvenation. All invited authors are well-known in their home country or region, and some of them are quite active in both ISAPS and WAPSCD as a teaching faculty for international aesthetic education. Several unique Asian aesthetic surgical procedures are first presented in English literature by those aesthetic plastic surgeons who have not had an opportunity to publish their excellent works.

In this a twenty-article issue, the first seven articles focus on facial rejuvenation. Two articles focus on Botox and fillers for facial rejuvenation and contouring, and this is followed by a fat-grafting article for facial rejuvenation and contouring. One article focuses on facial rejuvenation with fast recovery suspension technique, and another focuses on radiofrequency-assisted procedures for facial rejuvenation and contouring. One article focuses on an endoscopically assisted procedure for facial rejuvenation that can be a preferred technique for many Asian patients. One unique article focuses on facial rejuvenation

Clin Plastic Surg 50 (2023) xiii–xiv
https://doi.org/10.1016/j.cps.2022.08.011
0094-1298/23/© 2022 Published by Elsevier Inc.

with open techniques after previous filler injections. There are two articles on facial bone modifications. One article from the renowned Shanghai Ninth People's Hospital focuses on current practices for aesthetic facial skeletal contouring surgery, and another article from the renowned Chang Gung Memorial Hospital describes orthognathic surgery for improvement of the smile. One popular article introduces common techniques for periorbital rejuvenation in Asians. Three articles primarily describe advanced techniques in Asian upper blepharoplasty, revision of Asian upper blepharoplasty, and refined techniques in Asian lower blepharoplasty. There are two articles on Asian rhinoplasty; one focuses on primary rhinoplasty and the other focuses on revision of Asian rhinoplasty. Two articles on the breast represent some unique features of Asian aesthetic breast surgery. One article introduces advanced techniques of endoscopic-assisted transaxillary breast augmentation, and the other describes primary breast augmentation with fat grafting. The last three articles focus on the current trend and fast development in Asian body-contouring procedures as well as gynecologic cosmetic procedures. One article focuses on endoscopically assisted abdominoplasty, and another article focuses on gluteal augmentation with fat grafting. The last article focuses on vaginal rejuvenation with a relatively simple approach.

I believe this twenty-article issue covers almost the entire spectrum of Asian aesthetic surgery. It represents the recent advances and refinements of many aesthetic surgical procedures for Asians. With tireless efforts from all the authors, the current issue represents an excellent summary of advances and refinements in Asian aesthetic surgery.

As guest editor, I sincerely hope that you will enjoy reading this special issue of *Clinics in Plastic Surgery* and find it useful for your busy practice. It represents a true team effort from many world-renowned expert surgeons from the membership of WAPSCD. I would like to express my heartfelt gratitude to all contributors for their expertise, dedication, and responsibility to produce such a world-class issue of plastic surgery focusing on Asian aesthetic surgery. It is certainly my privilege to work with these respected authors in this special subspecialty of plastic surgery. Last, I would also like to express my special appreciation to the publication team of Elsevier, who put this remarkable issue together with the highest possible standard.

Lee L.Q. Pu, MD, PhD, FACS, FICS
Division of Plastic Surgery, Department of Surgery,
University of California, Davis, 2335 Stockton
Boulevard, Room 6008, Sacramento, CA 95817,
USA

E-mail address:
llpu@ucdavis.edu

Minimally Invasive Approach to Facial Rejuvenation
The Authors' Preferred Approach

Haiyan Cui, MD*, Guobao Wang, PhD

KEYWORDS

• Minimally invasion • Facial rejuvenation • Injection procedure • Esthetic design

KEY POINTS

- The highest level of esthetic treatment serves not only as a procedure but also as an artistic creation under the limitations of medicine, to discover and create the potential, personalized, and vivid beauty with nature.
- Based on oriental esthetic and anatomic features, the authors have proposed "未来 Future Codes" design in Chinese calligraphy describing the art of facial rejuvenation in Asians to help doctors perform well.
- The "Future Codes" concept encompasses a systematic overall design for the art of facial rejuvenation in Asians.
- This method is associated with beautiful meanings and is easy to learn and perform safely, including the 5 principles of minimally invasive facial rejuvenation: adding, subtracting, tightening, brightening and flexing.

 Video content accompanies this article at http://www.plasticsurgery.theclinics.com.

INTRODUCTION

In the past decade, there has been an increase in nonsurgical cosmetic procedures worldwide. Many patients choose dermal fillers,[1] botulinum toxin, thread rejuvenation,[2] and energy-based devices (EBDs),[3] such as fiber laser, and radio frequency (RF), to alter their appearance and restore tissue loss.[4,5]

Dermal fillers and botulinum toxin are the 2 most popular nonsurgical cosmetic procedures performed globally to treat age-associated changes and are often used in combination.[6] There are many kinds of filler materials for volume replacement and enhancement, such as hyaluronic acid,[7] collagen, polycaprolactone, poly-L-lactic acid,[8] and calcium hydroxylapatite.[9,10] These fillers can be used for cheek and chin augmentation, nose reshaping, midface volumization, and lip enhancement. Especially for Asians, fillers can improve facial contours with better contrast and a more dimensional effect. On the other hand, to reduce the appearance of wrinkles, many people choose injections of botulinum toxin. Botulinum toxin relaxes certain muscles on the face to make wrinkles less noticeable for a period.[1] The market for nonsurgical, energy-based facial rejuvenation techniques has increased exponentially since lasers were first used for skin rejuvenation in 1983. Improvements in safety and efficacy for energy-based treatment have expanded the patient base considering these therapies viable

Department of Plastic and Cosmetic Surgery, Tongji Hospital, Tongji University School of Medicine, 389 Xincun Road, Shanghai, 200065, China
* Corresponding author.
E-mail address: u2beauty1@sina.com

Clin Plastic Surg 50 (2023) 1–9
https://doi.org/10.1016/j.cps.2022.09.002
0094-1298/23/© 2022 Elsevier Inc. All rights reserved.

options.[11] In the authors' department, patients with mild and moderate degree of prominent fat bulging underwent 980-nm laser-assisted lipolysis via lower eyelid stab incision. The results show that patients with mild to moderate degree of bulging fat pads who resist surgery are good candidates for EBDs, for example, RF and laser-assisted technology (**Figs. 1–4**).

The use of nonsurgical esthetic facial treatments is also increasing in Asia.[1] To date, most studies of facial rejuvenation therapy have evaluated Western populations, although Asian populations differ in terms of culture, anatomic structure, perceptions of beauty, and signs of aging.[12,13] For the aforementioned reasons, there are many differences in desired outcomes between Caucasians and Asians. A thorough understanding of the key esthetic concerns and requirements for the Asian face is required to instruct appropriate facial esthetic treatments. Existing published guidelines cannot be directly applied to Asians. Thus, recommendations that are suitable for Asian populations are needed.

Special Considerations

As a biopsychosocial medical model is advocated, physicians' esthetic perception and humanistic care are required in addition to surgical techniques, especially in the field of plastic surgery. Cosmetic rejuvenation should follow the principle of overall design. Many patients have reported being unsatisfied with results, even if the operations were performed very well, because their doctor only solved the focal problem and neglected the relationships between the parts and the whole.[1,14] For instance, a perfect nose must have a good proportional esthetic relationship with the entire face, as well as a patient who originally intended to correct his or her nasolabial folds. After the injection, the nasolabial fold problem was solved, but the face became fat. Such cases demonstrate that it is particularly important to improve esthetic perception and humanistic care, especially among cosmetic surgeons.[15] Before performing a cosmetic rejuvenation, the overall design and construction of the human esthetic image must be considered, which will lead to better therapeutic outcome, psychological satisfaction, and social recognition of the patients. Furthermore, care should be taken to maintain the patient's psychological state throughout the treatment according to the biopsychosocial medical model.[16]

Procedures

In the summary of thousands of teaching and training cases, the authors have proposed "未来 Future Codes" design from Chinese calligraphy describing the art of facial rejuvenation in Asians to help doctors perform well. "未来" (see **Fig. 1**A) are pictographs of 2 Chinese characters, translated into English as "Future," which represent beautiful meanings and vividly describe the procedure and operating area of the design methods. The "Future Codes" is a method of assessment and operative system based on oriental esthetic and anatomic features, describing a concept of systematic overall design that is easy to learn and can help doctors obtain a satisfying result. The rejuvenation method in this article, which is simple, convenient, safe, effective, and easy to master with good clinical effect, is hidden in the Chinese calligraphy of the two characters, consisting of the following lines and reflecting the aging characteristics of the Asian face (Video 1, Video 2). This method is associated with beautiful meanings and is easy to learn and perform safely, including the 5 principles of minimally invasive facial rejuvenation: adding, subtracting, tightening, brightening, and flexing.

The middle line of the face (see **Fig. 1**B) passes through the forehead, the glabella complex, the nose, the lips, and the chin. This line is highly important and can affect the success or failure of the whole procedure because it determines the contour, symmetry, balance, coordination, proportion, stereo, light, and shadow on both sides of the face. Therefore, this is a key line in the "Future Codes" design.

The first horizontal line (see **Fig. 1**C) passes the arch of the temper region, the eyebrow, and the glabella complex. The second horizontal line (see **Fig. 1**D) passes through the cheeks or the "apple muscle." If an injection is applied inside this line, the cheekbone will appear narrower, helping reduce the width of the cheekbones in Asians. The horizontal lines of the eyebrow and the "apple muscle" are also considered aging criteria. Obvious lacrimal sulcus and nasolabial folds are considered signs of aging. On the other hand, the other 2 oblique lines run along the nasolabial folds (see **Fig. 1**E). The patient will appear younger if the nasolabial folds are treated with injection fillers. Finally, 2 nasojugal folds and the tear trough are added (see **Fig. 1**F), which combine the 2 Chinese characters and the "Future Codes." The "Future Codes" design includes the important esthetic points and lines of facial contour and encompasses the core principles of facial rejuvenation and esthetics (see **Fig. 1**). All these lines make up the word "Future" in Chinese characters. Therefore, Chinese calligraphy of the two characters represents the core of esthetic facial rejuvenation in Asian patients. And our esthetic concept of

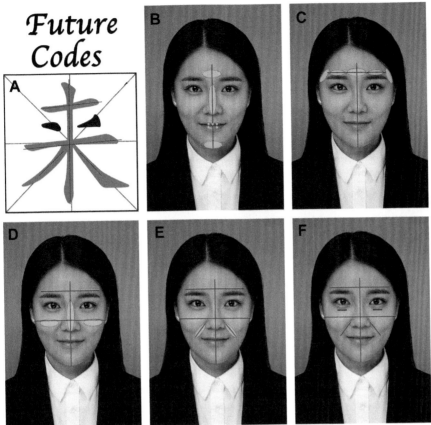

Fig. 1. Dr Cui's "Future Codes" design based on Chinese calligraphy. (*A*) Two Chinese characters "未来," which means "Future" in English. The concept encompasses the systematic overall design for the art of facial injection in Asians. The middle line of the face (*B*, 26-year-old woman) passes through the forehead, the glabella complex, the nose, the lips, and the chin. (*C*) The first horizontal line passes the arch of the temper region, the eyebrow, and the glabella complex. (*D*) The second horizontal line passes through the cheeks or the "apple muscle." (*E*) The other 2 oblique lines run along the nasolabial folds. (*F*) Finally, 2 nasojugular folds, tear trough, are added. Photo by Oliver Johnson on Unsplash

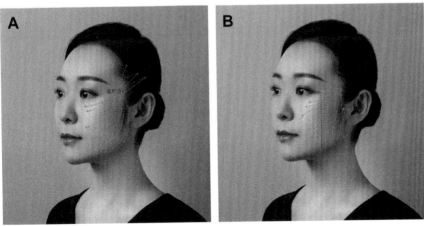

Fig. 2. (*A*) Thread rejuvenation. Bilayer continuous thread implantation with multiple Z sharped technique. (*B*) Bilayer, 2 entry points, 3 fan-shaped thread implantation technique. Watch the video for more details: Video 3 and Video 4.

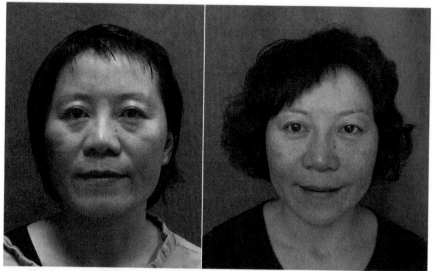

Fig. 3. Case 1. A 48-year-old woman underwent the assessment and injection procedures according to the authors' "Future Codes" design method: preoperative (*left*) and 1-week postoperative (*right*) views.

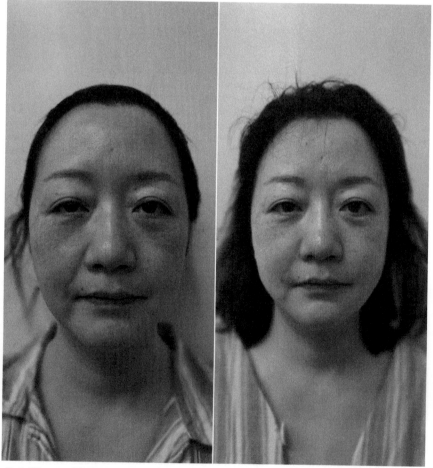

Fig. 4. Case 2. A 37-year-old woman: preoperative (*left*) and 2-week postoperative (*right*) views.

facial rejuvenation is overall design of the facial rejuvenation combined with 5 principles of minimally invasive facial rejuvenation: adding, subtracting, tightening, brightening, and flexing. The fillers (see Video 1, Video 2), fat grafting, and thread rejuvenation are adding and flexing method, including bilayer continuous thread implantation with multiple Z sharped technique (**Fig. 2**A, Video 3) and bilayer, 2 entry points, 3 fan-shaped thread implantation technique (see **Fig. 2**B, Video 4). Botulinum toxin, optical fiber laser (Video 5), and RF (Video 6) are reduction and tightening methods.

The appearance of aging is mainly due to relaxation of the skin and soft tissue, displacement of the tissue structure, the appearance of skin folds, changes in the texture of the skin, and the lack of tissue capacity and elasticity. These features are also reflected in the "Future Codes." The operation is feasibly performed with knowledge of anatomy, and complications can be effectively avoided by following this rejuvenation protocol.

Postoperative Care and Expected Outcome

Through the systematic comprehensive "Future Codes" design, the patient acquired a face with harmonious ratios, a contouring structure, clear light and dark contrast, tightened skin, and flattened eye bags. The procedures resulted in the appearance of more spirited eyes, a stereo and natural nose structure, rounded apple muscles, narrow cheekbones, shallow and round nasolabial folds, and enhanced length, convexity, and radius of the chin. The entire facial appearance was perceived as younger.

The following features are commonly considered to be pleasing: (1) elegant bearing, (2) slim figure, (3) beautiful face, (4) slender neck, (5) proportional breasts, (6) narrow waist, and (7) round hips. In the authors' opinion, cosmetic doctors can be divided into 3 levels as follows: the ones on the first level are those who use various products and equipment and just master basic techniques and basic knowledge of anatomy to solve basic problems. At the second level are the ones who are experienced in facial rejuvenation and can prevent and manage complications. At the third level, the highest level of esthetic treatment, not only serving as a procedure but also mastering the principal techniques and deepening their fundamental knowledge, doctors regard injection therapy as an artistic creation conducted under medical restrictions to create beauty in individuals; the creation of beauty will be achieved through systematic and overall design instead of a single method of treatment.

Management of Complications

Complications include signs of local reactions such as bruising and swelling, infections, allergies, nodules, Tyndall effect, vascular adverse events, and serious systemic adverse reactions. The authors have done statistics in their own department, demonstrating that 9 of 147 patients experienced minor local reactions such as bruising and swelling 3 days after "Future Codes" procedure. The issue resolved itself shortly; none of them presented any signs of infection, allergies, local nodules, vascular adverse events, or serious systemic adverse reactions.

Revision or Subsequent Procedures

Adjuvant therapy: After the injection treatment, the following procedures can also be applied to achieve better effects: (1) a fiber laser can be used to dissolve eye bag fat, (2) RF can be used to tighten the skin of the lateral corner of the mouth and the mandibular margin, and (3) hair can be trimmed.

Case Demonstrations

Case 1

A 48-year-old woman underwent the injection process according to the authors' "Future Codes" design method.

1. Injection at the middle line: (a) The glabella complex is injected with 1 mL hyaluronic acid by puncturing with a sharp needle until the tip touches the periosteum, ensuring no blood is withdrawn, and then pushing slowly. The area is massaged while injecting. (b) The nose is injected with 1 mL hyaluronic acid plus 1% lidocaine for local anesthesia by puncturing the tip of the nose with a 23G blunt needle. (c) The lips are injected with a total of 0.4 mL hyaluronic acid with a 30G sharp needle: 3 points on the upper lip and 2 points on the lower lip are injected with 0.08 mL each. (d) The chin is injected with 1 mL hyaluronic acid with a 27G to 30G sharp needle by puncturing with the sharp needle until the tip reaches the periosteum.
2. Injection of the first horizontal line: (a) The eyebrows are injected with 0.6 mL hyaluronic acid with a 23G blunt needle by subcutaneously puncturing with a blunt needle at the eyebrow tail. Hyaluronic acid is injected into the eyebrow while subcutaneously retracting the needle. (b) The temporal region is injected with 2 mL hyaluronic acid using a sharp needle by touching the needle tip to the periosteum, ensuring no blood is withdrawn, and then pushing slowly.

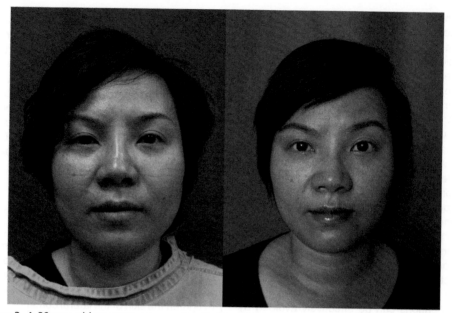

Fig. 5. Case 3. A 36-year-old woman: preoperative (*left*) and 8-week postoperative (*right*) views. Case 4. A 29-year-old man: preoperative (*left*) and 4-week postoperative (*right*) views.

Each side of the temporal region is injected with 1 mL hyaluronic acid while massaging.

3. The second horizontal line for the "apple muscle" is injected with 1 mL hyaluronic acid. For the apple muscle, the nasolabial folds, and the tear trough, a 23G blunt needle is used to puncture 1.5 cm away from the outer corner of the mouth, subcutaneously or on the periosteum, and 0.8 mL hyaluronic acid is injected on each side. The needle tip can reach the apple muscle, the tear trough, and the nasolabial folds.

4. The nasolabial folds are injected with 2 mL hyaluronic acid by puncturing 1.5 cm away from the outer corner of the mouth, with 1 mL injected on each side.

The tear trough is injected with 0.3 mL hyaluronic acid by puncturing 1.5 cm away from the outer corner of the mouth, with 0.15 mL injected on each side (see **Fig. 3**).

Case 2

A 37-year-old woman underwent the comprehensive use of multiple methods of hyaluronic acid injection, thread rejuvenation, and botulinum toxin treatment according to the authors' "Future Codes" design method. The preoperative and

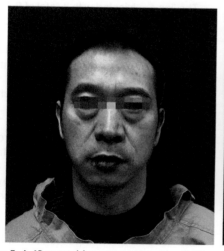
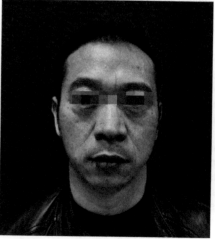

Fig. 6. Case 5. A 42-year-old man: preoperative (*left*) and immediately postoperative (*right*) views.

2-week postoperative follow-up views are provided in **Fig. 4**; more details are provided in Videos 2–4.

Case 3

A 36-year-old woman underwent minimally invasive laser-assisted lipolysis and skin tightening on lower face. The results were satisfactory during the 2-month follow-up visit (**Fig. 5**).

Case 4

A 29-year-old woman underwent minimally invasive laser-assisted lipolysis and skin tightening on lower face. The results were satisfactory during the 1-month follow-up visit (**Fig. 5**).

Case 5

A 42-year-old man underwent minimally invasive laser-assisted lipolysis and skin tightening on

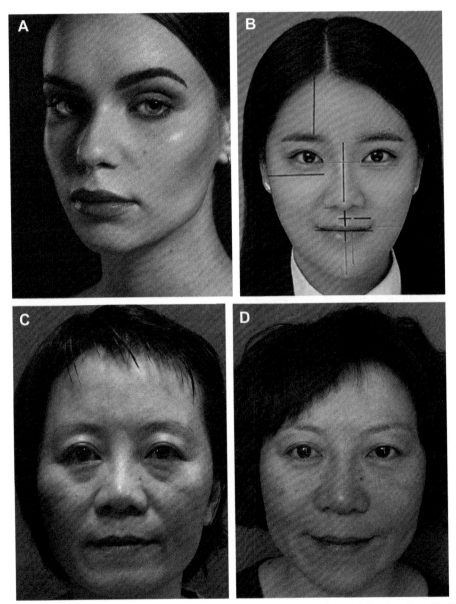

Fig. 7. (*A, B*) Western and oriental faces. The proportion markers on a beautiful Asian face (*B*, 26-year-old woman). The green line is the baseline X, then the blue line is 1.618 X, the black line is 0.618 X, the orange line is 0.382 X, and all the same color lines are the same length. 1.618, 0.618, and 0.382 are all gold ratios (The theory of proportion markers from Dr Arthur Swift[21]). (*C, D*) 48-year-old woman, before (*lower left*) and 3 months after injection (*lower right*) according to "Cui Codes" design method (Photo by Oliver Johnson on Unsplash [see **Fig. 7A**].)

lower eyelids. The results were satisfactory immediately postoperatively (**Fig. 6**); more details are provided in Video 5.

DISCUSSION

Most Asian patients, regardless of age, prefer to avoid surgery as much as possible and seek natural results. Therefore, patients' expectations should be evaluated, and innovative procedures should be proposed to meet Asian patients' esthetic needs, including the facial shape, structure, and proportion, as well as the effects of aging on their faces. The esthetic standards of Eastern and Western populations remain different. Westerners possess clear facial contours, narrow cheekbones, contouring structures, and obvious light and shadow effects. Oriental faces are plump, with large cheekbones, unclear contours, and delicate skin (**Fig. 7**). Facial filling is commonly performed to restore vitality and resist aging in Western countries. Orientals focus on filling and contouring. As Asians differ from Westerners in facial appearance and anatomic structure, noninvasive esthetic treatments are appropriate for Asians.[1] However, to date, most studies and recommendations regarding facial rejuvenation have referred to Western populations.[17–19] Regardless of national and cultural differences, some esthetic principles, including symmetry, balance, proportion, coordination, and unity of diversity, are shared in common between Eastern and Western populations (see **Fig. 7**). In addition to these basic principles, the following features are also commonly considered to be pleasing: (1) elegant bearing, (2) slim figure, (3) beautiful face, (4) slender neck. (5) proportional breasts, (6) narrow waist, and (7) round hips.[1,14] The highest level of esthetic treatment serves not only as a procedure but also as an artistic creation under the limitations of medicine, to discover and create the potential, personalized, and vivid beauty with nature.

Researchers have discovered that the human perception of physical beauty is closely related to the golden ratio (as rounded to 1.618). The ratio of the distance between certain regions of the face relative to the distance of another defined region is considered ideal at 1.618.[20]

Most faces regarded as beautiful or attractive have a significant number of markers whose proportions are very close to the golden ratio. As shown in **Fig. 7**B, the green line is the baseline X, the blue line is 1.618 X, the black line is 0.618 X, and the orange line is 0.382 X; lines of the same color are the same length. 1.618, 0.618, and 0.382 are all gold ratios, and there are golden ratios between various lines.

Therefore, proportional esthetics is an important feature of beauty and occupies an important position in formal esthetics.[21]

The authors[14,16,22] have published papers since 2007 putting forward the concept of overall esthetic design, which includes a systematic overall design and esthetic evaluation before the treatment procedure, psychological counseling during the peritreatment period, and the comprehensive use of multiple methods. After treatment, making up, clothing, modeling, and etiquette training are necessary complements to create a beautiful appearance that would be deemed to exude charm and vitality.

In the authors' opinion, cosmetic doctors can be divided into 3 levels as follows: the ones on the first level are those who use various products and equipment and just master basic injection techniques and basic knowledge of anatomy to solve basic problems. At the second level are the ones who are experienced in facial rejuvenation and can prevent and manage complications. At the third level, mastering the principal rejuvenation techniques and deepening their fundamental knowledge, doctors regard rejuvenation therapy as an artistic creation conducted under medical restrictions to create beauty in individuals; the creation of beauty will be achieved through systematic and overall design instead of a single method of treatment.[2,23]

SUMMARY

An increasing number of Asian people are seeking nonsurgical facial esthetic treatments. Ethnic Asians differ from Western populations in both facial appearance and baseline structural facial anatomy. However, there is a lack of clinical instruction to doctors who provide facial esthetic treatment of Asian patients. Therefore, there is an urgent need for instruction to guide physicians in performing cosmetic rejuvenation treatments for Asian patients, and these procedures should be easy to learn and perform safely. The authors' "Future Codes" design is derived from Chinese calligraphy of 2 Chinese characters, which means "Future" in English. The concept encompasses a systematic overall design for the art of facial rejuvenation in Asians. The author H.C. has thousands of cases of treatment experience and has extensive teaching experience of training more than 10,000 practitioners. This method is associated with beautiful meanings and is easy for clinicians to master. This is the first systematic solution available in the clinic that can be used to design facial esthetics and rejuvenation in Asians through Eastern philosophy and culture.

CLINICS CARE POINTS

- The concept of overall esthetic design, which includes a systematic overall design and esthetic evaluation before the treatment procedure, psychological counseling during the peritreatment period, and the comprehensive use of multiple methods.
- "Future Codes" design in Chinese calligraphy describes the art of facial rejuvenation in Asians to help doctors perform well.
- 5 principles of minimally invasive facial rejuvenation: adding, subtracting, tightening, brightening, and flexing.

DISCLOSURE

The authors have no financial interest to declare in relation to the drugs, devices, and products mentioned in this article.

SUPPLEMENTARY DATA

Supplementary data related to this article can be found online at https://doi.org/10.1016/j.cps.2022.09.002.

REFERENCES

1. Cui H. Aesthetic facial injection in asians[M]. China: Peking University Medical Press; 2017. p. 163.
2. Cui H. Aesthetic thread rejuvenation in asians[M]. China: Peking University Medical Press; 2019. p. 211–4.
3. Cui H. Minimally invasive body sculpting in asians [M]. China: Peking University Medical Press; 2022.
4. Pu Lee LQ. Aesthetic plastic surgery in asians: principles & techniques[M]. CRC Press; 2015.
5. Tijerina JD, Morrison SD, Nolan IT, et al. Predicting public interest in nonsurgical cosmetic procedures using google trends[J]. Aesthet Surg J 2020;40(11):1253–62.
6. Roman J, Zampella JG. Demographics of men and minorities in cosmetic clinical trials of botulinum toxin and hyaluronic acid fillers[J]. Dermatol Surg 2019;46(9):1164–8.
7. Percec I, Bertucci V, Solish N, et al. An Objective, quantitative, dynamic assessment of hyaluronic acid fillers that adapt to facial movement[J]. Plast Reconstr Surg 2020;145(2):295e–305e.
8. Jabbar A, Arruda S, Sadick N. Off face usage of poly-l-lactic acid for body rejuvenation[J]. J Drugs Dermatol 2017;16(5):489–94.
9. Chang JW, Koo WY, Kim EK, et al. Facial rejuvenation using a mixture of calcium hydroxylapatite filler and hyaluronic acid filler[J]. J Craniofac Surg 2020;31(1):e18–21.
10. Phillips KS, Wang YUS. Food and drug administration authors publish articles on dermal filler materials, injections, methods, and skin preparation[J]. Plast Reconstr Surg 2017;140(4):632e–3e.
11. Britt CJ, Marcus B. Energy-based facial rejuvenation: advances in diagnosis and treatment[J]. JAMA Facial Plast Surg 2017;19(1):64–71.
12. Liew S, Wu WT, Chan HH, et al. Consensus on changing trends, attitudes, and concepts of asian beauty[J]. Aesthet Plast Surg 2016;40(2):193–201.
13. Nouveau-Richard S, Yang Z, Mac-Mary S, et al. Skin ageing: a comparison between Chinese and European populations. A pilot study[J]. J Dermatol Sci 2005;40(3):187–93.
14. Cui Haiyan. Overall design and construction of facial injection cosmetology[J]. Dermatol Bull 2018;35(6):621–6.
15. Nerini A, Matera C, Di Gesto C, et al. Exploring the links between self-compassion, body dissatisfaction, and acceptance of cosmetic surgery in young Italian women[J]. Front Psychol 2019;10:2698.
16. Cui Haiyan, Zhao Haiguang, Xu Haisong, et al. An innovative approach for facial rejuvenation and contouring injections in asian patients[J]. Aesthet Surg J Open Forum 2021;3(2):1–6.
17. Haddad A, Menezes A, Guarnieri C, et al. Recommendations on the use of injectable poly-l-lactic acid for skin laxity in off-face areas[J]. J Drugs Dermatol 2019;18(9):929–35.
18. Freytag DL, Frank K, Haidar R, et al. Facial safe zones for soft tissue filler injections: a practical guide[J]. J Drugs Dermatol 2019;18(9):896–902.
19. Lin MJ, Dubin DP, Goldberg DJ, et al. Practices in the usage and reconstitution of poly-l-lactic acid [J]. J Drugs Dermatol 2019;18(9):880–6.
20. Prokopakis EP, Vlastos IM, Picavet VA, et al. The golden ratio in facial symmetry[J]. Rhinology 2013;51(1):18–21.
21. Stein R, Holds JB, Wulc AE, et al. Phi, fat, and the mathematics of a beautiful midface[J]. Ophthalmic Plast Reconstr Surg 2018;34(5):491–6.
22. Cui H, Chen J-An. Overall design and construction of aesthetic human body[J]. Chin J Med Aesthet Cosmet 2007;13(1):43–4.
23. Cui H. Art of Facial Injection In Asian. International Master Course on Aging Skin, IMCAS. Paris, France; 2016. p 163.

Facial Beautification and Rejuvenation with Injectables: My Preferred Approach

Wilson W.S. Ho, MBChB, FRCSEd

KEYWORDS

- Younger asian patients • Asian facial characteristics • Oval facial shape
- Preserve esthetic individuality • Customized approach • Combined treatment modalities

KEY POINTS

- Combined use of hyaluronic acid and botulinum toxin is more frequent in young Asian patients.
- Treatment target in Asians is to aim at an oval, small and narrow looking face with well projected midline structures and medial cheeks.
- Customized approach to create a natural and safe result while maintaining discrete Asian ethnic features and esthetic individuality.
- Combined treatment modalities for volume loss and tissue migration.

INTRODUCTION

The esthetic market in Asia has been blooming for the past 15 years. In line with the global decrease in average age for noninvasive cosmetic procedures, esthetic patients in Asia are younger than Western world and approximately 50% of them are aged 18 to 40 years.[1] The dense population with increasing disposable incomes, the growing awareness of treatment options available, increasing social acceptability and accessibility of noninvasive cosmetic enhancements, and inclination toward beauty and looking young are the main propelling factors in the market growth in the region.

Botulinum toxin and hyaluronic acid (HA) injections, either alone or in combination, are used extensively for beautification and rejuvenation among Asians. Just like the Western countries, botulinum toxin injection is the top of noninvasive cosmetic procedure in Asia. More younger Asian patients are having botulinum toxin injections for wrinkle removal especially on upper face expressive lines as wrinkles are less tolerable to them. As it is common among Asians to have a heavy and short lower face, botulinum toxin injection is frequently used to improve facial shape by slimming down the strong masseters and to relax the hyperactive mentalis muscle caused by the poor structural support from a retruded chin.[2,3] Body contouring like leg contouring and trapezius slimming by injecting botulinum toxin are popular in East Asia as well.[4,5] Apart from the intramuscular injection, intradermal injection of microdroplet of botulinum toxin is common in Asia for a more subtle result in wrinkle removing. In addition, it can also enhance skin quality by improving the skin tone, shrinking down of pore size, and reducing sebum production and erythema.[6,7]

Once again, more younger Asian patients are having HA injections to deal with their facial structural issues. HA is the workhorse to shape the esthetically undesirable flat, wide and short Asian face into a more attractive oval, well projected, and balanced face. Hence, more young Asian patients are having HA injections to enhance the projection of central facial features including forehead, glabella, nose, chin, and medial cheeks for beautification. In mature Asians, it is more challenging to address the undesirable facial structural deficiencies compounded by skin atrophy, volume depletion, and tissue migration caused by aging.

The Specialists: Lasers, Aesthetic and Plastic Surgery, Private, Room 601, Prosperity Tower, 39 Queen's Road Central, Hong Kong
E-mail address: howsclinic@yahoo.com.hk

Clin Plastic Surg 50 (2023) 11–17
https://doi.org/10.1016/j.cps.2022.08.006
0094-1298/23/© 2022 Elsevier Inc. All rights reserved.

Under such circumstance, combination therapy of HA injection with other treatment modalities like botulinum toxin injection, radiofrequency, high intensity focused ultrasound and thread will be a better option for an optimal rejuvenation. Furthermore, combined injection of HA and botulinum toxin in highly mobile areas like forehead and glabella, or area like chin with hyperactive mentalis helps to reduce muscle activity and hence facilitates tissue integration of HA and perhaps prolong the duration of the filler.

ESTHETIC GOALS FOR ASIAN PATIENTS

Different people have different definitions of beauty and attractiveness. Although some physicians try to quantify and standardize beauty by anthropometric measurements and proportions, others respect the differences and similarities between beauties of all races. One gender-specific global similarity of beauty in women is facial shape.[8] An oval facial shape represents femininity, youthfulness, and attractiveness. It runs a smooth course from the forehead to the temples, posterior cheeks, mandibular angles, jawlines to the chin. In aging process, this youthful attractive oval shape will gradually become more rectangular with broken lines and angulations. Unfortunately, Asians typically have wide bitemporal, bizygomatic, and bigonial width with short vertical facial height and flat or even concave faces from profile view (**Fig. 1**).[9,10] All these characteristics end up in a wide, short and flat face that is masculine, aged, tense and esthetically unappealing. Even worse when these inherent facial deficiencies aggravated by the structural and morphological changes in aging process with loss of volume and sagging. Hence, the goals of beautification and rejuvenation with injectables for both young and mature Asians are to create an oval facial shape, to increase the facial height and three-dimensionality. Beware of applying the golden ratio or phi proportion principles when injecting Asians which sometimes can end up with ridiculous results (**Fig. 2**). In general, the ultimate target in treating Asians is to aim at a balanced, small, and narrow-looking face with well-projected midline structures and medial cheeks while preserving their discrete Asian ethnic features and esthetic individuality. Most of these are achievable by injectables without any downtime.

INJECTION PRINCIPLE AND STRATEGY

It is not easy to deliver a promising result by injectables as they appear to be. The usual problem among new injectors is that they are too eager to

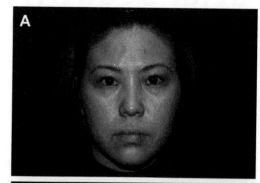
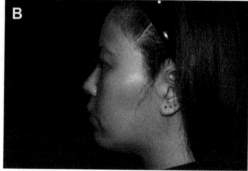

Fig. 1. (*A*) An Asian woman illustrating the typical morphological features with a short and wide face. (*B*) Lateral view revealing poorly projected nose, medial maxilla and chin resulting in a flat face.

inject. Injectables should be regarded as serious as all other medical procedures. Likewise, it should be started by taking a comprehensive medical history, paying particular attention to history that may jeopardize the result or give rise to adverse events like record of allergy to injectables, previous cosmetic surgery over the injection area, autoimmune disease, active inflammation or infection at or near the injection site. Spend adequate time in patient communication and expectation management. A thorough holistic total facial assessment, with and without facial animation, is a must before making a customized treatment plan. As treatment of one area can have impact on other areas, a list of treatment priority is needed. Frequently, combined treatment modalities is required to achieve the optimal result that may be better to deliver in different treatment sessions to avoid unexpected side effects and downtime.

As an oval facial shape is salient in beautification and rejuvenation, HA fillers are frequently used to remove the depression or shadow over forehead, temples and preauricular areas in Asians. This is often conjoined with lower face width reduction by slimming down the masseters with botulinum toxin. The retruded chin is enhanced by HA and

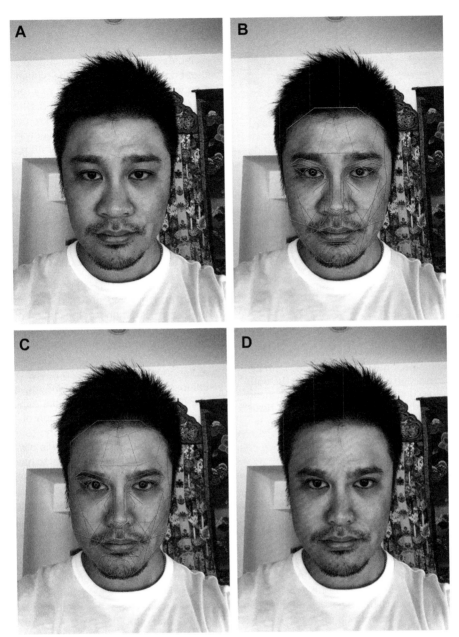

Fig. 2. (*A*), (*B*), (*C*) Dr Siew Tuck Wah MD applying the golden ration portion on his face for rejuvenation by using Photoshop. (*D*) An unnatural result which was deviated from his ethnic origin with loss of his unique facial characteristics. (*Courtesy of* Siew Tuck Wah, MD, Singapore, SG.)

may sometimes combine with botulinum toxin to relax the hyperactive mentalis. In addition to contributing an oval facial shape, the augmented chin also improves the facial height and projection. Facial three-dimensionality can be further improved by HA fillers injection to glabella, nose, and medial cheeks in most circumstances. With better-projected nose and medial cheeks, and the removal of hollow over temples and preauricular regions, this will create a visual perception of a

narrower midface. All these HA fillers should be injected either supraosteally or in deep fat compartment in order to provide the structural support for facial contouring.

INJECTION TECHNIQUES

Procedure is performed in clinic setting with patient in supine position for marking and injection under good lighting (**Fig. 3**). Apply topical

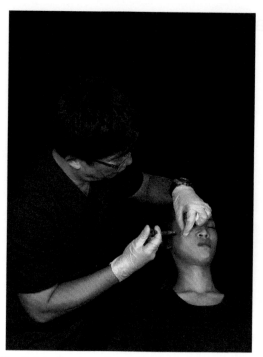

Fig. 3. Injection is performed in clinic setting with patient in supine position under good lighting. Use both hands when injecting, with the non-injecting hand guiding the needle and product into the tissue without spreading.

anesthetic cream in the patient who is sensitive to pain. Otherwise, simple ice pack application can offer reasonable numbing effect and also reduce the chance of bruising. Cleanse the injection area with 0.05% chlorhexidine thoroughly, avoid using agent like alcohol that may cause unnecessary skin irritation. Whether to use a needle or a cannula depends on personal preference and the area to be injected. Injection should be done slowly with low injection force and the smallest amount of product necessary. Use both hands when injecting, with the noninjecting hand guiding and controlling the needle or cannula and product into the desirable tissue plane without spreading. Small boluses injection, limited to 0.1 mL per bolus, should be used when injecting deep into the periosteum or deep fat compartments, whereas linear threading technique is preferred when injecting into the superficial tissue layer. Stop injecting if there is excessive pain, especially pain outside injection area, and injection site blanching that may suggest intravascular event. Gentle massaging and molding sometimes are required to smooth out the uneven contour after injection. Finally, apply antibiotic cream to those needle entry points to finish the procedure.

POSTOPERATIVE CARE AND EXPECTED OUTCOME

Injectables are regarded as lunchtime procedures without downtime. However, the patient is advised not to wear makeup and avoid any form of massage over the injected area for 24 h. Strenuous exercise and alcohol consumption are generally not recommended on the day of injection. Hot and spicy food should be avoided for 48 h after injection of the lips to prevent overwhelming swelling. Gentle cleansing over the injected site is allowed if needed. Mild swelling over the injected area is common but in general what you see is what you get.

MANAGEMENT OF COMPLICATIONS

Although the majority of HA filler complications like swelling and bruising are mild and self-limiting, other less common complications including irregularity, nodules, and hypersensitivity reaction usually resolve after hyaluronidase and anti-inflammatory treatments. The most serious intravascular complication can lead to tissue necrosis, visual loss, and even cerebral infarct, and hence warrants more detailed discussion. Although early recognition and prompt intervention of a vascular occlusion can reduce the long-term consequences significantly, prevention is always better than cure. Therefore, it is essential to have a sound knowledge of facial vascular anatomy before injection. However, intravascular injection can occur even at the hands of experienced injectors. Fortunately, uneventful healing was the usual outcome after immediate hyaluronidase treatment on diagnosis, with 86% being resolved within 14 days and only 7% suffered moderate scarring requiring surface treatments.[11] Measures to minimize intravascular injection include low-pressure small bolus injection, keep the needle moving while injecting, and stop injection if there is severe pain, especially pain outside injection site, or blanching over injection area. There are high-risk zones and low-risk zones for vascular occlusion, but there is no risk-free zone. Because of anatomical variations and distorted anatomy from previous filler injection or surgery, intravascular injection cannot be ruled out completely and ultrasound assistance may play a role in improving the safety of HA injection.[12] There are lot of controversies about aspiration before each injection but if one practices aspiration, it should be done with proper needle size and aspiration duration.[13,14] Furthermore, a negative aspiration does not mean the needle tip is not inside a blood vessel and may offer a false sense of security. Another controversy perhaps, is a blunt cannula has less intravascular complications than a needle. Although some experts recommend blunt cannulas,[15] one published article revealed that blunt cannulas cause the majority of severe vascular complications in HA injection.[16]

SUBSEQUENT PROCEDURES

Injectable are often combined with other treatment modalities such as thread lift and energy-based devices in one treatment session without compromising the results. It is recommended not to inject more than 4-mL HA filler for a hollow face in one session to avoid excessive and prolonged swelling and discomfort. Touch-ups can be done in 2 weeks. HA fillers nowadays can last 12 to 18 months and therefore injection for maintenance is commonly performed on yearly basis.

CASE DEMONSTRATIONS
Case 1

A 29-year-old Asian woman with boxy forehead, flat medial cheeks, and poorly projected midline facial structures (**Fig. 4**A). She had HA injection of 1 mL to forehead, 0.4 mL to nasal dorsum, 0.3 mL to columella, 1 mL to medial cheeks, and 0.8 mL to chin without any downtime. She looked more balanced with improved facial shape and three-dimensionality while preserving her discrete Asian ethnic feature and esthetic individuality immediately after the injection (**Fig. 4**B).

Case 2

A 35-year-old Asian lady with high cheekbones, a wide and flat midface (**Fig. 5**A). Result of a smaller facial appearance with narrower looking midface 8 weeks after uneventful HA injection of 1 mL to temples, 1.2 mL to preauricular regions, 0.5 mL to nasal dorsum, 0.8 mL to medial cheeks, and 1 mL to chin (**Fig. 5**B). There was an additional improvement of under-eye shadow after HA enhancement of medial cheeks.

DISCUSSION

The attitude of injection should be conservative, under-correct rather than overfill, respect and preserve patient's anatomical structure, and inject safely. Most of the unnatural results are caused by unawareness of esthetic ideal, poor patient assessment, inappropriate injection techniques like large bolus injection and placement of the product in wrong tissue layer, wrong choice of product, and overfilling. Repeated large-volume HA injections will not only end up in overfilling with distorted facial features and permanently

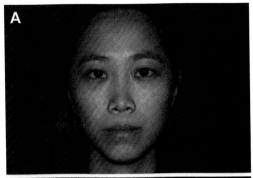
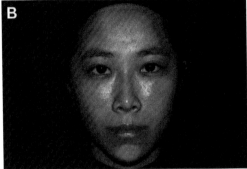

Fig. 4. (*A*) A young Asian woman with boxy forehead, flat medial cheeks and midline structures. (*B*) Immediately after HA injection to forehead, nasal dorsum, columella, medial cheeks and chin showing improved facial shape and three-dimensionality while preserving her discrete Asian ethnic feature and esthetic individuality.

damaged the normal anatomical structures, but also increase the risk of filler adverse events. Aging process involves multiple facial layers and it is the combination of bone resorption, atrophy of deep fat compartments, and malpositioning of superficial fat compartments that contribute to a hollow face.[17] The problem of volume-based injection (VBI) is to solve the issue of the hollow face resulting from volume loss and tissue malpositioning by volumization alone. It involves repeated large bolus of big volume injection to replenish the depleted volume and lift up the ptotic tissue. According to VBI, the more volume being injected, the more projection and lifting will be achieved. This kind of injection will not only end up in overfilling with a distorted appearance, but also carry higher risk of vascular occlusion, product migration, and delayed inflammatory hypersensitivity reaction.

The principle of tissue-targeted filling (TTF) is to use combined treatment approach to tackle the pathophysiological changes of aging in volume loss and tissue migration. It is a rheology-based injection concept focusing on injecting a smaller amount of filler, which is resilient to repeated facial

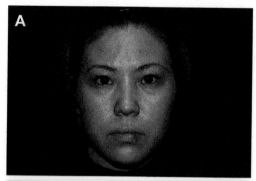

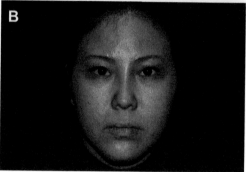

Fig. 5. Result of a narrower midface appearance after removal of hollow over temples and preauricular regions with enhanced projection of nose and medial cheeks. Note the additional improvement of under-eye shadow after injection of medial cheeks. (*A*) Before, (*B*) after treatment.

movements, at the right tissue layer with the filler rheology similar to the tissue that is being replaced. In other words, the philosophy of TTF is to replace "the like with the like" in volume depletion. TTF is often combined with other treatment modalities such as thread and energy-based devices like microfocused ultrasound for tissue repositioning. Biostimulants like calcium hydroxyapatite and poly-l-lactic-acid (PLLA) for neocollagenesis and skin quality improvement, lasers, and intense pulsed light for skin pigmentation and radiance can also be incorporated into the treatment plan. This holistic approach gives rise to a more natural result and avoids the problems of VBI including disproportionate face, overfilled appearance, surface irregularity, and lumpiness.

Although the injection principle and technique in Asians are basically the same, the treatment strategies and treatment endpoints are quite different from treating Caucasians as the facial structures, aging process, esthetic ideal, and concept of beauty are not the same. All esthetic procedures should be customized in regard to gender, age, ethnicity, culture background, medical history, and patient's desire to achieve a safe and balanced result while maintaining esthetic individuality and discrete ethnic features. Applying one standardized treatment approach for all will only end up in poor outcomes and unhappy patients.

SUMMARY

An oval facial shape with good projection and proportion is regarded as the ideal attractive youthful face across all nations. Treating mature Asians with the hollow face is challenging for a physician who needs to combine sound anatomical knowledge, detailed patient assessment with a holistic treatment plan, understanding of Asian facial structures and aging process, artistic sense, safety consideration, proper injection technique, and right product selection for a safe and promising result. Knowing the limitation of injectables, avoid solving all problems with injectables only or using a single standard treatment protocol on different faces. Combined holistic treatment approach is the benchmark of current esthetic medicine.

CLINICS CARE POINTS

- Beautification and rejuvenation with injectables in Asians can be challenging.
- Achieving an oval facial shape and enhancing the three-dimensionality is the ultimate treatment goal.
- Combined treatment approach is the standard in dealing with various problems of structural deficiencies and signs of aging.

DISCLOSURE

The author has no financial interest to declare in relation to the drugs, devices, and products mentioned in this article.

REFERENCES

1. Liew S, Wu WTL, Chan HH, et al. Consensus on changing trends, attitudes, and concepts of Asian beauty. Aesthetic Plast Surg 2016;40(2):193–201.
2. To EW, Ahuja AT, Ho WS, et al. A prospective study of the effect of botulinum toxin A on masseteric muscle hypertrophy with ultrasonographic and electromyographic measurement. Br J Plast Surg 2001; 54(3):197–200.
3. Yu CC, Chen PK, Chen YR. Botulinum toxin A for lower facial contouring: a prospective study. Aesthetic Plast Surg 2007;31(5):445–51.

4. Cheng J, Chung HJ, Friedland M, et al. Botulinum toxin injections for leg contouring in East Asians. Dermatol Surg 2020;46(Suppl 1):S62–70.

5. Zhou RR, Wu HL, Zhang XD, et al. Efficacy and safety of botulinum toxin type A injection in patients with bilateral trapezius hypertrophy. Aesthetic Plast Surg 2018;42(6):1664–71.

6. Park JY, Cho SI, Hur K, et al. Intradermal microdroplet injection of diluted incobotulinumtoxin-A for sebum control, face lifting, and pore size improvement. J Drugs Dermatol 2021;20(1):49–54.

7. Luque A, Rojas AP, Ortiz-Florez A, et al. Botulinum toxin: an effective treatment for flushing and persistent erythema in rosacea. J Clin Aesthet Dermatol 2021;14(3):42–5.

8. Goodman GJ. The oval female facial shape – a study in beauty. Dermatol Surg 2015;41(12):1375–83.

9. Le TT, Farkas LG, Ngim RC, et al. Proportionality in asian and north american caucasian faces using neoclassical facial canons as criteria. Aesthetic Plast Surg 2002;26(1):64–9.

10. Gu Y, McNamara JA Jr, Sigler LM, et al. Comparison of craniofacial characteristics of typical Chinese and Caucasian young adults. Eur J Orthod 2011;33(2):205–11.

11. Goodman GJ, Roberts S, Callan P. Experience and management of intravascular injection with facial fillers: results of a multinational survey of experienced injectors. Aesthetic Plast Surg 2016;40(4):549–55.

12. Schelke LW, Decates TS, Velthuis PJ. Ultrasound to improve the safety of hyaluronic acid filler treatments. J Cosmet Dermatol 2018;17(6):1019–24.

13. Van Loghem JA, Fouché JJ, Thuis J. Sensitivity of aspiration as a safety test before injection of soft tissue fillers. J Cosmet Dermatol 2018;17(1):39–46.

14. Torbeck RL, Schwarcz R, Hazan E, et al. In vitro evaluation of preinjection aspiration for hyaluronic fillers as a safety checkpoint. Dermatol Surg 2019;45(7):954–8.

15. de Maio M, DeBoulle K, Braz A, et al. Facial assessment and injection guide for botulinum toxin and injectable hyaluronic acid fillers: focus on the midface. Plast Reconstr Surg 2017;140(4):540e–50e.

16. Zhou SB, Chiang CA, Liu K. False sense of safety: blunt cannulas cause the majority of severe vascular complications in hyaluronic acid injection. Plast Reconstr Surg 2020;146(2):240e–1e.

17. Farkas JP, Pessa JE, Hubbard B, et al. The science and theory behind facial aging. Plast Reconstr Surg Glob Open 2013;1(1):E8–15.

Fat Grafting Combined with Liposuction Improves Cosmetic Facial Contours in Asians

Dong Wang*, Ming Ni, Min Gong, Chao Yang

KEYWORDS

• Liposuction • Fat grafting • Facial contours • Surgical design

KEY POINTS

- A surgical method for reshaping the contours of Asian faces is described.
- The method is based on a "three-line and nine-point" esthetic design suitable for Asians, aiming at increasing the "facial three-dimensional projection" and reducing the "Facial width."
- Fat grafting combined with liposuction can reflect the concept of our design for a potential good esthetic outcome.
- Our clinical results are satisfactory and a more attractive facial appearance can be achieved.

 Video content accompanies this article at http://www.plasticsurgery.theclinics.com.

INTRODUCTION

The application of autologous fat grafting in facial contour and rejuvenation of Asian people has been proven clinically for a long time and achieved satisfactory and lasting results.[1] With the development of the times, especially the rapid promotion of short videos, people need more delicate faces and like to have three-dimensional sense and obvious outline under the lens. However, Asians usually have a flat facial contour, broad cheekbones, and mandibles, including a narrow flat forehead, low-flat eyebrow arch, a low nasal back, a blunt nose tip, and a short chin.[2] Facial contour is usually mainly determined by subcutaneous fat and bones. Patients with bloated face caused by subcutaneous fat accumulation can undergo facial liposuction. Where the face is not full, fat transplantation will be performed. The combination of these two methods can meet higher demand. But up to now, there is no esthetic design idea

for Asian women. The effect made by doctors is influenced by esthetic preferences, and the esthetic effect after the operation is quite different.

In this article, the authors aimed to present a facial esthetic design that can be used to guide the combined operation of facial liposuction and facial fat grafting for Asians, that is, the "three-line and nine-point" design method. Based on the design idea of "three-line and nine-point," the authors combined facial liposuction and fat grafting to treat a large number of patients with esthetic facial contour issues and achieve visibly beautiful result as their face looks smaller, younger, and attractive with more three-dimensional definition.

INDICATIONS AND CONTRAINDICATIONS OF THE PROCEDURE

It is suitable for people whose facial contours are mainly affected by fat accumulation and skin sagging is not obvious. It is the contraindication of

Beijing Yimei Medical Cosmetology Plastic Clinic, No. 55, DongSanHuan North Road, Chaoyang District, Beijing 100020, China
* Corresponding author.
E-mail address: 646854688@qq.com

Clin Plastic Surg 50 (2023) 19–31
https://doi.org/10.1016/j.cps.2022.08.001
0094-1298/23/© 2022 Elsevier Inc. All rights reserved.

conventional surgery. People who have unrealistic expectations are also within the scope of surgical contraindications.

PREOPERATIVE EVALUATION AND SPECIAL CONSIDERATIONS

Nowadays, Asian women prefer a Westernized esthetic that preserves racial characteristics, that is, "mixed esthetics."[3] Combining the needs of "mixed esthetics" with the possibility of facial fat surgery, the author summarizes an esthetic design idea suitable for Asian women: "three-line and nine-point" (Fig. 1). Three lines: middle line (the central axis of the face) and the parapupillary lines (when the head is in a horizontal position and the eyes are looking straight ahead, a parallel line of 6 mm outward to the vertical lines of the pupils on both sides). Nine points (9 highlights): forehead top, forehead center, eyebrow arch on both sides, nose, anterior cheek on both sides, lip bead, and chin. The parapupillary lines are used as the dividing line for the types of facial fat surgery. The lateral areas of the parapupillary lines are the parts with reduced facial contour, mainly for facial fat aspiration, including the zygomatic arch area, cheek, and the jowl fat compartment. The areas between the two lines contain nine highlight areas, which are the parts with an increased facial stereoscopic impression, mainly for facial fat grafting. The role of the midline: (1) it can evaluate the left and right symmetry of the face and (2) the facial highlight expression line-the three-dimensional structure presented is the symbol of facial beauty.[4] Nine points: That is, nine facial esthetic highlights, which guide the key transplantation areas when facial fat grafting. After enhancing the nine highlights of the face through fat grafting, it can present an obvious three-dimensional sense. In addition to the area covered by the "three-line and nine-point," the obvious mandibular margin contour is also expected by patients. To enhance the mandibular edge contour, liposuction in the jaw-neck area should also be considered[5] (Fig. 2).

Before surgery, it is very important to explain the possible complications and precautions during recovery to the patients in detail, so as to avoid the early uneasiness after surgery. Patients with unrealistic expectations need to be treated with caution.

SURGICAL PROCEDURES
Fat Harvesting and Processing

The abdomen or thigh is usually chosen as the fat donor site, mainly because the fat in these areas is easily obtained and the concentration of adipose-

derived stem cells (ASCs) is higher.[6] Intravenous anesthesia and tumescent anesthesia are usually selected for surgical anesthesia. First, tumescent anesthesia was performed in the fat donor site, and 38°C swelling solution (500 mL normal saline, 15 mL 2% lidocaine, 0.5 mL 1: 1000 epinephrine, 5 mL 5% sodium bicarbonate) was used in the subcutaneous fat layer with a porous injection needle with an aperture of 2.0 mm (Fig. 3A). Tumescent anesthetic solution close to body temperature, when injected into the body, the less stress response produced by the body, and at the same time, it can reduce the destruction of adipocyte activity.[7] After the tumescent anesthesia injection is completed, wait for 10–15 min and connect the three-hole liposuction needle with an aperture of 2.5 mm to the 20-mL syringe (see Fig. 3A), manually reciprocate the subcutaneous fat layer to obtain the fat graft, and keep 10 mL of air in the syringe during exercise. Then, the obtained fat graft was left standing for a short time, and the liquid under the syringe was thrown away. The fat graft was transferred to a 10-mL syringe by Coleman centrifugation technology, and placed in a centrifuge for centrifugation at 2000 rpm for 3 min. After centrifugation, the fat graft has three layers, and only the central layer is retained. The treated fat graft was poured into a metal cup, and the fibrous tissue was manually removed and shredded and mixed with the fat graft. The fibrous tissue is not discarded because of the accumulation of ASCs, which may improve the survival rate of fat.[8] and transferred to a 1-mL syringe for later use.

Anesthesia for Facial Surgical Procedures

Immediately after the completion of tumescent anesthesia in the fat donor site, swelling solution anesthesia (500 mL 0.9% saline, 15 mL 2% lidocaine, 0.5 mL 1: 1000 epinephrine, 5 mL 5% sodium bicarbonate) was performed on the facial surgery area. The needle entry point was broken with a special metal tapered needle (Fig. 3B). This procedure can reduce the residence time of fat graft in vitro, which is beneficial to the activity of fat graft. Use a 1.0 mm porous injection needle (Fig. 3C) to inject a proper amount of swelling solution into the surgical level evenly, and the skin at the end of injection does not need to appear orange peel, so as to prevent excessive swelling from affecting the observation shape during operation. (Video 1) Injection of swelling solution can predict the amount of fat grafts needed in the fat receptor region. As the swelling solution infiltrates, it can constrict blood vessels and reduce the risk of bleeding and vascular embolism. Fat graft was

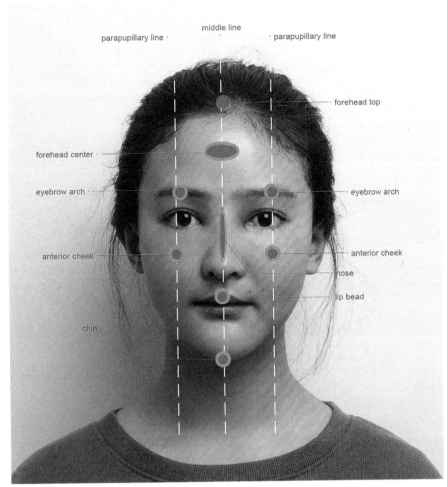

Fig. 1. "Three-line and nine-point"—an esthetic design idea suitable for Asian women.

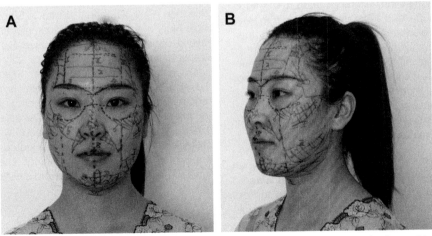

Fig. 2. Front view design drawing (*A*), the side view design drawing (*B*), the blue line is the fat grafting area, and the red line is the liposuction area. Liposuction area: the zygomatic arch area, cheek, and the jowl fat compartment, jaw-neck area; Fat grafting area: forehead, temporal part, brow arch, nose, tear trough, anterior cheek, nasolabial sulcus, and chin.

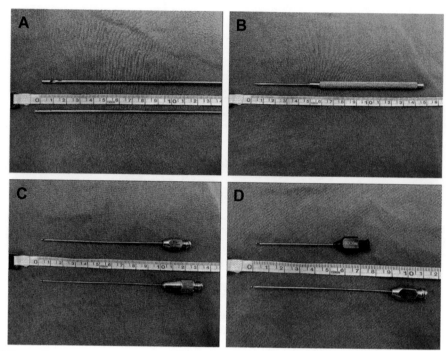

Fig. 3. A 2.0-mm diameter porous injection needle and a 2.5-mm diameter three-well liposuction needle (*A*). A metal tapered needle (*B*). A 1.0-mm diameter porous injection needle and a single-hole blunt liposuction needle with a pore size of 1.6 mm (*C*). A 1.0 mm × 50 mm single hole blunt needle and a 1.2 mm × 90 mm single hole blunt needle (*D*).

obtained from fat donor site after facial tumescent anesthesia was completed.

Facial Liposuction

The aspiration area is mainly located outside "the parapupillary line." The needle entrance of facial fat suction is usually located in hidden parts of the face, such as the hairline edge, front of tragus, front of earlobe, and submental skin fold (**Fig. 4**). A single-hole blunt liposuction needle with an aperture of 1.6 mm is connected with a 20 mL syringe to pump fat manually (see **Fig. 3**C). During the suction process, the syringe keeps 5 mL air and keeps the pinhole downward. The suction sequence is the zygomatic arch area, cheek, the jowl fat compartment, jaw, and neck area. The layer is limited to the subcutaneous fat layer, and is sucked in a multi-tunnel, uniform fan-shaped manner (**Fig. 5**, Video 2). Most Asian women have temporal depression, which is considered to affect their beauty. Obvious depressions are usually improved by fat grafting. However, mild depression can be visually improved or even corrected by aspiration to the zygomatic arch region.[4] When aspirating the zygomatic arch region, pay attention to the transition with temporal and cheek, and observe the overall fluency and contour. The

"mixed esthetic" pursued by Asian women—with clear mandibular edge and slightly sunken cheek outline, is achieved primarily by suction for zygomatic arch area, cheek, the jowl fat compartment, jaw, and neck area.[5]

Facial fat grafting

In fat grafting, 1-mL syringe is mainly used to connect 1.2 mm × 90 mm single-hole blunt needle for injection (**Fig. 3**D), and 1.0 mm × 50 mm single-hole blunt needle is used for finer injection if upper eyelid depression is improved (see **Fig. 3**D). The transplantation techniques were all combined with uniform retrograde linear injection and "peeling" filling. Another key point is multi-level and micro-transplantation. Depending on different recipient regions, the injection level selected from the periosteum to the subcutaneous will change. At the same time, the amount of injected fat should be controlled at 0.05–0.1 mL every time the cannula is pulled out, so as to avoid excessive local injection.

Frontal and Temporal Fat Grafting

The forehead needs selective fat grafting. As far as esthetics is concerned, the highlight area of frontal forehead should be located at the center and top of the forehead on the central axis, and gradually and fat graft evenly on the periosteum from the distal end to proximal end in the order of transition area-frontal center area-frontal parietal area, with the key grafting area located at frontal-parietal area, and pay attention to the smooth transition of frontotemporal junction area (**Fig. 6**, Video 3).

The visual flatness or even slight depression of the temporal part is more in line with the requirements of Asian women's pursuit of "small face," whereas the full temporal part will increase the outline visually. Because the zygomatic arch region was the first to complete liposuction, the temporal depression has been improved visually,[9] so the author is relatively cautious about the fat capacity of temporal depression transplantation. For the temporal region, choose the appropriate needle entry point from the hairline edge, and inject the fat grafts appropriately into the subcutaneous layer from the distal end to proximal end, whereas avoiding excessive injection, especially in the lateral area of the orbital bone margin (see **Fig. 6**, Video 3).

Eyebrow arch and nasal fat grafting

Asian women have the characteristics of a low nose and low flat eyebrow arch. Increasing the height of the nose and eyebrow arch can increase the three-dimensional sense of the face. The increase in the eyebrow arch can also make the eyes deeper. Controlling the nasal frontal angle from 115° to 125°, which is the ideal angle preferred by Asian women.[10] Another area that needs extra attention is the triangle area formed by the connection between the nasal root and the eyebrows on both sides. Western women have a three-dimensional triangle, just like a flying "wild goose"—the author named it "Wild goose style Beauty Horn," which is one of the symbols of "mixed esthetics."

Fat grafting of eyebrow arch is inserted from eyebrow tail (see **Fig. 4**). The injection level of

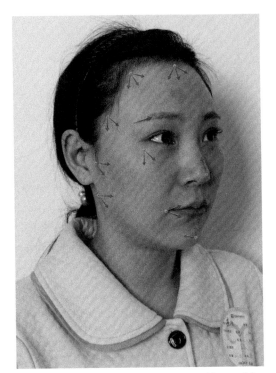

Fig. 4. Entry positions for liposuction and fat grafting.

decrease to both sides. However, the top of the forehead has not been paid attention to in the past. The authors believe that the frontal-parietal area is the most important area to be transplanted, and the highest area of the forehead is located on or above the horizontal line of frontal tubercle. From the side view, the forehead area has a soft vertical curve from the hairline to the eyebrow arch, and does not protrude. The key grafting area is between the parapupillary lines, and the transition area is outside the parapupillary lines. On the forehead, select the appropriate needle entry point from the edge of the hairline (see **Fig. 4**),

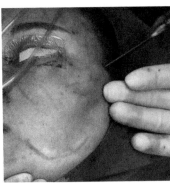
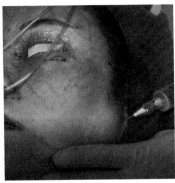
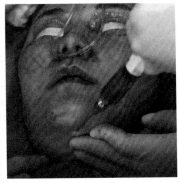

Fig. 5. Suction sequence is the zygomatic arch area, cheek, the jowl fat compartment, jaw and neck area and the layer is limited to the subcutaneous fat layer.

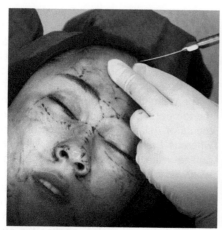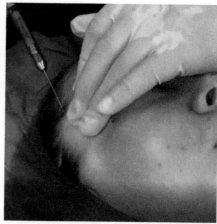

Fig. 6. Fat grafting of the forehead on the periosteum and fat grafting of the temples in the subcutaneous layer.

eyebrow arch is limited to subcutaneous fat layer, and fat graft is gradually injected from distal end to proximal end, paying attention to the shaping of "Wild goose style Beauty Horn" (**Fig. 7**, Video 4).

Nasal fat grafting is inserted from nasal tip (see **Fig. 4**), and the fat graft are injected step by step in the order of nasal root-back- tip-columella, mainly in the central part, mainly in the central part. The injection level of nasal root and nasal dorsum is limited to periosteum, and the nasal columella is mainly injected into the anterior nasal spine, which can properly raise the nasal base and increase the nasolabial angle, whereas the nasal tip needs proper injection, especially the full and soft nasal tip before operation (see **Fig. 7**, Video 4).

Middle Facial Fat Grafting

Fat grafting in the anterior cheek is usually concentrated in the area formed inside the parapupillary lines and above the horizontal line of the apex of alar sulcus, including the tear trough and zygomatic-buccal sulcus. In Asian women, the zygomatic process highlight area is lateral. If the highlighted area is moved to the nasal side without moving other parts of the face, the middle face will be visually narrowed.[11] Therefore, liposuction of zygomatic arch is performed to shorten the width of the middle face and weaken the highlighted area of the projection of the malar body.[9] Then, by transplanting fat into the target area of the anterior cheek, the highlighted area can be moved to the nasal side, which can further shorten the width of the middle face visually, which is a key step to achieve the "small face." Do not inject too much fat, and when the face is static, the area is preferably flat or slightly convex. Otherwise, once excessive fat is transplanted, a bloated feeling will

appear when making dynamic expressions, and an aging feeling will appear once drooping.

Anterior cheek fat grafting is injected from the lateral side of the infraorbital border (see **Fig. 4**), and injected from a deep fat pad to subcutaneous multi-level, with deep support as the main part. For tear troughs and zygomatic-buccal sulcus, more micro and deep injections are required, and linear injection must be moved and no more than 0.05 mL to avoid nodule formation (**Fig. 8**, Video 5).

Nasolabial sulcus fat transplantation is injected from the lateral side of the infraorbital border (see **Fig. 4**), and the injection level is subcutaneous and supraperiosteal, mainly supraperiosteal. As the needle is inserted from the outside of the infraorbital margin, the moving direction of the needle tube is perpendicular to the nasolabial groove, which can avoid aggravating the original static lines of the nasolabial groove (see **Fig .8**, Video 5).

Lower Facial Fat Grafting

Asian women prefer an oval chin, and the convexity of the chin should be slightly behind or just at the line drawn through nostrils, and perpendicular to Frankfort Horizontal plane.[2] During fat grafting it should be noted that the chin usually only increases convexity, not length, and too long chin will affect facial esthetics.

Lower facial fat grafting is inserted from the middle of chin (see **Fig. 4**). The injection levels are subcutaneous and supraperiosteal. First, the fat graft is injected into the periosteum of the chin to support it until the protrusion reaches the esthetic standard, and then injected subcutaneously on both sides of the chin, paying attention to the transition with the mandibular margin. Puppet lines, one of the key areas to be improved in facial

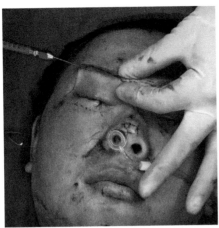
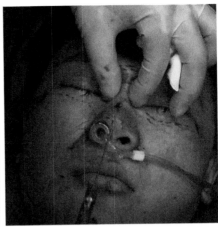

Fig. 7. Injection level of eyebrow arch is limited to subcutaneous fat layer and the injection level of nasal root and nasal dorsum is limited to periosteum.

rejuvenation, are caused by the atrophy of the mandibular fat pad, and also by the drooping and accumulation of the jowl fat compartment.[12] First, fat aspiration, which reduces the effects of sagging and accumulation, and then the fat graft was injected subcutaneously into the mandible through the moving direction of the needle tube perpendicular to the puppet pattern to supplement the capacity and further enhance the effect (**Fig. 9,** Video 6).

Postoperative Nursing

Elastic clothing is worn for 4 weeks in the donor area, the elastic mask can be worn in the facial liposuction area for 2 weeks, swelling can last for 1 or 2 weeks and there may be local hard lumps, which can be massaged appropriately. Avoid massage in the face fat grafting area for 3 months.

Expected Outcomes and Management of Complication

From 2017 to 2020, the lead author performed facial liposuction combined with fat grafting for 173 patients based on the esthetic design idea of " three-line and nine-point," all of whom were women, with an average age of 35.4 (21–49 years). All patients were followed up for more than 12 months. Among them, only eight (4.6%), because they felt that the facial stereoscopic sense was insufficient, were dissatisfied with the results, and all of them underwent a single facial fat graft after 6 months and the postoperative results were satisfactory. Both postoperative bruising and swelling recovered within 2 weeks. No serious complications such as hematoma, infection, nerve injury or fat necrosis occurred in all patients.

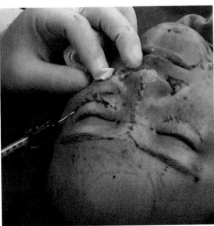
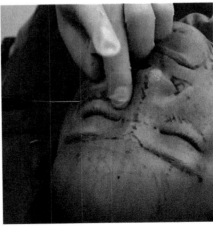

Fig. 8. Fat grafting of anterior cheek and nasolabial sulcus is injected from deep fat pad to subcutaneous multi-level.

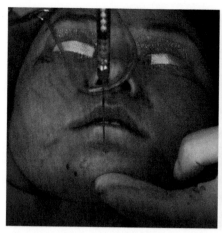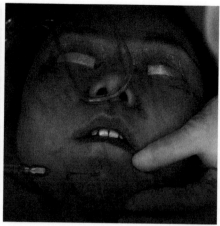

Fig. 9. Injection levels of the chin are subcutaneous and supraperiosteal and fat grafting of puppet lines is injected subcutaneously.

Revision or Subsequent Procedure

For those patients with insufficient facial contour or stereoscopic sensation, at least 6 months apart and after a second surgical adjustment, satisfactory results are obtained.

Case Presentation (Up to Four)

Photographs of four representative patients are illustrated in **Figs. 10–13**.

Case 1: A 22-year-old woman reshapes her facial contours through facial liposuction combined with fat grafting. Facial liposuction area: zygomatic arch, the jowl fat compartment, cheek, jaw-neck area; Facial fat grafting area: forehead, brow arch, nose, tear trough, nasolabial sulcus, chin, puppet pattern. In the preoperative views, facial contours are blurred (a, c); 14 months after the operation, the face is visibly stereoscopic (b, d) (see **Fig. 10**).

Case 2: A 29-year-old woman reshapes her facial contours through facial liposuction combined with fat grafting. Facial liposuction area: zygomatic arch, the jowl fat compartment, cheek, jaw-neck area; Facial fat grafting area: forehead, brow arch, nose, tear trough, anterior cheek, nasolabial sulcus, lip, chin, puppet pattern. In the preoperative views, facial contours are flattened and bloated (a, c); 12 months after the operation, the face is significantly narrowed and clearly contoured (b, d) (see **Fig. 11**).

Case 3: A 36-year-old woman reshapes her facial contours through facial liposuction combined with fat grafting. Facial liposuction area: the jowl fat compartment, cheek, jaw-neck area; Facial fat grafting area: forehead, brow arch, nose, tear trough, anterior cheek, nasolabial sulcus, chin, puppet pattern. In the preoperative views, facial contours are bloated (a, c); 13 months after the operation, the facial contours are clear (b, d). Especially in the forehead top fat grafting, its effect on the contours of the face can be seen (see **Fig. 12**).

Case 4: A 42-year-old woman reshapes her facial contours through facial liposuction combined with fat grafting. Facial liposuction area: zygomatic arch, the jowl fat compartment, cheek, jaw-neck area; Facial fat grafting area: forehead, brow arch, nose, tear trough, anterior cheek, nasolabial sulcus, chin, puppet pattern. In the preoperative views, facial contours are swollen (a, c); 14 months after the operation, The facial contours are clearer and younger (b, d) (see **Fig. 13**).

DISCUSSION

The "mixed esthetics," which combines the "small face" pursued by Asian women with the "three-dimensional sense" of Caucasian outline, is loved by Asian women. In the past, fat grafting turned the face into a "T" area, forming an inverted triangle on the face, confirming that it can make the face younger.[13] However, this esthetic design is vague. The authors propose the "three-line and nine-point" esthetic design method. The lateral side of the parapupillary lines is mainly liposuction. It is possible to narrow the contours of the middle of the face by reducing the volume of soft tissues without affecting the bone structure.[9] And it avoids complications of the middle faces which are narrowed by zygomatic osteotomy, re-immobilization, and poor reduction plasty.[14] If the patient's masseter muscle is hypertrophied, botulinum toxin can be injected postoperatively, which can further achieve the esthetic contour of the lower face.[15] Fat grafting is mainly used between

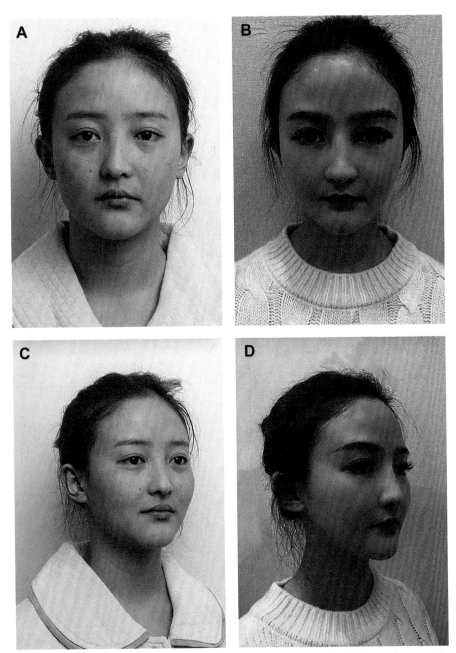

Fig. 10. Case 1: A 22-year-old woman reshapes her facial contours through facial liposuction combined with fat grafting. Facial liposuction area: zygomatic arch, the jowl fat compartment, cheek, jaw-neck area; Facial fat grafting area: forehead, brow arch, nose, tear trough, nasolabial sulcus, chin, puppet pattern. In the preoperative views, facial contours are blurred (*A, C*); 14 months after the operation, the face is visibly stereoscopic (*B, D*).

the parapupillary lines, especially the highlight areas on the central axis, which need to be strengthened during fat grafting.

Facial liposuction combined with fat grafting is more suitable for experienced plastic surgeons. Here, the authors share personal experiences of intraoperative judgment. First in the liposuction area of the face, the zygomatic arch area and temporal part are visibly flat during intraoperation, and the temporal part is not protruding. The cheek area is also flat. In the grafting area of the face, the forehead needs to be grafted appropriately and selectively, and the area of transplantation is focused on the middle

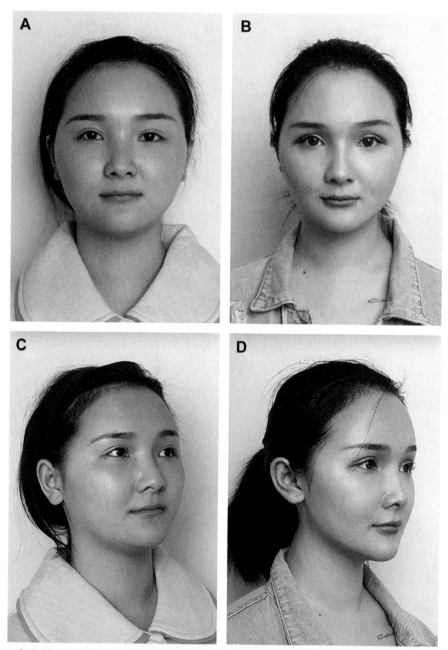

Fig. 11. Case 2: A 29-year-old woman reshapes her facial contours through facial liposuction combined with fat grafting. Facial liposuction area: zygomatic arch, the jowl fat compartment, cheek, jaw-neck area; Facial fat grafting area: forehead, brow arch, nose, tear trough, anterior cheek, nasolabial sulcus, lip, chin, puppet pattern. In the preoperative views, facial contours are flattened and bloated (*A, C*); 12 months after the operation, the face is significantly narrowed and clearly contoured (*B, D*).

line, and it is especially noticed that the area of 1 cm above the eyebrows should be filled with caution. Temporal transplantation should not be protruding. Anterior cheeks are transplanted in moderation. The reason for the dissatisfaction among the analysis study subjects was that the patients expected the face to be more three-dimensional, and after the secondary fat grafting, the face became more three-dimensional and satisfied.

Although based on the design idea of "three-line and nine-point," satisfactory results were obtained in the author's clinical practice. However, there are the following limitations, first of all, bone

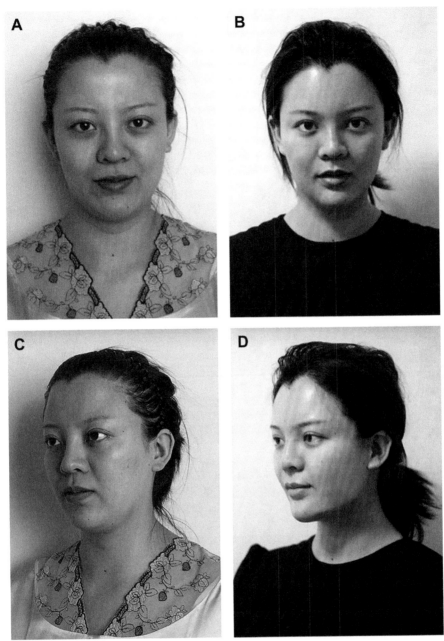

Fig. 12. Case 3: A 36-year-old woman reshapes her facial contours through facial liposuction combined with fat grafting. Facial liposuction area: the jowl fat compartment, cheek, jaw-neck area; Facial fat grafting area: forehead, brow arch, nose, tear trough, anterior cheek, nasolabial sulcus, chin, puppet pattern. In the preoperative views, facial contours are bloated (*A, C*); 13 months after the operation, the facial contours are clear (*B, D*). Especially in the forehead top fat grafting, its effect on the contours of the face can be seen.

contouring surgery is still recommended for patients with protruding cheekbones but less subcutaneous fat and expect a significant narrowing of the middle face. The endpoint of facial liposuction lacks an objective criterion and highly depends on the experience of the surgeon. Secondly, the survival rate of fat grafting is still uncertain, and further exploration is needed to improve the survival rate; in the end, the postoperative effect only stays in visual changes, lacking objective data such as three-dimensional volume measurement to support a more reliable evaluation.

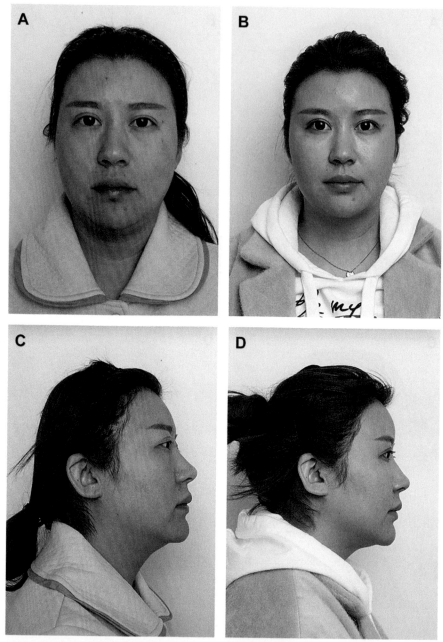

Fig. 13. Case 4: A 42-year-old woman reshapes her facial contours through facial liposuction combined with fat grafting. Facial liposuction area: zygomatic arch, the jowl fat compartment, cheek, jaw-neck area; Facial fat grafting area: forehead, brow arch, nose, tear trough, anterior cheek, nasolabial sulcus, chin, puppet pattern. In the preoperative views, facial contours are swollen (*A, C*); 14 months after the operation, the facial contours are clearer and younger (*B, D*).

SUMMARY

For Asian women, fat grafting combined with liposuction can cosmetically reshape facial contour based on the "three-line and nine-point" design. The facial contour in those patients can significantly be improved because of resulted "smaller face" and more "three-dimensional definition" and a more attractive appearance. Our technique can easily be learnt and can be mastered by the most well-qualified plastic surgeons for a satisfactory outcome.

CLINICS CARE POINTS

- For different people, it is very important to flexibly use the design idea of three-line and nine-point.
- To familiarize yourself with facial anatomy and select the appropriately positioned needle entrance.
- To inject an appropriate amount of tumescent anesthetic.
- Proficiency in facial liposuction and fat grafting surgery is required

DISCLOSURE

The author has nothing to disclose.

SUPPLEMENTARY DATA

Supplementary data related to this article can be found online at https://doi.org/10.1016/j.cps.2022.08.001.

REFERENCES

1. Egro FM, Coleman SR. Facial fat grafting: the past, present, and future. Clin Plast Surg 2020;47(1):1–6.
2. Samizadeh S, Wu W. Ideals of facial beauty amongst the Chinese population: results from a large national survey. Esthetic Plast Surg 2020;44(4):1173–83.
3. Liew S, Wu WTL, Chan HH, et al. Consensus on changing trends, attitudes, and concepts of asian beauty. Esthetic Plast Surg 2020;44(4):1186–94.
4. Xiong Z, Jiang Z, Liu K. Midline volume filler injection for facial rejuvenation and contouring in asians. Esthetic Plast Surg 2019;43(6):1624–34.
5. Keramidas E, Rodopoulou S. Radiofrequency-assisted liposuction for neck and lower face adipodermal remodeling and contouring. Plast Reconstr Surg Glob Open 2016;4(8):e850.
6. Geissler PJ, Davis K, Roostaeian J, et al. Improving fat transfer viability: the role of aging, body mass index, and harvest site. Plast Reconstr Surg 2014;134(2):227–32.
7. Wu YD, Li M, Liao X, et al. Effects of storage culture media, temperature and duration on human adipose-derived stem cell viability for clinical use. Mol Med Rep 2019;19(3):2189–201.
8. Yang Z, Jin S, He Y, et al. Comparison of microfat, nanofat, and extracellular matrix/stromal vascular fraction gel for skin rejuvenation: basic research and clinical applications. Aesthet Surg J 2021;41(11):NP1557–70.
9. Yang M, Gu Y, Wang D, et al. Liposuction of the zygomatic arch area: a novel concept to improve the midface contour. Esthetic Plast Surg 2022. https://doi.org/10.1007/s00266-021-02765-8. published online ahead of print, 2022 Jan 20.
10. Swift A, Remington K. BeautiPHIcation™: a global approach to facial beauty. Clin Plast Surg 2011;38(3):347, v.
11. Linkov G, Mally P, Czyz CN, et al. Quantification of the esthetically desirable female midface position. Aesthet Surg J 2018;38(3):231–40.
12. Gierloff M, Stöhring C, Buder T, et al. The subcutaneous fat compartments in relation to esthetically important facial folds and rhytides. J Plast Reconstr Aesthet Surg 2012;65(10):1292–7.
13. Yang Z, Li M, Jin S, et al. Fat grafting for facial rejuvenation in asians. Clin Plast Surg 2020;47(1):43–51.
14. Myung Y, Kwon H, Lee SW, et al. Postoperative complications associated with reduction malarplasty via intraoral approach: a meta analysis. Ann Plast Surg 2017;78(4):371–8.
15. Chang CS, Kang GC. Achieving ideal lower face esthetic contours: combination of tridimensional fat grafting to the chin with masseter botulinum toxin injection. Aesthet Surg J 2016;36(10):1093–100.

Facial Rejuvenation with Fast Recovery Suspension Technique

Dejun Zhu, MD[a,1,*], Haiyang Yu, MD[b,1], Kai Liu, MD, PhD[c,*]

KEYWORDS

- Local anesthesia • Minimally invasive surgery • Special instruments and thread
- Suspension technique • Facial rejuvenation

KEY POINTS

- This procedure causes little tissue trauma and has a short operation time.
- Using the principle of vector space mechanics, zygomatic ligament, and deep temporal fascia as fixation points are the key parts of facial lifting.
- The change of esthetic outcome is immediate and lasts for a long time.
- Aiming to restore the position of the deep fat compartment of the middle face and the corner of the mouth, this operation also produces good effects on the tightening and lifting of the superficial lateral buccal Superficial Muscular Aponeurotic System (SMAS) and the platysma muscle of the mandibular margin.

 Video content accompanies this article at http://www.plasticsurgery.theclinics.com.

INTRODUCTION

Aging is a natural process. After middle age, the surface tissues of the human body begin to age, especially in the form of wrinkles, loosening, and atrophic changes in the skin of the face and neck. The surgical technique to remove wrinkles on the face and neck is called facial rejuvenation surgery.[1,2]

To combat the trend of skin aging, the use of facial wrinkle removal has become increasingly rejuvenating. Traditional facial wrinkle removal surgery generally uses a long incision in the coronal shape of the scalp, in front of the ear to behind the ear, with a large peeling area and a long operation time, which may lead to complications such as obvious postoperative scarring, incisional alopecia, numbness, and abnormal sensation in the operated area, discouraging many candidates. In

recent years, the application of minimally invasive methods in facial wrinkle removal is increasing. Minimally invasive face-lifting with poly-p-dioxanone (PPD) absorbable threads, micro laser, and other facial implants are most prevalent, but the maintenance time of the wrinkle removal effect is short. To explore an effective minimally invasive lifting method, fast recovery suspension technique for facial rejuvenation has gained popularity, especially in Asia.[3–5] In this article, my preferred approach to facial rejuvenation with fast recovery suspension technique is described. Its indications and anatomic considerations are also described.

INDICATIONS AND CONTRAINDICATIONS

According to the condition of facial aging, especially the soft tissue descends of the middle and

[a] Nike Cosmetic Medical Clinic, 50 Guangfeng Industrial Avenue, Zhongshan City 523000, P.R.China; [b] Litchi Cosmetic Medical Clinic, 358 Juyuan Road, Hangzhou 310000, P.R. China; [c] Department of Plastic and Reconstructive Surgery, Shanghai Ninth People's Hospital, School of Medicine, Shanghai Jiao Tong University, 639 Zhizhaoju Road, Shanghai 200011, P.R. China
[1] These authors contributed equally to this study.
* Corresponding authors.
E-mail addresses: Chengxin515@126.com (D.Z.); drkailiu@126.com (K.L.)

Clin Plastic Surg 50 (2023) 33–41
https://doi.org/10.1016/j.cps.2022.09.001

lower face with some skin laxity, but the fat accumulation is still not obvious.

This procedure is mainly applicable to patients between the ages of 25 and 45 years old, who usually have obvious lacrimal grooves and zygomatic buccal groove, deepening of the nasolabial folds, the downward movement of the fat pad, flatted cheek, drooping of the corner of the mouth, and early jowling (**Fig. 1**). They should be healthy with no major medical issues.

PREOPERATIVE EVALUATION AND SPECIAL CONSIDERATIONS

We hope to achieve the best results by using the most minimally invasive methods. Therefore, we should first consider the volume and tissue displacement of facial soft tissues. The reduction or absence of volume will affect the esthetic appearance, and the facial soft tissue displacement makes tiredness and aged look. This procedure is able to quickly and immediately improve the middle facial descent, such as zygomatic buccal groove, lacrimal grooves, and poor lower eyelid position. In addition, this operation also has great advantages in improving the nasolabial folds, the drop and deepening of the corner of the mouth, the buccal concave, and the tightening and lifting of the mandibular margin. If there is a serious loss of volume in the temporal region and/or middle face with significantly depressed buccal fat, appropriate hyaluronic acid (HA) or autologous fat filling can be administered. In addition, the combination of Botox to relax the jaw and neck muscles can also enhance the outcome of this procedure.

Facial aging is caused by a combination of thinning of the facial skin base, loss of the number of elastic fibers in the dermis, loss of elasticity, laxity of muscle tissue, and reduction of total subcutaneous fat. These changes cause the outer corners of the eyes to sag, deepen the nasolabial folds, and visually flatten the cheekbone area.[6,7] The anatomic layers of the facial soft tissues from superficial to deep are skin, subcutaneous fat layer, SMAS layer (superficial fascial system), subfascial loose tissue layer, and muscle layer; the SAMS fascial layer is a subcutaneous fibrous membranous structure of

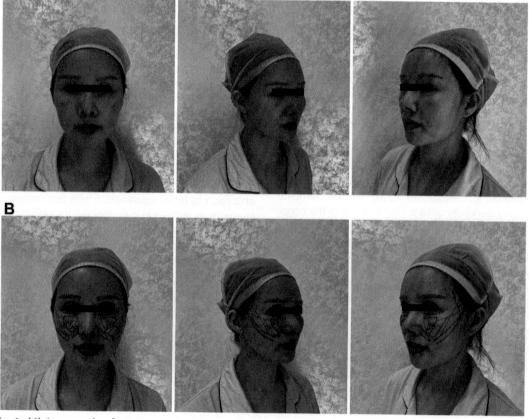

Fig. 1. (*A*) An example of a typical patient for the procedure. (*B*) Preoperative marking of the procedure for the same patient.

the face from the head to the neck, which is separated from the skin by delicate fat tissue above and from the deep fascia by lax connective tissue below.[8,9] The loose connective tissue layer allows the facial skin to slide up and down and is called the sliding layer. The sliding layer is the anatomic basis for minimally invasive facial skin lift. The skin, fat layer, SMAS fascial layer, subfascial sparse tissue layer, and muscle layer all have a certain degree of extensibility. This is an inherent characteristic of the soft tissue structure. The sliding layer of the facial soft tissue anatomy and the inherent ductile properties of soft tissues provide the anatomic basis for the application of minimally invasive submerged guided suspension surgery for facial rejuvenation.[10,11]

The SMAS layer, located about 4.5 mm deep under the skin, is between the subcutaneous fat and muscle. As we age, the elastin in the SMAS layer begins to be severely lost, and the lifting function becomes weaker, so the skin gradually becomes saggy, wrinkled, double-chinned, and other aging signs. Aging starts from the inside out, so the treatment of aging should also start from the inside out. To restore the delicate, smooth, and elastic skin, the first step is to work on the SMAS layer. Traditional facelifts only work on the top layer of the skin, so the results are short-lived and unnatural. An ultrasonic knife (Ulthera) can reach the SMAS layer directly through ultrasonic waves, stimulating the deep skin collagen restructuring and regeneration, thus comprehensively correcting the problems of sagging, wrinkles, and elasticity of facial skin.[12,13]

Fascia suspension lift is also a kind of wrinkle reduction surgery, using a special apparatus to do deep stripping and cutting of fascia, improving the fascia from a folding scheme to a shearing process. Theoretically, the pulling force is greater, but at the end, the epidermis and muscles are removed at the same time and then the counter skin suture is performed. Because of the special apparatus and sutures used during the surgery, it has no scarring and much less hair loss. This unique suture will not break even if the muscle and skin are under excessive tension and the SMAS is cut.[14,15]

In recent years, plastic surgeons have found, through a large number of clinical practices of facelift and wrinkle reduction surgery that the effect is quite different when the fascial layer on the periosteum is tightened and folded, and then the epidermis and muscles are lifted. In this way, the face can lift more sagging skin in the same sagging state, and by lifting and folding the SMAS, the skin is tightened from the deeper layers, so that the facial muscles and skin do not look tight and appear natural.

SURGICAL PROCEDURES

Fig. 1B shows the preoperative planning for the procedure. Local anesthesia and facial nerve block are performed at the riveting point, and then, appropriate local anesthetics (lidocaine + ropivacaine 1:1 with 1:100,000 of epinephrine) are infiltrated to the planned polydioxanone (PDO)-implanted areas in the fixation points to reduce pain (**Fig. 2**, Video 1).

One fixation point of over the zygoma (lateral margin of suborbicularis oculi fat pad [SOOF]) and three fixation points of the temporoparietal region near the hairline are used as the key points of vector elevation and lifting effect of this operation (**Fig. 3**).

The 90-cm PDO single-type reverse saw suture is placed into the special guide needle. The guide needle is entered the surface of the zygoma through the pre-prepared insertion point of the zygoma. It is then turned toward the zygoma and

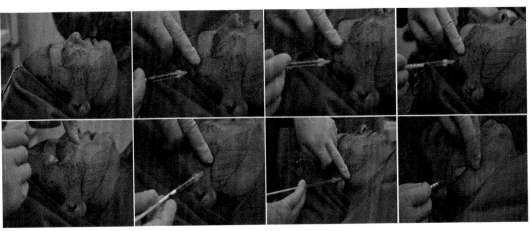

Fig. 2. Local anesthesia and facial nerve block were performed.

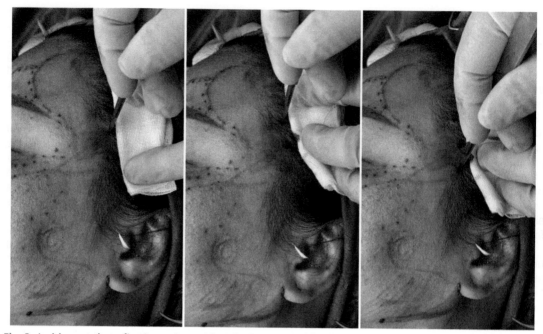

Fig. 3. Incisions at three fixation points within the hairline of the temporoparietal region were marked.

entered the deep fat pad above the zygoma. It is crossed the deep surface of the nasolabial fold according to the designed subcutaneous path. The needle is drawn back 0.5 cm and gently pressed and touched to the end of the suture with the finger. The distal end of the suture is tightened. If the suture is firmly grabbed, the needle can be pulled back to one-third. The thread is then implanted in the parallel direction or superficial to SMAS and can be placed back and forth to its original place. The thread is grasped tightly, and its proximal end is placed to the temporal region in a reverse fashion. This step can be repeated until complete equal power (vector mechanics) can be adjusted based on the angle. All these steps can be repeated. In the case of heavy corner of the mouth and zygomatic buccal groove with zygomatic ligament as an across the point combining with the "V" shape lifting, the effect of the deep tissue gathering can be achieved (**Fig. 4**).

To further stabilize and tighten the superficial layer of the SMAS, the "0" thread is cut to different lengths according to the distance to the application site. Three small incisions (1.5 cm apart for two-way approaches) are made within the temporal hairline with a guided needle. Two "0" inverted saw sutures are implanted parallel to the tip of each ear. All threads are placed and are connected with the forceps. The lifted height and the stability of the implant threads are adjusted parallel to the tip of each ear and tied at the fixation point. Then, a single root of the thread is advanced

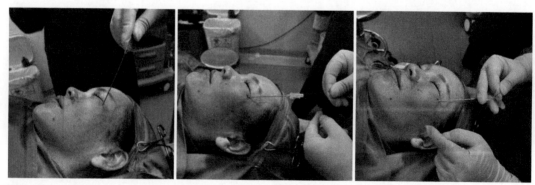

Fig. 4. The guide needle was inserted into the periosteum of the zygoma through the pre-prepared insertion point.

from the deep temporal fascia to the second fixation point through a two-way-guided device. The thread knot is adjusted and placed into the deep layer and fixed with a cross-knotted vascular clamp. In the highest point, the galea aponeurotica (epicranial aponeurosis) is riveted with a guided device and fixed with knots. Finally, the knot of each thread is buried deeply under the galea aponeurosis of the forehead toward the cheek. At the end of the operation, all incisions are closed with 7 to 0 silk suture except two small incisions of the face that are closed with 8 to 0 silk suture. At the end of the procedure, the nasolabial fold and temporal region are secured with elastic tapes (**Fig. 5**).

Postoperative Care and Expected Outcome

The postoperative care is the same as most facial rapid recovery thread lifts techniques, which requires strengthening the protection of the surgical incision and strengthening the dressing and tightening of the surgical area.

MANAGEMENT OF COMPLICATIONS

The common complications after the fast recovery suspension surgery are infection, bleeding, and so forth, which can be treated postoperatively with antibiotics. The author has experienced no significant complications in his case series.

REVISION OR SUBSEQUENT PROCEDURES

As our surgery is less invasive but effective, subsequent procedures are usually not necessary in the short term. However, further repeated procedures may be needed after 5 to 10 years.

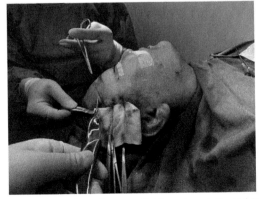

Fig. 5. Three threads were tightened and fixated in the temporal region.

CASE DEMONSTRATIONS
Case 1

In a case of a 44-year-old Chinese woman, we evaluated her facial condition before the operation. The aging and stiffness of her whole face were obvious, and the main characteristic manifestations were laxity around the eyes and in the middle and lower face, moving down of the apple muscle and aging changes of skin texture (**Fig. 6**A–C). The surgical scheme designed by us was aimed at the facial contour and strived to achieve the change of the youthful appearance of the face. Among them, the relaxation of the platysma muscle and the management of the chin and neck were crucial. It was also important to improve periocular aging, especially the formation of lower eyelid pouches. After surgery, we can see the disappearance of lower eyelid pouches, the elevation of the mouth angle, the restoration of the apple muscle, and a change in the overall fluidity of the mandibular margin (**Fig. 6**D–F). The change of the whole face curve is very obvious, and the state of the face is significantly younger. As shown in **Fig. 6**G–I, 2 years after the operation, the patient's face still maintained a good state of rejuvenation.

Case 2

A 34-year-old Chinese woman presented with some of the early signs of aging in her midface, which were characterized by flattening of the midface, exposure of the zygomatic buccal groove, overall downward movement of the fat pad, shallow nasolabial folds, and loose skin at the mandibular margin, combined with a feeling of tiredness around the eyes (**Fig. 7**A–C). As her basic condition was relatively good, during the operation, we focused on improving her whole face fat pad, zygomaticus major muscle, zygomaticus minor muscle, upper lip levator muscle, nasal alar muscle, and so on. It not only improves the fullness of the whole middle face, so that the displaced tissue can return to its original shape, but also improves the shape of the outer corner of the eye (**Fig. 7**D–F). As shown in **Fig. 7**G–I, 1 year after the operation, the patient's facial contour was clear, and the whole eye area and mandibular margin remained in a good state of rejuvenation.

Case 3

A 40-year-old Chinese woman presented with a flat midface with less volume, deep nasolabial folds, loose medial superficial buccal fat pad, and a less fluid mandibular margin. The whole

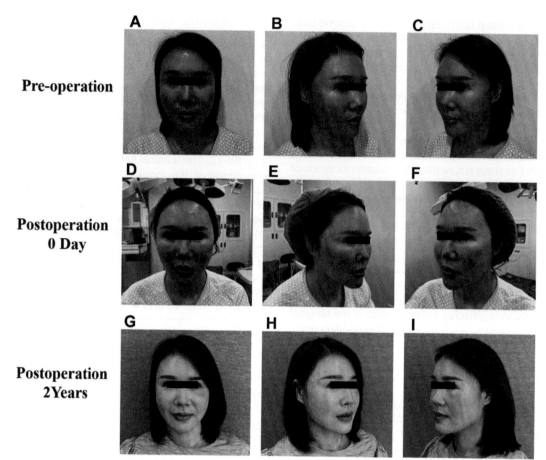

Fig. 6. Preoperation: the front (*A*), right (*B*), and left (*C*) sides of the patient's face. Immediate postoperative: the front (*D*), right (*E*), and left (*F*) sides of the patient's face. Two years postoperative: the front (*G*), right (*H*), and left (*I*) sides of the patient's face.

face looked tired, not soft enough and not tight enough (**Fig.** 8A–C). After this operation, the patient changed significantly (**Fig.** 8D–F). The patient, a doctor, was an early adopter of the procedure and only had periocular wrinkle removal after surgery. After 20 months of clinical observation, the patient showed good long-term follow-up without other adverse reactions (**Fig.** 8G–I).

DISCUSSION

The author has proposed several considerations for the choice of this procedure. Selecting the lateral part of zygomatic SOOF for restoration of the middle facial deep fat compartment has the following advantages: The riveting point is SOOF that is closely attached to the periosteum, with limited mobility and stable tissue structure. It is relatively safe because there are less blood vessels and nerves in this area. As a deep fat pad reduction, the protrusion of the weakened SOOF in the zygomatic region is avoided by direct rivet

lifting of the temporal region, which results in the projection of the zygomatic region. Because of this change, the esthetic appearance of the middle face can be optimized.

Fixing points in the temporal region in this procedure have two main advantages. First, lifting and stabilization of the middle face and improvement of its contour but excessive facial width, caused by weakening high lifting, can be avoided. As three points are fixed to the deep temporal fascia and the galea aponeurosis and the multiple knotting is fixed to lift the face rather than a single line and single point for lifting force, such a stabilization time would last relatively long. Second, as this particular area of the face is rich in blood vessels and nerves, selected small incisions, blunt tissue dissection with scissors, and two-way-guided surgical approaches are very important to avoid any injuries to those structures.

PPD is an absorbable thread and commonly used as an individual thread that is placed under the facial skin to form a linear lifting force, which

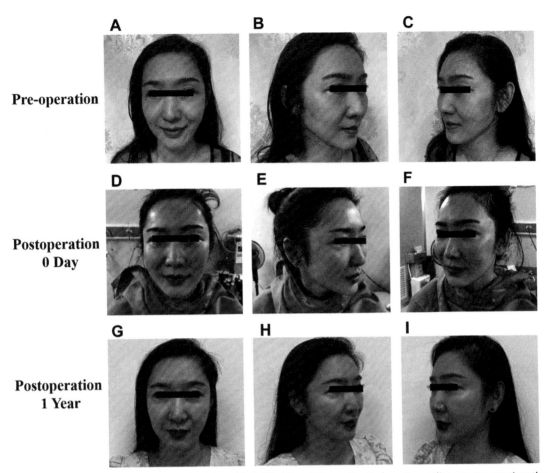

Fig. 7. Preoperation: the front (*A*), right (*B*) and left (*C*) sides of the patient's face. Immediate postoperative: the front (*D*), right (*E*), and left (*F*) sides of the patient's face. One year postoperative: the front (*G*), right (*H*), and left (*I*) sides of the patient's face.

is scattered and uneven. As it is absorbable, its lifting effect may only last a short time, generally in 3 to 6 months. The large number of foreign bodies placed under the facial skin at one time can also lead to complications such as inflammatory reactions, scarring strips, and even granulomas. Therefore, it is extremely important to explore an effective way for minimally invasive facial rejuvenation with less surgical dissection and thread lifts. A good minimally invasive facial rejuvenation technique should maintain relatively long-term postoperative results while being able to reduce trauma to the patient with less scar as possible and minimal impact on the patient's daily life.[16]

The minimally invasive suspension technique for facial rejuvenation using buried guide needles provides a new way of thinking for minimally invasive facial rejuvenation surgery. The principle is to lift the face as a unit, unlike only suture sculpting, which uses nonabsorbable braided threads to maintain any attempted relatively long-lifting

effect. The early appearance of the lift can be overcorrected because of excessive skin tightening and tissue edema. The skin buildup at the hairline will gradually subside within 1 to 3 months after surgery and the relatively stable surgical result can be achieved 3 months after surgery and may be maintained for 3 to 5 years. This procedure is less invasive, faster recovery, easy to perform, and no need for postoperative wrapping, and can be more acceptable by the patient. The limitation of this method is only suitable for patients with mild or moderate facial aging with less noticeable skin laxity, not for patients with severe facial aging with more noticeable skin laxity. The early postoperative effect is obviously stronger, and its effect becomes more stable 3 months after surgery.[17]

One suspension technique can be used to correct forehead wrinkles and excess skin. During the procedure, a skin incision in the middle of the forehead is made according to the preoperative design to enter the galea aponeurosis. A special

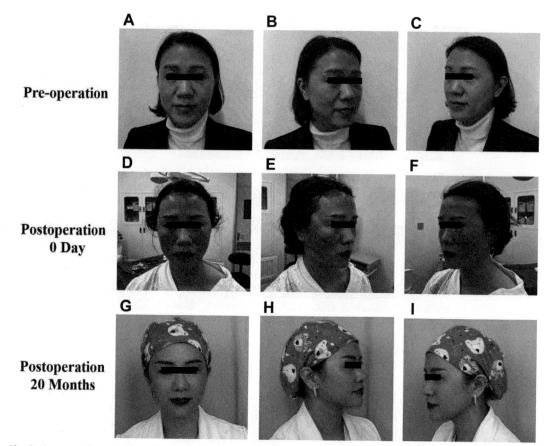

Fig. 8. Preoperation: the front (*A*), right (*B*), and left (*C*) sides of the patient's face. Immediate postoperative: the front (*D*), right (*E*), and left (*F*) sides of the patient's face. Postoperative 20 months: the front (*G*), right (*H*), and left (*I*) sides of the patient's face.

dissector is used to separate the subgaleal space and to reach the upper part of the eyebrow and the root of the nose. A special small-tipped knife is used to incise the frontalis muscle, corrugator muscle, and procerus muscle. During the dissection, the bleeding can be stopped by electrocoagulation, and the sharp separation along the SMAS fascia is performed to reach the root of the nose with a special instrument so that wrinkles at the root of the nose and Kawasaki lines can be corrected.[18]

Intermittent suspension is combining both "6"-shaped suspension and single-line suspension. This technique is generally indicated for patients who desire improvement of both forehead wrinkles and excess skin, and those who would need more extensive forehead lift for forehead aging. It is mostly suitable for middle-aged people aged 35 to 45, and the overall outcome after surgery may make those patients look about 10 years younger.[19]

Circumferential suspension is an extension of our technique for lifting a large area of the forehead. A circular incision is made within the frontal scalp along with both sides of the ear, without cutting the skin, muscles, and fascia. It is suitable for patients between 40 and 65 year. Its lifting effect is obvious and lasting, so that the forehead wrinkles and lose forehead skin can be effectively corrected. The surgery usually takes about 2 to 3 hours. It can completely restore the youthful look of the face.[20]

SUMMARY

With in-depth research on the mechanism of facial aging and rejuvenation, various new minimally invasive facial rejuvenation techniques have been discovered lately. The rapid recovery suspension technique has several advantages such as faster recovery, satisfactory results, and minimal or no surgical complications. Our surgical technique is minimally invasive and includes fixation of the relaxed tissue to achieve a stable and long-lasting result of facial rejuvenation. Its complications are relatively rare. With the combination of other facial rejuvenation techniques, the cosmetic outcome can be even more enhanced and long lasting. A clear understanding of different suspension techniques and the development of an individualized treatment plan based on the patient's aging can be the key for success.

CLINICS CARE POINTS

- Incision management is critical. We sutured the larger wound, applied repair gel to the wound site after suturing, and removed the suture in 5 to 7 days.
- During the operation, the suture's knot should be placed in the deep tissue, at the base of the incision.
- After the operation, proper management for the exposure of the suture's knot may be needed.

SUPPLEMENTARY DATA

Supplementary data related to this article can be found online at https://doi.org/10.1016/j.cps.2022.09.001.

REFERENCES

1. Tavares JP, Oliveira C, Torres RP, et al. Facial thread lifting with suture suspension. Braz J Otorhinolaryngol 2017;83(6):712–9.

2. Wattanakrai K, Chiemchaisri N, Wattanakrai P. Mesh suspension thread for facial rejuvenation. Aesthet Plast Surg 2020;44(3):766–74.

3. Wu W, Mendelson B. Invited discussion on: Mesh suspension thread for facial rejuvenation. Aesthet Plast Surg 2020;44(3):775–9.

4. Atiyeh BS, Chahine F, Ghanem OA. Percutaneous thread lift facial rejuvenation: Literature Review and Evidence-based Analysis. Aesthet Plast Surg 2021;45(4):1540–50.

5. Erol OO, Sozer SO, Velidedeoglu HV. Brow suspension, a minimally invasive technique in facial rejuvenation. Plast Reconstr Surg 2002;109(7):2521–32, 2533.

6. Swift A, Liew S, Weinkle S, et al. The facial aging process from the "inside out. Aesthet Surg J 2021;41(10):1107–19.

7. Mendelson B, Wong CH. Changes in the facial skeleton with aging: implications and clinical applications in facial rejuvenation. Aesthet Plast Surg 2012;36(4):753–60.

8. Whitney ZB, Jain M, Zito PM. Anatomy, Skin, Superficial Musculoaponeurotic System (SMAS) Fascia. 2022.

9. Surek CC. Facial anatomy for filler Injection: the superficial Musculoaponeurotic system (SMAS) is not Just for facelifting. Clin Plast Surg 2019;46(4):603–12.

10. Cotofana S, Fratila AA, Schenck TL, et al. The anatomy of the aging face: a Review. Facial Plast Surg 2016;32(3):253–60.

11. Mendelson B, Wong CH. Changes in the facial skeleton with aging: implications and clinical applications in facial rejuvenation. Aesthet Plast Surg 2020;44(4):1151–8.

12. Del TE, Aldrich J. Extended SMAS Facelift. 2022.

13. Khan HA, Bagheri S. Management of the superficial musculo-aponeurotic system (SMAS). Atlas Oral Maxillofac Surg Clin North Am 2014;22(1):17–23.

14. Byun JS, Hwang K, Lee SY, et al. Forces required to Pull the superficial fascia in facelifts. Plast Surg (Oakv) 2018;26(1):40–5.

15. Khan HA, Bagheri S. Surgical anatomy of the superficial musculo-aponeurotic system (SMAS). Atlas Oral Maxillofac Surg Clin North Am 2014;22(1):9–15.

16. Rammos CK, Mohan AT, Maricevich MA, et al. Is the SMAS Flap facelift safe? A Comparison of complications between the Sub-SMAS approach versus the subcutaneous approach with or without SMAS Plication in aesthetic Rhytidectomy at an Academic Institution. Aesthet Plast Surg 2015;39(6):870–6.

17. Guyuron B, Seyed FN, Katira K. The Super-high SMAS facelift technique with Tailor Tack Plication. Aesthet Plast Surg 2018;42(6):1531–9.

18. Santorelli A, Cerullo F, Cirillo P, et al. Mid-face reshaping using threads with bidirectional convergent barbs: a retrospective study. J Cosmet Dermatol 2021;20(6):1591–7.

19. Hau KC, Jain S. Malar reshaping technique using bidirectional barb thread suspension procedure for 3-dimensional aging in Asian faces. Int J Womens Dermatol 2021;7(5Part B):747–55.

20. Park YJ, Cha JH, Han SE. Maximizing thread usage for facial rejuvenation: a Preliminary patient study. Aesthet Plast Surg 2021;45(2):528–35.

Facial Rejuvenation and Contouring with Radiofrequency-Assisted Procedures in Asians

Yuneng Wang, MD, Bo Yin, MD, Facheng Li, MD, PhD*

KEYWORDS

- Radiofrequency technique • Liposuction • Facial rejuvenation • Minimal invasive surgery

KEY POINTS

- Radiofrequency (RF)-assisted liposuction treatment for facial skin tightening is suitable for patients who need to choose between skin excision surgery and facial liposuction, which has a wide range of potential applications in Asia.
- Combined liposuction–RF treatment, which provides a superimposed effect, is more effective than liposuction alone.
- It is crucial to obtain the desired surgical result by allowing adequate exposure and protection of the fibrous septal network (FSN) so that the RF energy directly works on the FSN as integrated as possible.

INTRODUCTION

Currently, more than ever, there are more treatment options for facial rejuvenation and contouring.[1] Excisional facial surgery, including multifarious rhytidectomy, is an effective procedure for patients with facial and neck skin laxity. Available treatment procedures are characterized by long downtime, prolonged scarring, and numbness, making them less popular among Asians. Facial liposuction is suitable for young patients with adipose accumulation and good skin texture and elasticity. However, three types of patients fall into the category of patients having to choose between undergoing a skin excision procedure or liposuction alone: (1) younger patients who increasingly desire facial contouring and soft tissue tightening; (2) patients with skin laxity that is neither severe enough to necessitate an excisional procedure nor good enough to be indicated for liposuction; and (3) patients who need to undergo an excisional procedure and are unwilling to accept the treatment option.[2] In these patients, minimally invasive or nonexcisional, skin-tightening techniques with minimal scarring are required for facial contouring and rejuvenation.[3]

In recent years, the use of radiofrequency (RF) technology in skin tightening has become popular. The technology treats skin laxity by heating the reticular dermis, which triggers a healing cascade, leading to collagen formation and soft tissue contraction.[4–6] FaceTite (InMode Corporation, Lake Forest, California) bipolar RF device achieves skin contraction and contouring through its thermal effect on the collagen in the dermis and subdermal fibrous septal network (FSN) tissue.[7] In the last decade, our team began to use FaceTite combined with facial liposuction for facial rejuvenation and contouring procedures, acquiring satisfactory and long-lasting results without any severe complications. Therefore, the authors recommend facial liposuction combined with the RF procedure

Conflict of Interest: The authors have nothing to disclose.
Plastic Surgery Hospital, Chinese Academy of Medical Sciences and Peking Union Medical College, No.33 Badachu Road, Shijingshan District, Beijing 100144, China
* Corresponding author.
E-mail address: drlfc@sina.com

Clin Plastic Surg 50 (2023) 43–49
https://doi.org/10.1016/j.cps.2022.08.009

for the treatment of skin laxity. Minimal-invasive liposuction creates working channels for RF treatment and sufficiently exposes the subdermal FSN tissue so that the RF energy can directly act on the collagen of the FSN for thermal shrinkage, leading to better surgical results. Herein, the authors describe the preferred techniques for facial rejuvenation and contouring.

Indications and Contraindications

The indications were as follows: early jowling, mild skin laxity of the face and neck, moderate and severe skin laxity of the face and neck, unwillingness to undergo surgery, awareness of the limitations of RF treatment, recurrence after excisional facial surgery, and unwillingness to undergo surgical revision. Contraindications were as follows: pregnancy or breastfeeding, severe skin laxity, severe chronic disease, severe broad neck banding, presence of a pacemaker or automatic internal cardioverter defibrillator, surgery within the last 3 months in the treatment area, and inability to complete postoperative care.

Preoperative Evaluation and Special Considerations

It is important to communicate with the patient carefully to determine their needs and concerns. In addition, surgeons need to educate patients on the surgical principles, results, and possible complications of facial liposuction combined with RF treatment. Particularly, surgeons have to explicitly discuss the limitations of RF treatment compared with a skin-excision surgery in achieving skin contraction.[8] An effective preoperative consultation helps prevent unrealistic patient expectations before the procedure and disappointments after the procedure.

Combined liposuction–RF treatment can be combined simultaneously with facial filler procedures including fat grafting or hyaluronic acid. Although these injections are in the deep subcutaneous and deep supraperiosteal plane, which is not affected by the thermal effects of the RF treatment, it is still recommended that they are performed after both liposuction and RF treatment are completed.

Surgical Procedures

Devices

The authors performed skin tightening using a first- and second-generation FaceTite RF apparatus (InMode Inc., Lake Forest, CA), which delivers energy to trigger immediate and extended contraction of dermal and subcutaneous collagen. The FaceTite system consists of a bipolar RF handpiece and a computer device. A special FaceTite handpiece, 10 cm in length and 1.7 mm in diameter, was used in our procedure. The internal electrodes were coated with Teflon, and RF was emitted only from the tip. The external electrodes received RF and closed the current circuit. Compared with the first-generation device with skin surface temperature control, the second-generation device included a temperature surge protection. The temperature surge protection does not only help in the real-time monitoring of the internal and external electrode temperature, but also proves useful in analyzing the rate of temperature increases to avoid thermal injury before dangerous temperature surges. When the internal and external electrodes exceed the set threshold, the device is automatically stopped. Reports showed that the overall complication rate for the second-generation FaceTite was 0.7%, which was significantly lower than that of the first-generation device (14.6%).[9]

Facial liposuction

Before the procedure, the liposuction area was marked with patients in the standing position (**Fig. 1**). The procedure is generally performed under intravenous or local anesthesia. The tumescent solution consisted of 600 mg lidocaine, 1 mg epinephrine, and 500 mg sodium bicarbonate in 1 L normal saline. Incision puncture was performed with a 14g needle, and the procedure was performed through four puncture incisions: two incisions behind each earlobe for the lower face and two under the chin for the neck. Thereafter, a tumescent solution was injected into the subcutaneous plane until inflation was achieved. Approximately 80 to 120 mL of solution was used in the lower face, and another 80 to 120 mL of solution was used for neck treatment. Afterward, the incisions were closed with temporary sutures to prevent the leakage of tumescent solution. Thereafter, the authors waited 10 to 15 min for epinephrine to produce a vasoconstrictive effect to reduce bleeding. A specially designed four-hole liposuction cannula with a 1.6 mm diameter and a smooth side-hole of 1 mm × 2 mm was attached to a 5 mL syringe, and the negative pressure of the withdrawn syringe was set at 1 to 2 mL. Of note, in regions near important blood vessels and nerves, the frequency of liposuction was reduced and the negative pressure of the withdrawn syringe did not exceed 1 mL. A very low negative pressure of 100 to 200 mm Hg was maintained in the syringe to preserve the integrity of the FSN maximally.[10] The liposuction plane was located in the subcutaneous adipose tissue. Fan-

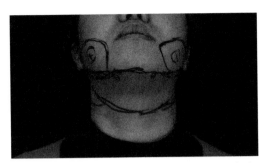

Fig. 1. Preoperative lower face and neck area design for treatment. The 1 to 2 cm area around the mandibular border was area that should be avoided to preserve marginal mandibular innervation.

shaped criss-cross channels were used during liposuction to ensure that the procedure was as uniform as possible. After achieving satisfactory liposuction results, the leftover tumescent solution was squeezed out.

Facial radiofrequency treatment

After liposuction, the parameters of facial RF were set to 20 W, external electrode cut-off temperature was 39.0 °C, and internal electrode cut-off temperature was set to 68 °C. The slow and gradual application of thermal energy to the soft tissue evenly distributes energy to avoid tissue necrosis caused by local energy accumulation.[11] Thereafter, a sterile ultrasound gel was placed on the treatment area, reducing the coefficient of friction to allow the external electrode of the handpiece to slide on, while increasing the contact area between the external electrode and the skin for better energy delivery. The internal electrodes of the FaceTite apparatus were placed in the subcutaneous adipose layer at a depth of approximately 3 mm to ensure that they are on the superficial side of the superficial musculoaponeurotic system (SMAS) to avoid damage to the facial nerve. Owing to the convexity of the treatment zone in relation to the straight FaceTite handpiece, caution should be paid to prevent end hits and a rapid increase in temperature that could lead to full-thickness injury of the dermis.[11] The prior liposuction procedure created working channels for the RF treatment at the appropriate treatment plane, and the surgeon was also able to confirm the depth by palpating the head of the handpiece externally. The inner electrode of the handpiece was inserted into the distal part of the treatment area and a stamp-like movement was applied. Each stamp lasted 1 to 2 s. When the desired temperature was reached, the FSN tissue contracted and the monitoring sensor automatically cut off the RF energy. To enhance the effect, the handpiece was moved

from the distal end to the proximal end, and each stamp was repeated for 30% to 50% of the stamped position to create an energy superposition effect. The thickness of the subcutaneous tissue after aspiration should be carefully evaluated. The stamping technique should not be used if the subcutaneous tissue is too thin, which can avoid the appearance of superficial dermal nodules or skin necrosis. Afterward, the superficial sliding technique was used that the handpiece was sliding slowly from the distal area of the treatment area to the proximal in a fan shape. It provided a uniform thermal effect on the tissue and smooth skin lifting. Temperature and treatment duration were precisely controlled to avoid excess temperature or prolonged action, which cause cell necrosis and stimulate inflammatory responses, leading to fibrosis, scarring, and hardening. In addition, the authors avoided the medial side of the marionette line and 1 to 2 cm around the mandibular border to preserve marginal mandibular innervation, which resulted in a smooth and clear jawline.[12,13]

Postoperative Care and Expected Outcome

After the operation, the elastic net cover was combined with a cotton pad for 1 day. The authors recommend the patient to wear a compression garment day and night for 5 days and thereafter, at night only for 2 weeks. For experienced surgeons, facial liposuction combined with RF treatment is a relatively safe technique, with a high rate of patient satisfaction and a low rate of complications.

Management of Complications

The procedure has few major postoperative complications requiring medical or surgical interventions. The authors have performed the technique for facial rejuvenation for many years and have obtained favorable long-term results without severe complications. Minor complications are subcutaneous tissue induration and localized skin depression. The subcutaneous tissue induration can be recovered by massage. Localized skin depressions can be improved by autologous fat grafting more than 3 months after our treatment.

Revisions or Subsequent Procedures

Few patients dissatisfied with the outcome are considered to have bilateral facial asymmetry. For these cases, small range liposuction combined with RF treatment using AccuTite device can be performed as the revision procedure.

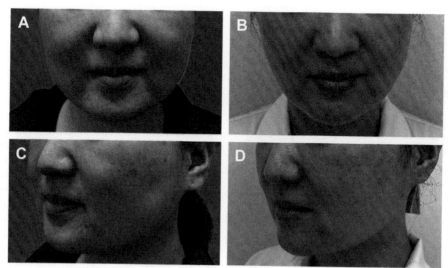

Fig. 2. Case 1. A 33-year-old woman presented for facial rejuvenation with liposuction combined with RF treatment, who was unsatisfied with the outcome of Ultherapy treatment(*A, C*). Intraoperatively, the manipulation was complicated by the resistance created by the scar tissue. Three months images after the procedure showed removal of shadows on both sides of the face and slim curved jawline (*B, D*).

CASE DEMONSTRATIONS

Photographs of three representative patients are provided in **Figs. 2–4.**

DISCUSSION

Asian women have become increasingly interested in facial rejuvenation and contouring. Facelifting is a mix of good results, high risk, severe scars, and a prolonged recovery period. Noninvasive treatments, such as Thermage and Ultherapy are easy to accept; however, the results are limited. In contrast, RF-assisted liposuction (RFAL) has a short surgery duration, small incisions, few complications, and short convalescence. Liposuction enables better sculpting of the lower face curves, whereas RF solves the issue of skin laxity after liposuction, which is precisely suitable for the Asian patient populations caught between surgical lifting and noninvasive treatments.[14] In addition, the procedure is an excellent option for patients with moderate aging changes

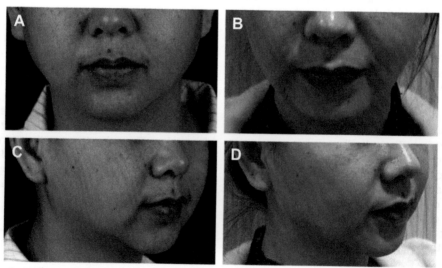

Fig. 3. Case 2. A 35-year-old woman presented for facial rejuvenation with liposuction combined with RF treatment (*A, C*). Preoperatively, this patient demonstrated mild skin laxity of the face. Seven months images after the procedure showed removal of shadows on both sides of the face (*B, D*).

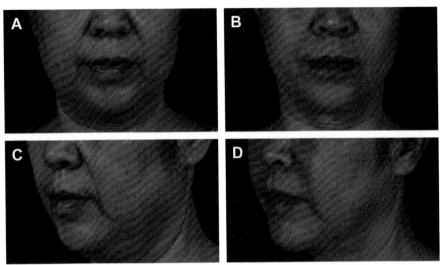

Fig. 4. Case 3. A 67-year-old woman presented with severe skin laxity of the lower face and neck, who was unwilling to undergo rhytidectomy (*A, C*). 1 year images after the liposuction combined with RF treatment showed good preservation of the tightening effect of the lower face and neck (*B, D*).

but who do not desire to undergo skin excision surgery. With the expanding indications of RF treatment, both patients and surgeons expect to achieve the best surgical results with minimal trauma. Therefore, it is important to enhance the outcomes of RFAL for wide application.

The conventional RFAL technique involves RF treatment after injection of the tumescent solution, followed by aspiration of the coagulated adipose tissue via the FaceTite handpiece. During RF treatment, the energy emitted by the RF device affects subcutaneous adipose tissue, FSN, tumescent solution, and other conductors (**Fig. 5**). The tightening principle works by the RF's thermal effect on the FSN to promote its contraction. The RF energy acting on other tissues reduces energy efficiency and increases tissue trauma. In the clinical practice of facial rejuvenation and contouring, our team proposed to perform facial

liposuction before RF treatment. With liposuction, the working channels of the RF treatment are created by the criss-cross movement of the liposuction cannula at the appropriate plane.[15] In addition, liposuction effectively removes the adipose tissue surrounding the FSN, which exposes the FSN and allows direct RF energy effect on the tissue, enhancing the effectiveness of RF energy usage and reducing the amount of energy required for RF, thus enhancing surgical results and resulting in less tissue trauma (**Fig. 6**).

With facial liposuction, the authors recommend a sufficient amount of tumescent solution, a small liposuction cannula, and a low-negative-pressure technique.[16] The tumescent solution, which exceeded the volume of the aspirated fat by more than ten times, was injected into the subcutaneous tissue to reduce intraoperative bleeding and postoperative skin bruising. In addition,

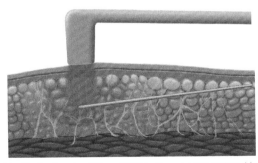

Fig. 5. During traditional RFAL, the energy emitted by the RF device works on the subcutaneous adipose tissue, FSN, tumescent solution and other conductors.

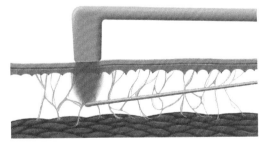

Fig. 6. With our technique, the thermal effect generated by RF is maximized on FSN and the energy loss is reduced.

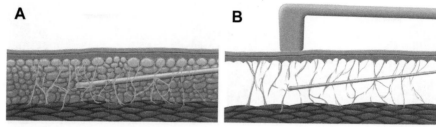

Fig. 7. The authors believe that high-negative-pressure liposuction destroys the integrity of the FSN (*A*), and that fracture of the FSN leads to worse contraction (*B*).

sufficient tumescent solution expands the space between the skin and SMAS layer, thereby preventing damage to the facial nerve branches and preserving the reticular fibrous septum. The use of a small cannula with a small hole on the side reduces the possibility of negative pressure grabbing and damage to the reticular fibrous septum. Facial liposuction should be performed gently with very low-negative-pressure, and the authors believe that high-negative-pressure liposuction destroys the integrity of the FSN and an FSN fracture leads to worse contractions (**Fig. 7**). Preservation of appropriate flat subcutaneous adipose tissue and an intact FSN are key to facial liposuction for RF treatment.

RF treatment should be performed at the appropriate layer and with proper manipulation approaches. The layer of RF treatment is determined by a prior liposuction operation, which allows the surgeon to focus better on RF treatment, avoiding treatment planes that are excessively deep or superficial, and reducing complications. The general principles of handpiece manipulation are treatment area zoning, uniformity of the stamped area, and control of the single-point treatment time and temperature, as energy is applied to the FSN in small, precise, and uniform amounts to obtain the best results. In addition, small areas should be treated with caution, as damage to these areas could lead to local depressions resulting from local tightening of the longitudinal fiber bundles connecting the deeper tissue to the skin.

SUMMARY

Facial liposuction combined with RFAL is a safe and effective facial rejuvenation and contouring procedure. This technique is an improvement on the traditional RFAL. It is important for surgeons to be professionally trained and familiar with procedural principles. Gentle facial liposuction and proper manipulation of the RF handpiece are key to obtaining desired surgical results and reduced surgical trauma.

CLINICS CARE POINTS

- Combined liposuction–radiofrequency (RF) treatment has better outcomes, which means liposuction first followed by RF treatment.
- It is crucial to inject a sufficient amount of tumescent solution, use small liposuction cannula, and adopt a low-negative-pressure technique in facial liposuction.
- The medial side of the marionette line and 1 to 2 cm around the mandibular border should be avoided to preserve marginal mandibular innervation, which resulted in a smooth and clear jawline.

DISCLOSURE

The authors declared no conflicts of interest with respect to the research, authorship, and publication of this article.

REFERENCES

1. Atiyeh BS, Chahine F, Ghanem OA. Percutaneous Thread Lift facial rejuvenation: Literature Review and Evidence-Based Analysis. Aesthetic Plast Surg 2021;45(4):1540–50.
2. Theodorou SJ, Del Vecchio D, Chia CT. Soft tissue contraction in body contouring with radiofrequency-assisted liposuction: a treatment Gap solution. Aesthet Surg J 2018;38(suppl_2):S74–83.
3. Dayan E, Chia C, Burns AJ, et al. Adjustable depth Fractional radiofrequency combined with bipolar radiofrequency: a minimally invasive Combination treatment for skin laxity. Aesthet Surg J 2019;39(Suppl_3):S112–9.

4. Ion L, Raveendran SS, Fu B. Body-contouring with radiofrequency-assisted liposuction. J Plast Surg Hand Surg 2011;45(6):286–93.

5. Irvine Duncan D. Nonexcisional tissue tightening: creating skin surface area reduction during abdominal liposuction by adding radiofrequency heating. Aesthet Surg J 2013;33(8):1154–66.

6. Chia CT, Theodorou SJ, Hoyos AE, et al. Radiofrequency-assisted liposuction compared with Aggressive superficial, subdermal liposuction of the Arms: a bilateral Quantitative Comparison. Plast Reconstr Surg Glob Open 2015;3(7):e459.

7. Swanson E. A systematic review of subsurface radiofrequency treatments in plastic surgery. Ann Plast Surg 2022;89(3):274–85. https://doi.org/10.1097/SAP.0000000000003093.

8. Rohrich RJ, Chamata ES, Bellamy JL, et al. Technique for minimally invasive face and neck contouring with bipolar radiofrequency devices. Plast Reconstr Surg 2022. https://doi.org/10.1097/PRS.0000000000009358.

9. Chia CT, Marte JA, Ulvila DD, et al. Second generation radiofrequency body contouring device: Safety and Efficacy in 300 local anesthesia liposuction cases. Plast Reconstr Surg Glob Open 2020;8(9):e3113.

10. Mezzles MJ, Murray RL, Heiser BP. In vitro evaluation of negative pressure generated during application of negative suction volumes by use of various syringes with and without thoracostomy tubes. Am J Vet Res 2019;80(7):625–30.

11. Theodorou SJ, Paresi RJ, Chia CT. Radiofrequency-assisted liposuction device for body contouring: 97 patients under local anesthesia. Aesthet Plast Surg 2012;36(4):767–79.

12. DiBernardo GA, DiBernardo BE, Wu D, et al. Marginal mandibular nerve Mapping prior to Nonablative radiofrequency skin tightening. Aesthet Surg J 2021;41(2):218–23.

13. Olivas-Menayo J. The MICRO-lift: a ligaments-based anatomic technique for lower face and neck rejuvenation using bipolar radiofrequency. Aesthet Plast Surg 2022. https://doi.org/10.1007/s00266-021-02719-0.

14. Cook J, DiBernardo BE, Pozner JN. Bipolar radiofrequency as an Adjunct to face and body contouring: a 745-patient clinical experience. Aesthet Surg J 2021;41(6):685–94.

15. Han X, Yang M, Yin B, et al. The Efficacy and safety of subcutaneous radiofrequency after liposuction: a New application for face and neck skin tightening. Aesthet Surg J 2021;41(3):NP94–100.

16. Yin B, Zhang X, Cai L, et al. Low negative pressure combined with Supertumescence Microliposuction as a New method for Repairing facial fat Overfilling: a Case Series of 32 patients. Aesthet Surg J 2022;42(4):NP193–200.

Advanced Endoscopic Techniques in Asian Facial Rejuvenation

Chia Chi Kao, MD[a],*, Dominik Duscher, MD, PhD[b,c]

KEYWORDS

- Endoscopic face-lift • Endoscopic midface-lift • Endoscopic brow lift • Ponytail lift
- Ponytail face-lift

KEY POINTS

- Asian anatomy differs from whites: eyes are naturally slanted and smaller; the skin is thicker; tissue is in general more fibrous; forehead is flatter; bridge of nose is flatter; cheek bones are wide; and the face is rounder or square shaped.
- However, the popular Asian concept of beauty is a heart-shaped tapered face with double eyelids (without a wide tarsal platform show).
- Traditional SMAS face-lifts are not ideal to achieve these aesthetic goals. The Asian population is prone to hypertrophic and keloid scars. Lateral pull and loss of fat after SMAS dissection flatten the face more.
- The characteristics of the ideal facial rejuvenation techniques for Asians comprise hidden incisions to avoid hypertrophic scarring and cultural stigma.
- Our approach addresses the Asian face in all dimensions using minimally invasive modalities. The authors call this surgical technique "Ponytail Lift" and "Ponytail Facelift" and combine it with skin regenerative methods.

 Video content accompanies this article at http://www.plasticsurgery.theclinics.com.

INTRODUCTION

Face-lift surgery corrects natural-occurring aging processes of the face and is increasingly becoming popular especially among Asians.[1] However, the operative techniques established in the last 3 decades focus on white patients, and these approaches need to be adjusted when treating the Asian face.[2] This is certainly owing to the fundamental anthropomorphologic differences in Asian faces,[3] which consequently modify beauty perception in these countries.[4] Therefore, alternative aesthetic criteria are important for patient evaluation before performing surgery.[5]

A currently popular technique for Asian facial rejuvenation is the composite or deep plane face-lift, which requires periauricular incision and deep plane sub-SMAS dissection.[2] This is important to efficiently lift the thicker and heavier soft tissues and create a rejuvenated result, which is said to be longer lasting. This technique also allows resection of the buccal fat pads of the cheeks, which is desired in Asians to reduce the more round-shaped face outline. In combination fat grafting has been demonstrated as an integral tool to elevate cosmetic results by adding prominence to the flattening forehead, midface, nose, and chin but avoiding protrusion of the zygomatic

[a] KAO Plastic Surgery Institute, 900 Wilshire Boulevard, Suite 100, Santa Monica, CA 90401, USA; [b] The Face and Longevity Center Munich, Herzogstrasse 67, Munich 80803, Germany; [c] Department of Plastic, Reconstructive, Hand and Burn Surgery, BG-Trauma Center, Eberhard Karls University Tübingen, Tübingen 72076, Germany
* Corresponding author.
E-mail address: kaoplasticsurgery@gmail.com

Clin Plastic Surg 50 (2023) 51–60
https://doi.org/10.1016/j.cps.2022.07.008

arch and mandibular angle.[2] Consequently, the sites for facial fat grafting are positioned more in the front of the face.

Despite the popularity of this technique, the authors think a modern face-lift in Asian patients should demand a minimally invasive approach without compromising the aesthetic results of the traditional face-lift, but simultaneously reduce visible scars. Their approach addresses the aging face in all dimensions using minimally invasive modalities combining endoscopic lifting of the forehead and midface, microfat grafting, and trichloroacetic acid (TCA) peeling. This approach is called the "Ponytail Lift" (PTL). This is a surgical technique that simulates the vertical lift of the face when having the hair pulled up in a high ponytail. When this approach is combined with a deep contouring of the anterior part and a limited-incision neck lift, the authors call this procedure a "Ponytail Facelift" (PTFL).

The aim of this article is to illustrate that PTL and PTFL are the ideal procedures for rejuvenating the Asian face. The authors share their clinical insights and technical details.

Preoperative Evaluation and Special Considerations

Analysis of facial characteristics in Asians show a much wider and flatter face, which is primarily caused by the prominent and wider cheekbones along with the prominent mandibular angle.[6] Particularly, the eyes and nose, which are 2 common ethnical facial features in Asians, are the most frequent subjects for cosmetic surgery, which also represent key modifications in terms of facial westernization.[1] Asian eyes are characterized by their simplified or absent upper eyelid crease and much larger orbital fat pad.[7] The Asian nose is described to have a wide and lower nasal bridge and less prominent nasal tip projection, which lead to a flatter nose appearance.[8] Therefore, double eyelid surgery and augmentation rhinoplasty are among the most common surgical procedures requested by Asian patients.[9] Soft tissue, especially skin, is thicker and heavier, and the buccal fat pads are larger, which together lead to an increased sagging of the mid and lower facial area when aging progresses.[10] Rhytids and skin laxity in contrast are less present in Asian patients than in whites, minimizing the need for excision of excess skin. It has to be stressed that the Asian skin is prone to produce keloid scars and hyperpigmentation after dermal injury.[11] Traditional face-lift techniques with periauricular incisions have been frequently reported to produce hypertrophic scars in Asians; therefore, incisions should

be kept minimally and concealed or even avoided altogether.[11] In addition to the less favorable outcomes of face-lift scars in the Asian population, visible scarring is also considered a social stigma in the Asian culture more so than in the western world.[12]

Different regions in Asia have exclusive preferences in facial attractiveness.[13] However, some characteristics can be summarized and considered favorable: large bright eyes, some degree of nasal dorsum and tip projection, an oval facial shape, and a smooth mandibular outline.[5] Given the mentioned anatomical characteristics, Asian rejuvenation requires a dedicated surgical approach in accordance to the favored facial appearance.[5] Traditional SMAS techniques are not ideal for several reasons. In addition to noticeable scarring in front of the ear, shortening of the sideburns, and distortion of the ear's anatomy,[14] also, the traditional face-lift separates the skin from the fat and lifts the fat tissues off the muscle. This will devascularize the skin and traumatize the fat that could potentially result in atrophy of the skin and fat, leading to an unnatural or even more aged appearance.[15] The lateral pull and loss of fat after classic SMAS dissection will flatten the face even more, and this is profoundly counterproductive for shaping the Asian face.

SURGICAL PROCEDURES

Surgical marking includes the bony architecture, Pitanguy line,[16] and the anticipated location of the sentinel vein in the temporal area 1 cm superior to the superior zygomatic arch and 1 cm lateral to the zygomatic process (**Fig. 1**). Monitored anesthesia care with propofol sedation is used in all cases. Intubation is avoided to prevent distortion of the face. The areas of dissection are infiltrated with local anesthesia solution (a mixture of 50 mL lidocaine 1% with epinephrine and 50 mL bupivacaine is diluted 1:4 with saline resulting in 500-mL solution).

Appropriate candidates for the ponytail procedure are screened based on clinical examination, including physical examination of skin excess and video assessment of facial features in movement, to determine the extent of treatment required to achieve optimal facial rejuvenation.

Overview of the Ponytail Lift

PTL is designed for patients presenting in their thirties and forties with signs of early aging, commonly seen in the upper two-thirds of the face. A combination of endoscopic brow and cheek lift, skin-only blepharoplasty, microfat grafting, and skin resurfacing using 15% to 20% TCA peel is performed in this patient cohort. This

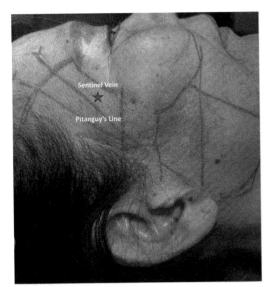

Fig. 1. Surgical marking. The bony architecture, Pitanguy line, and the anticipated location of the sentinel vein in the temporal area 1 cm superior to the superior zygomatic arch and 1 cm lateral to the zygomatic process are marked.

procedure is also suitable for younger female patients who have congenitally low-set masculine brows and cheek ptosis or hypoplasia who wish to soften and beautify their appearance.

Overview of the Ponytail Facelift

This procedure is indicated when there is enough laxity and redundancy of the neck skin that need to be resected. PTFL procedures include an extended posterior auricular incision. Correction of the anterior neck via plication and deep contouring as well as application of a posterior corset is necessary. Asian skin is typically thicker and more fibrous, so Asian patients do not develop excessive amounts of laxity or "turkey neck" so not a large amount of skin needs to be removed. The incision is perilobular into the posterior auricular sulcus and extends into the posterior mastoid hairline. The dissection of the neck is complete, all the way down to the clavicle and all the way back toward the anterior edge of the trapezius. The deep neck structures, such as submandibular glands, anterior belly of the digastric, and submental fat, are contoured. Laterally, the platysma muscle is tightened and sutured to the posterior neck fascia to further enhance the jawline. Importantly, there are no incisions in the pretragal area or temporal hairline.

OPERATIVE TECHNIQUES

1. *Limited incision lower face and neck lift:* A perilobular incision is made initially to avoid the pretragal incision, which will depend on the extent of skin that can be mobilized vertically after completing endoscopic dissection (Video 1 illustrates the surgical technique). The dissection plane is immediately superficial to the platysma, keeping all the subcutaneous fat with the skin flap and the posterior neck fascia down to the clavicle and extending posteriorly to the anterior border of the trapezius muscle. The subcutaneous fat is lifted with the skin to preserve cutaneous blood supply.

2. *Anterior neck deep contouring and anterior plication:* A submental curvilinear keyhole incision is made very anterior on the chin pad skin. Dissection proceeds along the platysma bands past the cricoid cartilage and connects the 2 sides of the neck dissection, working all the way down to the sternal notch. A horizontal incision is made at the level of the skin incision perpendicular to the platysmal muscle fibers to dissect and lift the platysma muscle. Subplatysmal fat is identified and then resected entirely to expose the anatomy of the anterior belly of the digastric muscle. The anterior belly of the digastric muscle is debulked as needed for contour[17] and then plicated with 4.0 Ethibond interrupted sutures. This will tighten the floor of the mouth. The anterior edge of the platysma is also plicated with 4.0 Ethibond interrupted suture, starting below the cricoid cartilage all the way up to the level of the skin incision to avoid cobra neck deformity. A 2-cm back-cut on the bands is made below the level of the cricoid. If the submandibular glands are enlarged and/or ptotic, the portion protruding below the level of the jawline is carefully resected. The cut surface of the submandibular gland is then sutured to the platysma muscle with 4.0 Vicryl mattress sutures to reduce dead space and the risk of sialocele.[18]

3. *Endoscopic forehead and cheek lift:* A 2-cm temporal incision is placed in an oblique orientation parallel to the hair follicles and a 1-cm paramedian incision is designed with a sagittal orientation. The temporal incision is placed lower than most incisions described for an endoscopic brow lift. Similarly, the vertically oriented paramedian incision is located to allow for the most aesthetically ideal brow elevation/rotation. In Asian patients, extensive brow rotation can lead to an angry appearance, so a conservative approach is advisable.

The dissection is performed between deep and superficial temporal fascia and done completely endoscopically. In the forehead and brow region, dissection is performed in the subperiosteal plane, all the way down passing the orbital rim.

In the temporal area, dissection proceeds endoscopically between the superficial and deep temporal fascia and continues down toward the zygomatic arch. The sentinel vein and the medial and lateral zygomaticotemporal neurovascular bundles are identified and preserved (**Fig. 2**). Dissection continues to the arch, and the arch ligament is sharply released. The zygomaticomalar ligament also needs to be released to gain access to the midface.

In the midface, the dissection plane is between the suborbicularis oculi fat (SOOF) and the orbicularis oculi muscle. The dissection continues along the zygomaticus major and minor muscle, down across the nasolabial fold. The zygomatic branch of the facial nerve must be preserved in this region. In order to minimize the risk of nerve injury, it is necessary to stay on the body of the zygoma and proceed medially, avoiding any lateral deviation.

The midface flap that is mobilized across the nasolabial fold is suspended from several fixation points to the deep temporal fascia. Nylon sutures, 3.0, are placed under direct endoscopic vision from the cheek fat pad and the lateral orbicularis oculi muscle to the deep temporal fascia.

4. *Posterior neck corset:* The posterior neck corset is performed by plicating the lateral edge of the platysma muscle to the posterior neck fascia down from near the clavicle up to the lower third of the face. This is done with a 4.0 interrupted Vicryl suture followed by 4.0 Vicryl running suture. In the lower face, the platysma SMAS is being pulled vertically by the jowl suspension sutures. A back-cut similar to the platysmal window[19] is performed to reorient the vector of pull in the neck posteriorly. Care is taken to avoid strangulating the great auricular nerve. This maneuver results in a longer and sleeker-appearing neck contour and a sharper jawline and allows more neck skin to be excised posteriorly.

5. *Contouring the neck skin flap:* Now that all of the muscle plication in the posterior corset is completed, the neck skin flap must be contoured evenly. In a heavy neck, usually, the skin flap is thick in the submental region and lateral jawline area. A direct excision thinning with scissors is preferred. Liposuction is minimized to avoid irregularity and scar band tethering.

For Asian patients, pretragal/perilobular skin can be distributed vertically with the endoscopic temporal and cheek lift, thus avoiding an extension of the incision up in the pretragal skin.

6. *Microfat grafting:* Fat is harvested from wherever the patient has excess, preferably accessible from the supine position. The inner thigh is most preferred followed by lateral thigh, lower abdomen, and upper abdomen. The approach taken is a classic Coleman technique (hand suction with a 10-cc syringe).[20] Injection is performed using Tulip gold micro-blunt tip cannulas adding prominence to the flattening forehead, midface, nose, and chin but avoiding protrusion of the zygomatic arch and mandibular angle.

7. *Skin resurfacing:* Depending on the skin thickness, 20% TCA peel is recommended.

Postoperative Care and Expected Outcome

Skin closure is performed in layers and begun in the postauricular space. Interrupted 4-0 nylon sutures are placed deep and subcutaneously, and 5-0 PDS interrupted sutures are placed 5 mm apart. The skin is closed with a 6-0 Prolene running suture. In the scalp, 5-0 nylon is used. Drains are placed across the forehead and diverted to the

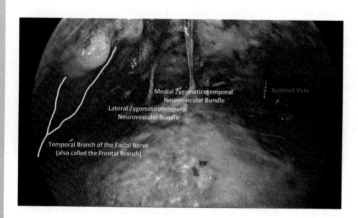

Fig. 2. Endoscopic anatomy of the temporal region (left side). The sentinel vein and the medial and lateral zygomaticotemporal neurovascular bundles need to be identified and preserved. The temporal branch of the facial nerve lies directly above in the temporoparietal fascia.

mastoid area. Another drain is placed underneath the chin and bottom of the neck dissection. Drains come out after 5 days; sutures in the auricular area and the lower eye lids are removed after 4 days, and all other sutures are removed after 7 days. The authors' standard postoperative regimen includes taping for the cheek, forehead, and brow area to reduce periorbital edema. For the same reason, the authors advise their patients to lie flat in bed for 2 days as well as lymphatic drainage. Hyperbaric oxygen therapy is advised to improve wound healing.

Management of complications
Hematoma is the most common face-lift complication requiring operative intervention.[21] However, this is only very rarely seen in the authors' cohort thanks to the endoscopic approach, allowing for meticulous dissection avoiding blood vessel injury.

The temporal branch of the facial nerve (also called the frontal branch) is the most commonly injured facial nerve in facial surgery.[22] The frontal branch crosses the zygomatic arch in the temporal region, supplying the auriculares anterior and superior. The more anterior branches supply the frontalis, the orbicularis oculi, and corrugator supercilii muscles. A neuropraxia of this nerve occasionally occurs transiently and can last typically from 3 days after the operation until 3 months postoperatively. The majority will resolve after 3 to 6 weeks. The usual reason is postoperative swelling potentially worsened or caused by fat grafting. The authors recommend balancing the facial expression if there is a noticeable difference with contralateral neurotoxin injections until the situation is resolved.

Revision or subsequent procedures
After extensive fat grafting to the face, lumpiness of the transplant can be a complication requiring revision or subsequent procedures. The authors usually approach this issue with a 20-gauge needle to try to disrupt the fat lump in an office setting. If this is impossible, the authors conduct a micro-liposuction under intravenous sedation to correct the fat irregularities.

CASE DEMONSTRATIONS
Case 1

Ponytail Lift in a 35-year-old Chinese woman
The patient presented initially with the request for lower eye lid fat removal. For overall facial beautification, the authors performed an endoscopic brow rotation, a midface-lift, a very conservative transconjunctival fat resection, and a free fat augmentation of frontal orbital rim/upper lid

junction, cheeks, nasoradix, and chin. For skin resurfacing, a 20% TCA peel was added. The results shown are 6 months postoperatively. The hypoplastic frontal bone and maxilla as well as the proptotic eyes were effectively corrected via PTL (**Fig. 3**).

Case 2

Ponytail Lift in a 52-year-old Japanese woman
The patient presented initially with a concern about looking tired. For overall facial beautification, the authors performed an endoscopic brow rotation, a midface-lift, a conservative transconjunctival lower blepharoplasty, and a free fat transfer to brows upper eyelids, nasoradix, and cheeks. For skin resurfacing, a 20% TCA peel was added. The results shown are 3 months postoperatively. The classical signs of the aging Asian periorbita, such as fat atrophy in the upper eyelid, and the contour deformity underlying the brow at the orbital rim were effectively corrected via PTL (**Fig. 4**).

Case 3

Ponytail Facelift in a 56-year-old Korean woman
The patient presented initially requesting an Asian blepharoplasty and facial rejuvenation. Importantly, she was strictly unwilling to accept preauricular incisions. The authors performed a limited incision lower face and neck lift with anterior neck deep contouring and anterior plication, an endoscopic forehead and cheek lift, a conservative transconjunctival lower blepharoplasty, and a free fat transfer to brows upper eyelids, nasoradix, and cheeks. For skin resurfacing, a 20% TCA peel was added. The results shown are 6 months postoperatively. The eyes, the drooping jowls as well as the neck contour were effectively corrected via PTL without any preauricular incisions (**Fig. 5**).

Case 4

Ponytail Facelift in a 67-year-old Chinese woman
The patient presented initially requesting general facial rejuvenation. The authors performed a limited incision lower face and neck lift with anterior neck deep contouring and anterior plication, an endoscopic forehead and cheek lift, a conservative upper and lower blepharoplasty, and a free fat transfer to brows, upper eyelids, nasoradix, and cheeks. For skin resurfacing, a 20% TCA peel was added. The results shown are 2 months postoperatively. The authors were able to achieve a complete rejuvenation of the face

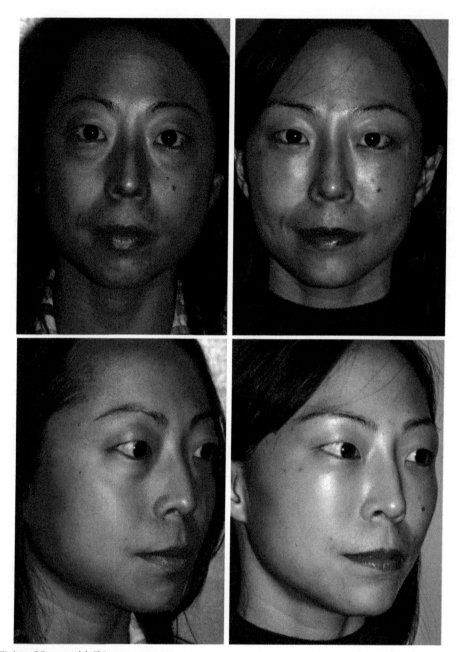

Fig. 3. PTL in a 35-year-old Chinese woman.

and neck without preauricular incisions applying the PTL technique (**Fig. 6**).

DISCUSSION

In terms of pearls for the success of the procedure, the authors strongly recommend patience during the whole operation. Follow the procedure step by step and avoid using electrocautery as much as possible during dissection, especially in the neck and lower face.

In the temporal dissection, it is very critical to first locate the sentinel vein. Only proceed with small spreads of your dissection scissors in this area. Lateral of the sentinel vein, the medial and lateral zygomaticotemporal neurovascular bundles need to be identified and preserved. These structures are sensory nerves and indicate the location of the temporal branch of the facial nerve, which lies directly above in the temporoparietal fascia. This structure must be preserved (see **Fig. 2**).

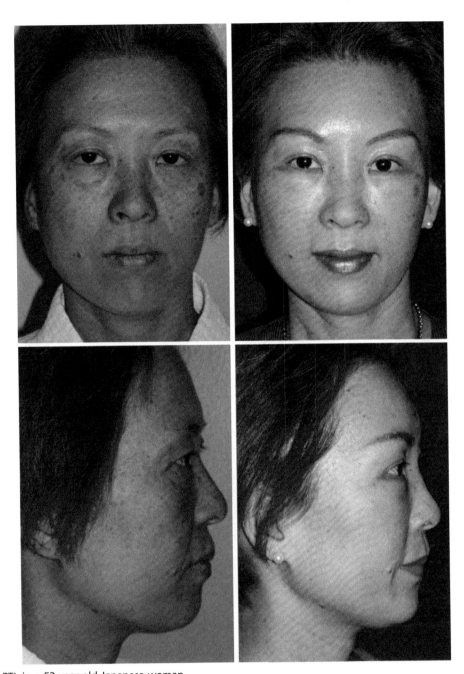

Fig. 4. PTL in a 52-year-old Japanese woman.

To ensure optimal outcome of fat grafting, harvest the fat with a very small canula (3 mm width, 1 mm side hole) and inject only retrograde around the eyes. Particularly in the Asian patients, the authors needed to avoid fat grafting in the lateral zygomatic area, not to widen the cheeks. Also specific to the Asian population and for the same reason, stitching to lift the lower face should not be placed at the height of the zygoma but rather in adjacent areas. Not all Asian patients are looking for a more western appearance; however, the frequently requested more dramatic expression of the eyes that many white patients are looking for at the moment should be avoided. The lateral canthal ligament should therefore almost never be released in Asian patients, averting an even more slant-eye look.

Although the authors frequently add CO_2 laser treatments for skin resurfacing to the Ponytail procedures, the authors strictly recommend 20% TCA peels only for their Asian patients because of their tendency to develop hyperpigmentation.

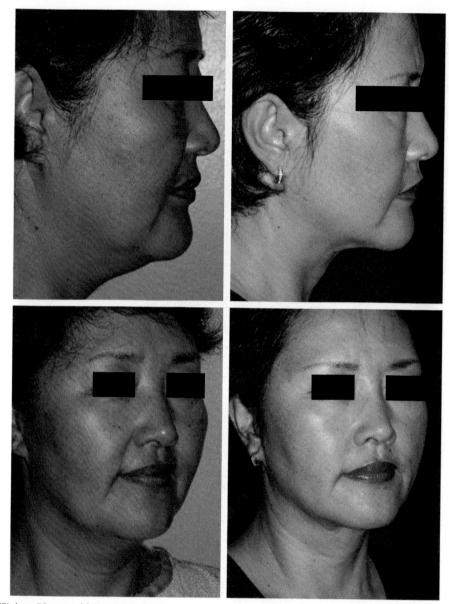

Fig. 5. PTFL in a 56-year-old Korean woman.

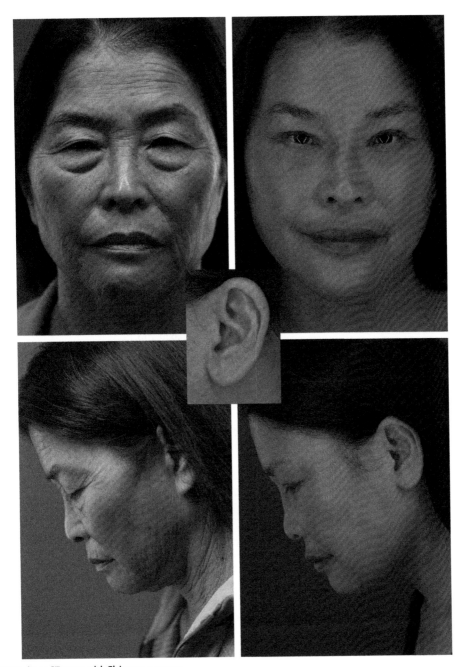

Fig. 6. PTFL in a 67-year-old Chinese woman.

SUMMARY

The Ponytail approach addresses the Asian face in all dimensions using minimally invasive modalities combined with skin regenerative methods. Offering the opportunity to tailor the facial profile, shape, and expression in addition to rejuvenation makes the PTL and PTFL ideal procedures for Asian patients.

CLINICS CARE POINTS

- Preoperatively, steroids are given to prevent swelling (Medrol Dosepak). In addition, 10 mg/kg tranexamic acid is infused to minimize bleeding.

- Intraoperatively, the authors have a picture of the patient at a younger age in the operating room. Also, an example of the desired eyebrow configuration can be very helpful in deciding on the final eyebrow positioning.
- Postoperatively, a head dressing and facial taping are applied to prevent swelling around the eyes. The head dressing is removed after 12 hours to avoid swelling of the face. For the same reason, patients are kept lying flat for 2 days after surgery. To enhance healing, the authors use a hyperbaric oxygen chamber daily for 3 to 5 days after surgery.
- Patients are kept on a soft diet for 3 days after surgery to protect the sutures that are put into the temporalis fascia and to reduce pain on mastication.

DISCLOSURE

Ponytail Lift and Ponytail Facelift are trademarks owned by Chia Chi Kao. The authors have no further disclosures.

ACKNOWLEDGMENTS

We thank Dr. Jun Jiang from the Technical University of Munich for valuable input for the introduction of the article.

SUPPLEMENTARY DATA

Supplementary data related to this article can be found online at https://doi.org/10.1016/j.cps.2022.07.008.

REFERENCES

1. Aquino YS, Steinkamp N. Borrowed beauty? Understanding identity in Asian facial cosmetic surgery. Med Health Care Philos 2016;19(3):431–41.
2. Wong CH, Hsieh MKH, Mendelson B. Asian face lift with the composite face lift technique. Plast Reconstr Surg 2022;149(1):59–69.
3. Yang X, Li D, Xue H, et al. Anatomical characteristics of the perpendicular plate of the ethmoid: an analysis of paranasal sinus computed tomography via three-dimensional reconstruction. J Craniofac Surg 2019;30(2):604–6.
4. Rhee SC. Differences between Caucasian and Asian attractive faces. Skin Res Technol 2018;24(1):73–9.
5. Bergeron L, Chen YR. The Asian face lift. Semin Plast Surg 2009;23(1):40–7.
6. Shirakabe Y, Suzuki Y, Lam SM. A new paradigm for the aging Asian face. Aesthetic Plast Surg 2003;27(5):397–402.
7. Lim WK, Rajendran K, Choo CT. Microscopic anatomy of the lower eyelid in Asians. Ophthal Plast Reconstr Surg 2004;20(3):207–11.
8. Suhk J, Park J, Nguyen AH. Nasal analysis and anatomy: anthropometric proportional assessment in asians-aesthetic balance from forehead to chin, part I. Semin Plast Surg 2015;29(4):219–25.
9. Gao Y, et al. Comparison of aesthetic facial criteria between Caucasian and East Asian female populations: an esthetic surgeon's perspective. Asian J Surg 2018;41(1):4–11.
10. Wong JK. Aesthetic surgery in Asians. Curr Opin Otolaryngol Head Neck Surg 2009;17(4):279–86.
11. Lv K, et al. Chinese expert consensus on clinical prevention and treatment of scar. Burns Trauma 2018;6:27.
12. Saetermoe CL, Scattone D, Kim KH. Ethnicity and the stigma of disabilities. Psychol Health 2001;16(6):699–713.
13. Soh J, Chew MT, Wong HB. An Asian community's perspective on facial profile attractiveness. Community Dent Oral Epidemiol 2007;35(1):18–24.
14. Hashem AM, et al. Facelift part II: surgical techniques and complications. Aesthet Surg J 2021;41(10):NP1276–94.
15. Hashem AM, et al. Facelift part I: history, anatomy, and clinical assessment. Aesthet Surg J 2020;40(1):1–18.
16. Pitanguy I, Ramos AS. The frontal branch of the facial nerve: the importance of its variations in face lifting. Plast Reconstr Surg 1966;38(4):352–6.
17. Marten T, Elyassnia D. Neck lift: defining anatomic problems and choosing appropriate treatment strategies. Clin Plast Surg 2018;45(4):455–84.
18. Auersvald A, Auersvald LA. Management of the submandibular gland in neck lifts: indications, techniques, pearls, and pitfalls. Clin Plast Surg 2018;45(4):507–25.
19. Cruz RS, O'Reilly EB, Rohrich RJ. The platysma window: an anatomically safe, efficient, and easily reproducible approach to neck contour in the face lift. Plast Reconstr Surg 2012;129(5):1169–72.
20. Coleman SR. Structural fat grafting. Aesthet Surg J 1998;18(5):386–8.
21. Sinclair NR, et al. How to prevent and treat complications in facelift surgery, part 1: short-term complications. Aesthet Surg J Open Forum 2021;3(1):ojab007.
22. Hendi A. Temporal nerve neuropraxia and contralateral compensatory brow elevation. Dermatol Surg 2007;33(1):114–6.

Facial Rejuvenation with Open Technique After Previous Filler Injection

Daping Yang, MD

KEYWORDS

- Facelift • Facial rejuvenation • Polyacrylamide hydrogel • Removal of injected material

KEY POINTS

- Complications arising from polyacrylamide hydrogel are well-documented in the literature.
- Complete removal of injected material is seldom possible.
- Patients who underwent removal of injected material were significantly more likely to express interest in facelift surgery.
- An open surgical technique with facelift incision to manage removal of polyacrylamide hydrogel and complication due to volume deflation and tissue descent is described.

INTRODUCTION

Polyacrylamide hydrogel (PAAG: Amazingel; Nan-Feng Medical Science and Technology Development Co., Ltd., Shijiazhuang, People's Republic of China) was used in breast augmentation and facial soft-tissue augmentation in China in 1999. Because complications of PAAG injections for breast augmentation were continuously reported,[1-3] the products were banned in China in 2006.[4] However, illegal use in facial augmentation continued. Because of illegal PAAG injections in cosmetic clinics, there have been more complications than previously reported in China.

The complications associated with PAAG injection including tissue infection, nodular formation, and migration along tissue planes have been well-documented.[5-8] Patients with complications in site of injected area came to our hospital for removal surgery. Complete removal of injected material is seldom possible. It is possible to perform excision together with local tissue such as partial mastectomy in the case of breast injection, when dealing with the complication of injection for breast augmentation. A major concern on polyacrylamide hydrogel injection in facial augmentation is that the injected material is not readily removable once complication arises

because facial structure is very complex, and more severe local complications such as facial nerve injury should be controlled. Therefore, facial lift with open technique for the removal of injected material in cheek and temporal regions has been used in our practice, which has not been reported in the literature. This article presents 22 cases of severe complications associated with PAAG injection in facial augmentation and provides an open surgical technique to manage the complication due to volume deflation and tissue descent.

Indications and Contraindications

For patients who have received injection filling in cheek and temporal regions with clinical symptoms, we recommend that patients receive aggressive procedure for surgical removal.

If patients with moderate or severe aging such as malar fat pad descent with nasolabial folds, jowls, and cervical skin laxity, we recommend that patients receive aggressive procedure for surgical removal and facelift simultaneously (**Fig. 1**).

Contraindications are including patients with high risk, such as those with advancing age, extrinsic skin damage (eg, sun exposure, cigarette smoke), and history of massive weight loss.

First Beijing BCC Plastic Surgery Hospital, No. 37, Guangqu Road, Chaoyang District, Beijing 100022, China
E-mail address: dapingyang@outlook.com

Clin Plastic Surg 50 (2023) 61–69
https://doi.org/10.1016/j.cps.2022.07.005
0094-1298/23/© 2022 Elsevier Inc. All rights reserved.

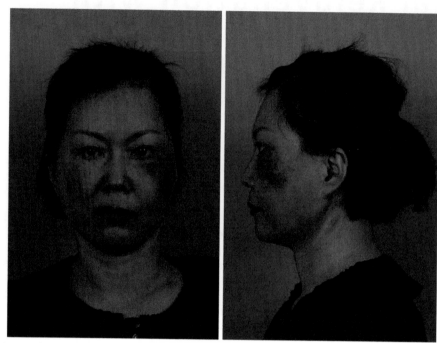

Fig. 1. Patient with moderate aging.

Preoperative Evaluation and Special Considerations

Preoperative discussion about what to expect not only helps prepare the patient but also facilitates postsurgical communication. Surgeons should communicate with the patient as to what to expect and what areas may be more difficult to fully correct.

Patients who have received injection filling in cheek and temporal regions with clinical symptoms seek improvement on both removal of injected material and face aging. They have a range of options available to them depending on the problems present; the degree of improvement they seek; and the time, trouble, and expense they are willing to undergo to obtain the improvement they desire. Although it is essential to discuss these options and the advantages and disadvantages of each, patients are also seeking our guidance as to what is possible, what is practical, and what is really best.

The important structures of the injection site, such as the facial nerve and the difficulty of the operation, should be considered, as well as the change of the local facial shape after removal because this type of injection is mostly performed on the facial deep plane, and the change of shape after the removal can cause new psychological trauma to the patient. Iatrogenic jowling can be an unintended consequence of removal of injected material in cheek due to volume deflation and tissue descent.

The removal of injected material can lead to a redundant and deflated soft tissue envelope, requiring a facelift to address jowling, cervicofacial laxity, and/or lower facial rhytids.

Patients who underwent the removal of injected material were significantly more likely to express interest in facelift. Before removal, the authors recommend comprehensive patient counseling that includes a discussion need for a facelift. When performing a facelift after removal, technical considerations include the mechanism of jowling (different from normal facial aging). The authors thought that these considerations can set more realistic expectations for patients.

Surgical Procedures

Surgical removal involves simultaneous facelift procedure. Facelift procedure that we performed includes lateral SMASectomy technique (Baker's technique)[9] and high-SMAS suspension technique (Barton's technique).[10] We have patients agree to allow us to option which technique we use during surgery, depending on the degree of facial tissue damage from injected material, such as tissue infection, nodular formation, and migration along tissue planes.

Lateral SMASectomy Technique

As Baker described, the outline of SMASectomy was marked on a tangent from the lateral aspect of the malar eminence to the angle of the mandible, essentially in the region along the anterior edge of the parotid gland. The deep fascia along the SMASectomy line was exposed to keep the dissection superficial to the deep fascia and avoid dissection into the parotid parenchyma. Then, a strip of the superficial musculoaponeurotic system (SMAS), 2 to 3 cm in width, was usually excised, depending on the degree of SMAS laxity and site of injectables. The SMAS flap was raised in the same plane parallel to the nasolabial fold, to explore gel masses and injected material, along a trajectory toward the lateral canthus and overlying the anterior portion of the parotid gland. Continuous with the lateral SMASectomy was the resection of a strip of posterior platysma muscle several centimeters long over the tail of the parotid and anterior border of the sternocleidomastoid. The malar fat pad dissection was performed with 1 to 2 cm undermining on the deep plane to explore and remove injected material. We performed two interrupted sutures in oblique vector at the deep temporal

fascia to suspender the malar fat pad, and other two interrupted sutures in vertical vector at near the front of the earlobe when closing the SMAS, then, 5 to 6 interrupted sutures were used to close the SMAS overlying the parotid which vectors were perpendicular to the nasolabial fold. The last 2 sutures advanced the platysma at the angle of the mandible to the retroauricular area in a posterosuperior direction to lift the cervical platysma postauricularly and to fix it to the mastoid fascia.[11–13]

High-SMAS Suspension Technique

The subcutaneous dissection above the zygomatic arch in the lateral orbital area was performed to release the cutaneous attachments of the crow's feet and to facilitate a smooth redraping of the temporal skin. A transverse SMAS fasciotomy above the zygomatic arch was performed. Using Barton's technique, the main SMAS flap was suspended to the deep temporal fascia vertically above the zygomatic arch to elevate the

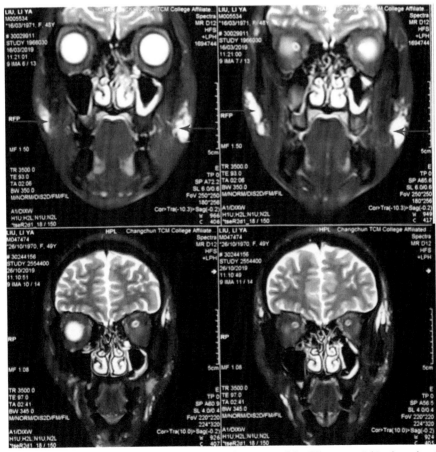

Fig. 2. (*Above*) Facial coronal T2 W slices of MRI showed infiltration of the filler material in the subcutaneous and SMAS layers (*arrows*). (*Below*) Six months after removal surgery with simultaneous facelift procedure.

malar and zygomatic soft tissues and an SMAS transposition flap from the SMAS flap was incised posteriorly, with the preauricular strip suspended superolaterally to the mastoid fascia to improve neck and jaw contour.

Postoperative Care and Expected Outcome

Drains are usually removed on the second day after surgery, and sutures are removed 7 days after surgery. If healing is progressing well, drain output is minimal, and no fluid collections are present, and if it seems that the patient is following dietary and other instructions, drains are removed at that time.

When sutures are removed will vary depending on the type of procedure performed. If a "short scar" facelift has been performed, a submental incision only will be present, and sutures are removed on the fifth day. If a facelift has been performed, 6-0 nylon sutures are removed on the seventh day. Half-buried vertical mattress sutures of

4-0 nylon with the knots tied on the scalp side are removed on the seventh to ninth day.

When patients return to work will depend on their tolerance for surgery, their capacity for healing, the type of work they do, the activities they enjoy, and how they feel overall about their appearance. Patients are asked to set aside 7 to 10 days to recover depending on the extent of their surgery, and additional time off is recommended if a facelift and related procedures are simultaneously performed.

Patients are advised to avoid all strenuous activity during the first 2 weeks after surgery. Two weeks after surgery, patients are allowed to begin light exercise and gradually work up to their presurgical level of activity. Four weeks after surgery, they are allowed to engage in more vigorous activities.

Chinese women are increasingly requesting procedures with minimal recovery, minimal cost, minimal risk, and maximal benefit with a natural-appearing and long-lasting result. We feel that procedures must be individually determined. Patients who have received injection filling in cheek

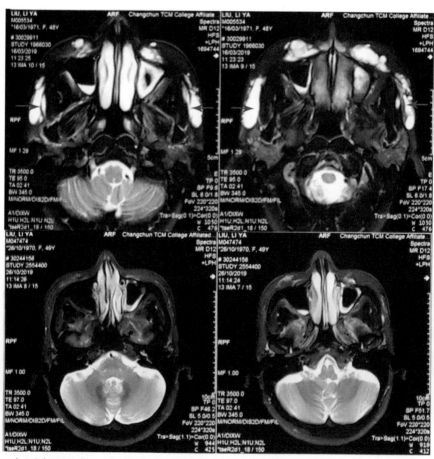

Fig. 3. (*Above*) Axial T2 W slices of MRI showed a mass lesion of injected material in the NLF and cheek regions (*arrows*). (*Below*) Six months after removal surgery with simultaneous facelift procedure.

and temporal regions with clinical symptoms seek improvement on both removal of injected material and face aging. We provide an open surgical technique with facelift incision and the deep plan dissection to explore and remove injected material. Complications of PAAG (such as granuloma formation, unsatisfactory contours, and gel migration), and complications after surgical removal (such as volume deflation, tissue descent) can be improved with the open surgical technique.

Management of Complications

Complications after PAAG injections including infection, inflammation, granuloma formation, uneven contours, abnormal skin sensations, and gel migration still occur. Patients with complications at the site of the injected area came to our hospital for removal surgery.

Due to the lack of a unified national treatment method, many doctors use needle aspiration to deal with it. It is difficult to completely aspirate PAAG due to the presence of separate capsules of gel. However, this method of aspiration may make things even worse, due to spreading gel into surrounding normal tissue.

Because aspiration fails to remove the PAAG, incision is needed. The incision directly on the skin at the site of the injection mass is the last choice because most patients are worried about visible scars. Intranasal incision, intraoral incision, hairline incision, or conjunctival incision can usually be used for local injected gel. However, due to the complex structure of the cheeks, the small incisions mentioned above cannot adequately explore gel masses in the deep plant of face. Complete removal of PAAG is almost impossible. Therefore, we provide an open surgical technique with facelift incision to deal with the removal of polyacrylamide hydrogel and complication due to volume deflation and tissue descent.

Revision or Subsequent Procedures

PAAG mingle with the local tissue. Therefore, when a complication arises, local tissue has to be excised together with the injected material, which results in significant morbidity to the injection site, such as volume deflation, tissue descent. Fat grafting can provide significant improvement for the correction of face deficiencies. More studies are required to support

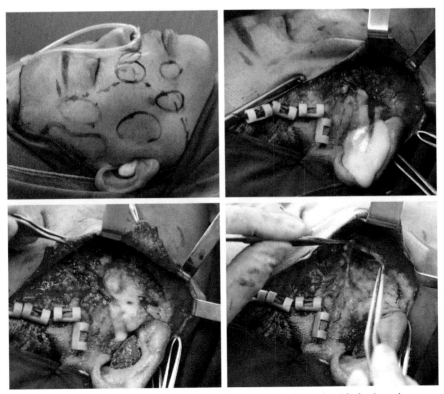

Fig. 4. Intraoperative view showing the extirpation of the injected polyacrylamide hydrogel.

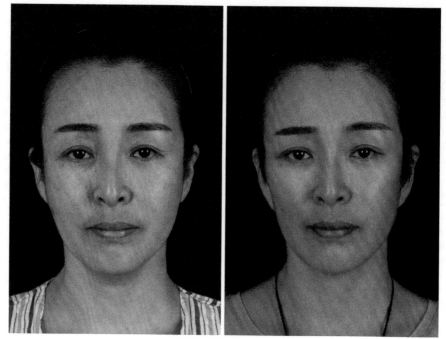

Fig. 5. A 48-year-old woman who underwent PAAG injected into her bilateral NLF and cheek regions for augmentation purpose 18 years ago. Preoperative photograph (*left*) and postoperative photograph of 6 months after removal surgery with simultaneous facelift procedure (*right*). The appearance of the lower two-thirds of her face had been improved.

the safety of management of complications after PAAG removal.

CASE DEMONSTRATIONS
Case 1

A 48-year-old woman had PAAG injected into her bilateral nasolabial folds (NLF) and cheek regions for augmentation purpose 18 years ago. She complained of nodularity and local inflammation in the injected site. MRI of the NLF and cheek regions showed a mass lesion of injected material. MRI showed infiltration of the filler material in the subcutaneous and SMAS layers in cheeks. The mass was hyperintense in T2 images, which was suggestive of inflammatory changes (**Figs. 2** and **3**). Debridement was performed with facelift incision. Removal surgery involves simultaneous facelift procedure (**Figs. 4** and **5**).

Case 2

A 39-year-old woman presented with lower face sagging due to history of heavy-filler injections using PAAG 10 years ago. The descent of the fillers in combination with laxity of facial tissues resulted in jowl formation. After filler removal (**Fig. 6**) and facelift, the appearance of the lower two-thirds of her face had been improved (**Fig. 7**).

DISCUSSION

Due to the lack of a unified national treatment method, many doctors use needle aspiration to deal with it. It is difficult to completely aspirate PAAG due to the presence of separate capsules of gel. However, this method of aspiration may

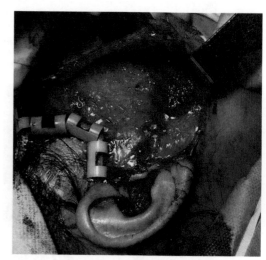

Fig. 6. Intraoperative view showing the injected polyacrylamide hydrogel was removed surgically.

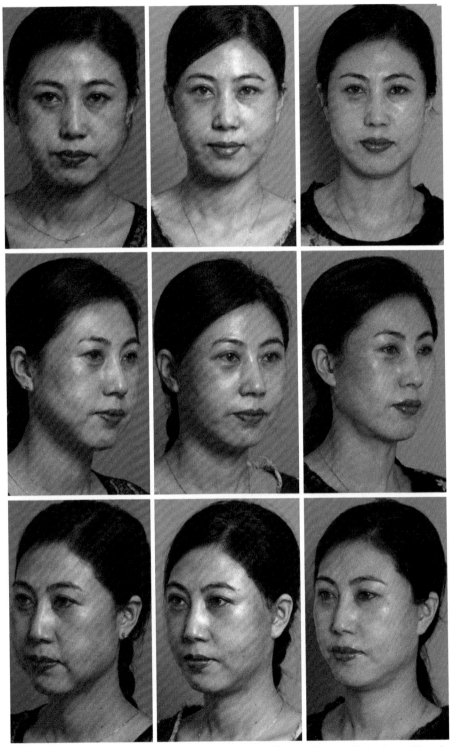

Fig. 7. A 39-year-old woman presented with lower face sagging due to history of injection with polyacrylamide hydrogel 10 years ago. Photographs obtained preoperatively (*left*), 3 months postoperatively (*center*), and 6 months (*right*) after removal surgery with simultaneous facelift procedure, demonstrating improvement in cheek and jowling.

make things even worse, due to spreading gel into surrounding normal tissue.

It is difficult to completely aspirate polyacrylamide hydrogel due to the presence of separate capsules of gel. Since aspiration fails to remove the polyacrylamide hydrogel, incision is needed. However, due to the complex structure of the cheeks, the small incisions mentioned above cannot adequately explore gel masses in the deep plant of face. Complete removal of polyacrylamide hydrogel is almost impossible. Therefore, we provide an open surgical technique with face lift incision to deal with removal of polyacrylamide hydrogel and complication due to volume deflation and tissue descent.

It is common knowledge that ideal soft tissue filler should be safe and should achieve a cosmetic effect that is sustainable and correctable. To be a safe material, the filler should be inert, noncarcinogenic, and readily removable once complication arises. To achieve a good cosmetic effect, the filler should be confined to the site into which it was injected (ie, migration-free). The material should also be readily removable on the patient's wish. Complications arising from PAAG are well-documented in the literature in which migration of material and local inflammation is commonly reported. Complete removal of injected material is seldom possible and excision together with local tissue (ie, mastectomy in the case of breast injection) is almost always required for the control of severe local complications.

We describe our armamentarium of facelift techniques for addressing the specific concerns of the aging Chinese face. We feel that each facelift must be individually determined. The adjustments necessitated by each patient's unique anatomy are the key factors to a natural-appearing result. We advocate a fresh and natural look after the facelift procedure and a reasonably fast recovery.

The anatomy of Chinese face does not necessitate substantial modification of the surgical techniques for successful facial rejuvenation. In our practice, various facelift techniques can produce excellent results.[11,12] It is impossible for each surgeon to be proficient in all procedures but it is necessary to adopt a technique that serves patients well and is, ideally, safe, consistent, easily reproducible, and applicable to various anatomic problems. In addition, every surgery is customized to the patient's anatomy and concerns. Therefore, the surgeon must have the versatility to individualize the technique according to the needs and desires of each patient. Our large case series of 1026 patients demonstrate consistent safety and effective esthetic results.[13]

SUMMARY

Complications arising from polyacrylamide hydrogel are well-documented in the literature. Long-term complications after PAAG injections in facial correction including infection, inflammation, granuloma formation, unsatisfactory contours, abnormal skin sensations, and gel migration still occur. Complete removal of injected material is seldom possible. Patients who underwent removal of injected material were significantly more likely to express interest in facelift. We provide an open surgical technique with facelift incision to deal with the removal of polyacrylamide hydrogel and complication due to volume deflation and tissue descent.

CLINICS CARE POINTS

- Ideal soft tissue filler should be safe and should achieve a cosmetic effect that is sustainable and correctable.
- The material should also be readily removable on the patient's wish.
- Complete removal of polyacrylamide hydrogel is seldom possible and excision together with local tissue is almost always required for the control of severe local complications.

PATIENT CONSENT

Patients provided written consent for use of their images.

REFERENCES

1. Cheng NX, Wang YL, Wang JH, et al. Complications of breast augmentation with injected hydrophilic polyacrylamide gel. Aesthet Plast Surg 2002;26:375–82.
2. Wang X, Qiao Q, Sun J, et al. The periareolar approach management of postoperative complications of breast augmentation by injected polyacrylamide hydrogel (in Chinese). Zhonghua Zheng Xing Wai Ke Za Zhi 2005;21:332–4.
3. Yue Y, Luan J, Qiao Q, et al. Retrospective analysis of complications of breast augmentation with injected polyacrylamide hydrophilic gel in 90 cases (in Chinese). Zhonghua Zheng Xing Wai Ke Za Zhi 2007;23:221–3.
4. State Food and Drug Administration (Web site) Available at: http://www.sda.gov.cn/WS01/CL0493/53328.html. Accessed June 26, 2012.

5. Ono S, Ogawa R, Hyakusoku H. Complications after polyacrylamide hydrogel injection for soft-tissue augmentation. Plast Reconstr Surg 2010;126: 1349–57.

6. Liu HL, Cheung WY. Complications of polyacrylamide hydrogel (PAAG) injection in facial augmentation. J Plast Reconstr Aesthet Surg 2010;63:E9–12.

7. Qiao Q, Wang X, Sun J, et al. Management for postoperative complications of breast augmentation by injected polyacrylamide hydrogel. Aesthet Plast Surg 2005;29:156–61 [discussion: 162].

8. Shen H, Lv Y, Xu J, et al. Complications after polyacrylamide hydrogel injection for facial soft-tissue augmentation in China: Twenty-Four cases and their surgical management. Plast Reconstr Surg 2012; 130:340e.

9. Baker DC. Lateral SMASectomy. Plast Reconstr Surg 1997;100:509–13.

10. Barton FE Jr, Hunt J. The high-superficial musculoaponeurotic system technique in facial rejuvenation: an update. Plast Reconstr Surg 2003;112:1910–7.

11. Zhang P, Sui B, Ren L, et al. The individualized facelift technique in improving facial asymmetry for Asian patients. Ophthalmic Plast Reconstr Surg 2018;34:516–21.

12. Gong M, Yu L, Ren L, et al. Lateral superficial muscular aponeurotic system stacking/superficial muscular aponeurotic systemectomy with orbicularis-malar fat repositioning: a procedure tailored for female Asian Patients. Dermatol Surg 2020;46:934–41.

13. Yang D, Yang J. Special considerations in Chinese face-lift procedure. Insights from a 15-year Experience of 1026 cases. Ann Plast Surg 2021;86. S244–S25.

Current Practices for Esthetic Facial Bone Contouring Surgery in Asians

Li Lin, MD, PhD, Wenqing Han, MD, PhD, Mengzhe Sun, MD, PhD,
Byeong Seop Kim, MD, Xiaojun Chen, MD, PhD, Zin Mar Aung, MD, PhD,
Ziwei Zhang, MD, PhD, Yanchun Zhou, BA[1], Xianxian Yang, MD, PhD,
Gang Chai, MD, PhD*, Haisong Xu, MD, PhD*

KEYWORDS

- Facial bone contouring surgery • Mandibular reduction • Malarplasty • Computer-assisted surgery
- Three-dimensional printing • Esthetic craniofacial surgery • Digital osteotomy template

KEY POINTS

- Asian esthetics is the culture and beauty foundation of Asian facial esthetic surgery.
- Facial bone contouring surgery is a surgical procedure to address the appearance of the facial structures by various craniofacial techniques, such as osteotomy, bone reconstruction, bone graft, and fixation.
- Digital medicine and three-dimensional printed customized osteotomy guider can improve the safety and effectiveness of facial bone contouring surgery.
- Facial bone contouring surgery combined with minimally invasive soft tissue cosmetic procedures makes facial contour surgery more minimally invasive and effective.

 Video content accompanies this article at http://www.plasticsurgery.theclinics.com

INTRODUCTION

Facial bone contouring surgery is a surgical procedure to address the appearance of the facial structures by various craniofacial techniques, such as osteotomy, bone reconstruction, bone graft, and fixation.[1] Oval shape faces are more popular and attractiveness facial contours in Asians, which means that prominent mandibular angle and malar complex are considered less esthetic anatomic features. Since 1980s, many authors have performed bone shaving or reduction in the zygomatic arch and/or mandibular angle region for technical modification of osteotomies to address the esthetic face contour. With the development of culture and economy, as well as the improvement of surgery techniques, facial bone contouring surgery became more and more popular in the last 20 years.

Currently, we use intraoral approach to avoid the skin scar and obtain the minimal invasive cosmetic result. However, this approach exposes the surgical area insufficiently, resulting in a limited field of vision and a small operating space. So, it is difficult to handle because surgeons may not be able to see the margin of the bone during the operation with a reciprocating saw. It is also difficult to accurately determine the osteotomy line, which is prone to cause vascular and nerve bundle injury, bilateral asymmetry, and other complications.

Department of Plastic and Reconstructive Surgery, Shanghai 9th People's Hospital, School of Medicine, Shanghai Jiao Tong University, 639 Zhi Zao Ju Road, Shanghai 200011, China
[1] Department of Nursing, Shanghai 9th People's Hospital, School of Medicine, Shanghai Jiao Tong University, 639 Zhi Zao Ju Road, Shanghai 200011, China
* Corresponding authors.
E-mail addresses: chaig1081@sh9hospital.org.cn (G.C.); xuhaisongmd@qq.com (H.X.)

Clin Plastic Surg 50 (2023) 71–80
https://doi.org/10.1016/j.cps.2022.08.002
0094-1298/23/© 2022 Elsevier Inc. All rights reserved.

With the wide application of digital technology in craniomaxillofacial surgery, three-dimensional (3D) computed tomographic (CT) reconstruction can provide surgeons presurgical plan with more comprehensive and intuitive preoperative evaluation of facial bone morphology.[2] Currently, we use the customized digital osteotomy template (DOT), which can be used to guide osteotomy during operation, so as to improve the safety and accuracy of facial bone contouring surgery.[3,4]

This article introduces the experience and progress of facial bone contouring surgery, especially mandibular reduction and malarplasty in East Asians based on craniofacial surgery technique used in the Department of Plastic and Reconstructive Surgery, Shanghai Ninth People's Hospital, Shanghai Jiao Tong University, Shanghai, China.

INDICATIONS AND CONTRAINDICATIONS
Indications

1. With clear surgical motivation
2. In good physical and mental health
3. Require improving the facial contouring by reducing the mandibular angle and/or malarplasty.

Contraindications

1. Psychological disorders, unreasonable requirements for surgery
2. Severe mouth opening restriction
3. Those who cannot tolerate surgery
4. With systemic chronic diseases that have not yet been controlled
5. Diseases that affect bone function and development, such as rheumatoid arthritis or genetic diseases that can cause asymmetric facial development
6. Acute and chronic infections in the skin of the facial region or in the mouth
7. Severe facial trauma or deformity
8. The location of the inferior alveolar nerve canal is too low, affecting the osteotomy.
9. Simple masseter muscle hypertrophy
10. Craniofacial tumor
11. Pregnant women
12. Age under 16 years old

PREOPERATIVE EVALUATION AND SPECIAL CONSIDERATIONS

Preoperative surgical plan should be considered on the general situation of the patient, including psychological needs and cultural identity and clinical manifestations.

Patient Selection and Consultation

Asians and Caucasians have vastly different ideal looks, according to studies.[5,6] Facial esthetic treatments in Asians are not aimed at Westernization, but rather the optimization of intrinsic Asian ethnic features, or correction of specific underlying structural features that are perceived as deficiencies (**Fig. 1**)[7]. Before performing surgery, the surgeon should thoroughly assess and understand the patient's motivation for requesting surgery. Patients may be persuaded to contact a plastic surgeon on the spur of the moment and make an impulsive choice to have surgery, especially if they meet someone who has. However, because their expectations may be significantly higher than the actual results, this population is not an ideal candidate for surgery.

Preoperative Assessment

Preoperative cephalometric imaging and a CT scan were performed in all patients. Three-dimensional software (Mimics 21.0, Materialise, Belgium) was used to open the DICOM format file, and 3D reconstruction was carried out for presurgical plan. Patients and surgeons can instantly discuss the 3D model planning if necessary. This preoperative evaluation was useful in assessing the severity of the malar complexes' prominence and lower facial look, which helped in accurately predicting the amount of bone reduction required (**Fig. 2A**). Attention should be paid to preoperative communication with the patient, and external incision is prohibited for those with scar constitution.

Customized Digital Designed and 3D-Printed Osteotomy Template

The accuracy and safety of osteotomies can be greatly improved with the use of a customized digital designed and 3D-printed osteotomy template. The authors innovated a surgical design system and 3D-printed metal osteotomy template to assist during the surgery. As an example, parameters related to mandibular angle osteotomy, which can reflect the morphology of the mandible, were selected to carry out the design. In addition, the distance between the inferior alveolar nerve and the osteotomy surface and the volume of the mandibular angle bone were also measured, as shown in **Fig. 2B**. In the 3D reconstructed image, to ensure the stability of the saw, the thickness of the outer side of the surgical template was set to be greater than 5 mm, whereas the thickness of the inner side was set to be 2 mm for the convenience of embedding the template into the mandibular angle. In addition, given that the

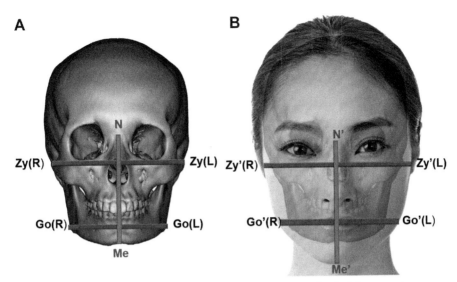

Fig. 1. Facial aesthetic proportion index measurements.Anatomy points for facial contouring surgery (Condyle (Co); Gonial (Go); Zygomatic point (Zy); Meton (Me); Mandibular ramus height (Co-Go); Midplane width (ZyL-ZyR); Intermandibular angle width (GoL-GoR); Facial width ratio (ZyL-ZyR/GoL-GoR)); A. Hard tissue; B. Soft tissue

ligaments at the attachment point of the masseter muscle of the mandibular angle are very tough, some space should be reserved to prevent

incomplete dissection resulting in residual soft tissue. The barb angle of the surgical template needs to be personalized according to the actual

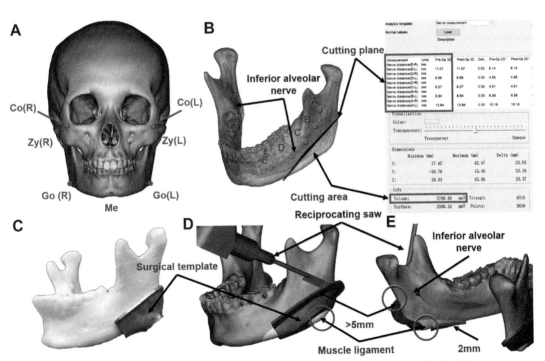

Fig. 2. Preoperational surgical design with CAD/CAM technology. (*A*) Anatomy points for facial contouring surgery. Co, condyle; Go, gonial; Zy, zygomatic point; Me, meton; Co-Go, mandibular ramus height; ZyL-ZyR, midplane width; GoL-GoR, intermandibular angle width; ∠Co-Go-Me, mandibular angle; ZyL-ZyR/GoL-GoR, facial width ratio. (*B*) IAN nerve distance and cutting bone volume measurement. (*C*) Computer-assisted manufacturing (CAM) 3D printing mandible. (*D*) Computer-assisted design (CAD) lateral of mandible. (*E*) Computer-assisted design (CAD) medial of mandible. IAN, inferior alveolar nerve.

situation of each patient. Generally, the reserved depth is 10 mm, as shown in **Fig. 2**C–E. The facial skeleton and skull model can be printed as a reference throughout the operation if necessary.

SURGICAL PROCEDURES
Malarplasty or Zygomatic Reduction

The surgical approach and technique for reduction malarplasty was introduced chiseling and/or shaving method to reduce the protruding portion of the malar bone through intraoral incision in 1980s.[8] After that, various surgical techniques have been devised, such as bone shaving, infracture of the zygomatic arch, and osteotomy/ostectomy of the zygomatic body.[9–13] Currently, there are two major procedures for the malarplasty we use. One is the bone shaving, and the other one is osteotomy, which usually we use I-shaped or L-shaped zygomatic reduction. For bone shaving, after intraoral incision and soft tissue stripping, burring, chiseling, and chipping can shave the outer cortex of the cheekbone and flat out the protruding zygomatic process. For I-shaped or L-shaped osteotomy, the incision for the intraoral part is same with the bone shaving. The zygomatic arch is cut obliquely and the repositioned superoposteriorly by sliding it back and fixing it with miniplate or wires (**Fig. 3**, Video 1). In addition, this method needs 1.5 cm long incision in the preauricular area to facilitate the fracture of the post zygomatic arch.[14]

Key technical points

1. Reduce the stripping range as far as possible to reduce the impact on soft tissue ptosis.
2. Osteotomy pieces require solid internal fixation to prevent segment displacement or nonunion due to facial motion imaging.
3. The anterior auricular incision is concealed as far as possible, and the posterior end can be made with greenstick fracture, so as to avoid facial nerve frontal branch injury.
4. After intraoperative osteotomy, mouth opening should be checked to avoid excessive internal push resulting in limited mouth opening of the temporomandibular joint.

Mandibular Reduction

Mandibular reduction is performed under general anesthesia. Either nasotracheal or endotracheal intubation can be used. Surgery was performed by an intraoral approach: the upper and lower dentition was separated, and the mucosa was incised 5 to 10 mm at the buccal sulcus of the gingival of the lower lip, from the anterior edge of the mandibular ascending ramus forward to the corresponding position of the first premolars. The mucosa, submucosal tissue, and muscle were cut layer by layer until the bone surface. The masseter muscle attachment was dissected under the periosteum to expose the mandibular angle, part of the ascending ramus and part of the lower margin of the mandible (**Fig. 4**).

The mandibular DOT prepared before the operation was inserted through the incision to maintain good contraption. A surgical saw was used to cut the bone close to the upper edge of the DOT (Video 2).

There are three main methods for mandibular osteotomy:

1 Mandibular angle shaving: For moderate hypertrophy or eversion of the mandibular angle, mark the part to be removed at the mandibular angle and apply grinding and drilling.[15]
2 Mandibular angle split osteotomy: For mild hypertrophy or varus of the mandibular angle, longitudinal split of the outer plate cortex is performed. The outer plate incision was perpendicular to the lower edge of the mandible, and the thickness of the osteotomy was one-third of the middle part of the mandible.[16]
3 Mandibular angle-body curved ostectomy: Mandibular angle-body curved ostectomy. For patients with severe hypertrophy or varus of the mandibular angle, a reciprocating saw or swing saw was used to complete the osteotomy after the osteotomy line at the marked mandible.[17]

Key technical points

1. The height of osteotomy was taken as the initial reference of occlusal plane.
2. Try to make a long arc osteotomy close to the lower part of the mental foramen to avoid the second mandibular angle and protect the inferior alveolar nerve and mental nerve.
3. Component dissection of mandibular angle, ascending branch and periosteum of body can avoid accidental arterial bleeding caused by intraoperative injury of facial artery and branches. If bleeding is surging, timely compression should be applied to stop bleeding, and bleeding site should be found quickly or under the guidance of endoscope to stop bleeding. Avoid systemic coagulopathy caused by massive and prolonged bleeding, such as disseminated intravascular coagulation (DIC).

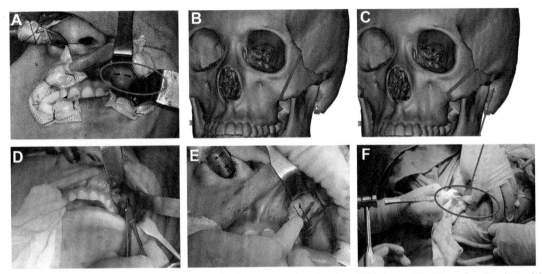

Fig. 3. Surgical procedures and osteotomy lines for zygomatic reduction. (*A*) Intraoral incision of malarplasty. (*B*) "I"-shaped osteotomy. (*C*) "L"-shaped osteotomy. (*D*) Osteotomy line marking. (*E*) Zygomatic osteotomy. (*F*) Cut off the zygomatic arch.

POSTOPERATIVE CARE AND EXPECTED OUTCOME

Pressure bandage dressing of head and face is very important after procedures. After surgery, anti-infection and fluid rehydration are usually used for 3 days. Semiliquid food is taken through a straw, and chlorhexidine mouthwash is used to clean the mouth. Elastic facial mask is recommended for one month after surgery. After one month, the swelling usually reduced by 80% and almost

by 3 months. After 3 months, the atrophy and stabilization of soft tissues, including the masseter muscle, resulted in a beautiful and stable facial contour.

MANAGEMENT OF COMPLICATIONS

Based on the study from 2010 to 2016,[14] there were 510 patients undergoing facial contour surgery are retrospective analysis in the Department of Plastic and Reconstructive Surgery, Shanghai

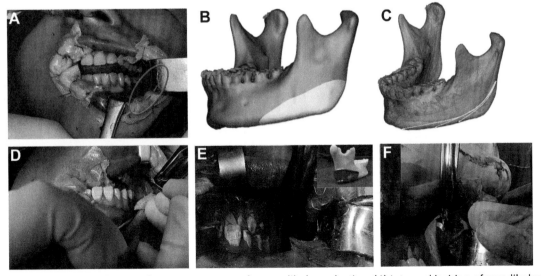

Fig. 4. Surgical procedures and osteotomy pattern for mandibular reduction. (*A*) Intraoral incision of mandibular reduction. (*B*) Mandibular reduction area. (*C*) Difference range of mandibular reduction. (*D*) Mucosal incision and periosteal stripping. (*E*). DOT placement. (*F*) Reciprocating saw perform osteotomy in guidance with DOT.

Ninth People's Hospital, Shanghai Jiao Tong University, including 93 males and 417 females, with an average age of 27.3 years. There were 316 cases undergoing mandibular reduction surgery and 194 cases undergoing malarplasty. The clinical complications are shown in **Table 1**.

Common complications and their managements are as follows.

Intraoperative Hemorrhage and Postoperative Hematoma

During the operation, blind and rough operation should be kept in mind for the dissection of muscles and other soft tissues and hemostasis while separation. If intraoperative hemostasis is not complete, it is easy to cause postoperative hematoma. The key to prevent hematoma is sufficient hemostasis during operation and perfect compression dressing after operation.

Parotid Duct and Facial Nerve Injury

Dissection of the masseter muscle is too shallow or too high. The separation and resection of part of the masseter muscle are mainly carried out in the inner layer of the masseter muscle, not involving the surface layer, and the range of muscle removal should not be too high.

Infection

Postoperative hematoma formation is an important cause of infection, and it is necessary to pay attention to aseptic operation to prevent the formation of hematoma during surgery.

Asymmetry

Careful preoperative examination and design are very important, and the patient should be clearly explained. If obvious asymmetry is found during the operation, part of the bony structure can be removed on the side with less osteotomy.

Case Demonstrations

- Case 1

    A 25-year-old woman, who was not satisfied with the contour of her mandible, underwent 3D digital design before surgery and then underwent mandibular reduction surgery. There were no postoperative complications, and she was very satisfied with the surgical results (**Fig. 5**).

- Case 2

    A 28-year-old man presented to our clinic due to dissatisfaction with his lower facial contours. Digital 3D-aided design was performed before surgery, and 3D-printed surgical DOT was used during surgery. After the operation, anti-infection and other symptomatic treatment, no obvious complications discharged. He was very satisfied with the results of the operation (**Fig. 6**).

Case 3

    A 30-year old woman presented to our clinic due to dissatisfaction with her facial contours. Computer-assisted design (CAD) and computer-assisted manufacturing (CAM) were performed before surgery. Three-dimensional printed surgical DOT was used during surgery. After the operation, anti-infection, and other symptomatic treatment, no obvious complications discharged. She was very satisfied with the results of the operation.

DISCUSSION

Asian people's appearance, esthetic and anatomical characteristics are different from those of westerners.[5,6,18] Cultural identity and psychological evaluation of facial contour surgery are very important in the whole process of facial bone contour surgery. Body image is an important part of personality theory and a core psychological

Table 1
Comparison procedure in mandibular angle surgery and zygomatic plastic surgery

Surgical Procedures	Cases	Surgical Time Hours	Blood Loss ml	Recovery Time Weeks	Complications N(%)
MBS	22	1.1	110	2	4 (18.2)
MASO	48	1.2	130	2	8 (16.7)
MAO	246	1.5	150	2	48 (19.5)
MS	38	0.8	90	3	4 (10.5)
LSZO/ISZO	156	0.9	100	3	11 (7.1)

Abbreviations: LSZO, L-shaped or I-shaped zygomatic osteotomy; MAO, mandibular angle osteotomy; MASO, mandibular angle split osteotomy; MBS, mandibular bone shaving; MS, malar shaving.

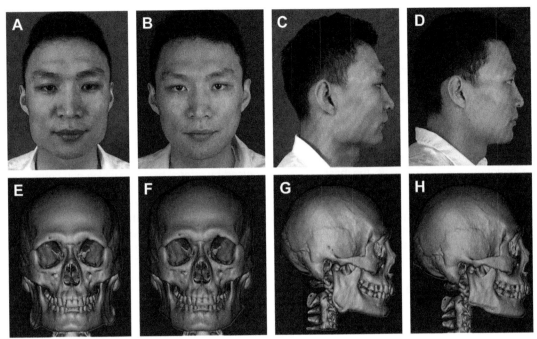

Fig. 5. Case 1 for mandibular reduction surgery.A,C: Preoperative views of a 28-year-old patient; B,D: Postoperative views after mandibular angle osteotomy 6 months later; E,G: 3D model of a 28-year-old patient; F,H: 3D model of after mandibular angle osteotomy 6 months later.

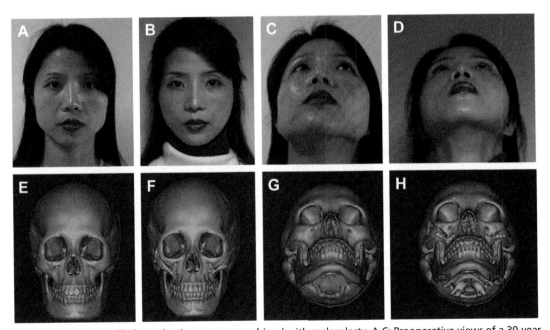

Fig. 6. Case 2 for mandibular reduction surgery combined with malarplasty. A,C: Preoperative views of a 30-year-old patient; B,D: Postoperative views after mandibular angle osteotomy combined with malarplasty 6 months later; E,G: 3D model of a 30-year-old patient; F,H: 3D model of after mandibular angle osteotomy combined with malarplasty 6 months later.

concept of cosmetic medicine. It changes with the change of individual psychology, environment, and physical experience. Patients' personality characteristics have a significant impact on their medical purposes, surgical expectations, and self-attention. Our previous published literature can give references for assessment experience based on Asian esthetics which can better assist doctors in the design of facial esthetics and psychological assessment of facial bone contouring surgery based on self-identity.[7,14,18] Comprehensive perioperative evaluation is the basic guarantee for obtaining good satisfaction in facial bone contouring surgery.

Facial bone contouring proceeds innovated start form Western countries while developed vigorously in the Asian. Adams[19] introduced a surgical technique for resecting mandibular bone and masseter muscle via the transcutaneous approach. Since then, a variety of improved correction methods for mandibular hypertrophy cosmetic procedures have been developed, including those in Asia.[15,20–23] These surgical approaches are from the earliest external approach updated to the intraoral approach.

In recent years, due to the new technology, new equipment, new materials, and other scientific innovations promoted the development of facial bone contouring surgery to minimally invasive surgery. Intraoral incision and the narrow field for surgical procedure will increase the complexity and risk. Therefore, the craniofacial fellowship training is necessary in performing facial bone contouring surgery for academic surgeon. Among Asian facial contouring proceeds, mandibular angle reduction and malarplasty or zygomatic arch reduction surgery are two common facial bone contouring procedures. If mandibular hypertrophy is accompanied by chin retrusion or asymmetric chin deformity, we can do genioplasty at the same time.[24,25]

Malar complex prominence usually appears as a protruding cheekbone in anterior, lateral, and oblique directions, and therefore, the zygomatic bone arch junction is the key element in reducing the sharp cheekbone. Inward alteration of the zygomatic arch is also an important element in narrowing the facial width in the frontal view. There are two commonly used osteotomy techniques for malarplasty reduction: I-shaped osteotomy and L-shaped osteotomy.[14]

Baek and colleagues[26] introduced I-shaped osteotomy. This osteotomy is placed lateral to the maximal malar projection and, thus, usually does not include the volume of malar projection. The osteotomized segment may be moved downward as the masseter muscle pulls the fragment.

The L-shaped osteotomy which we usually used has the advantage of including the volume of the malar projection. The displacement of fragment can be prevented as the masseter muscle cannot drag the fragment downward because the L-shaped fixing and mortise and tenon joint structure.

In the previous literature reports, the most concerned and serious complications of mandibular angle reduction are the intraoperative and postoperative hematomas and postoperative asphyxia caused by arterial bleeding which can course patient death.[14,17] The other common complications reported such as secondary mandibular angle after osteotomy, the result of unexpected fracture, or the inferior alveolar nerve injury. Currently, we use intraoral long-curved ostectomy mandibular reduction with an oscillating saw. Through the standardized perioperative procedures, in our experience, the incidence of severe complications has been reduced.

The DOT is the choice we have standardized for all facial bone contouring patients in recent years. In our experience, adequate preoperative computer-aided surgical design, osteotomy template, and accurate printing play a very important role in ensuring the satisfaction of surgical accuracy after completion. Our previous studies have shown that surgeons can use a precise preoperative design to reduce the operative time, reduce bleeding during surgery, and enable young surgeons to master facial contouring more quickly and safely. In particular, some new navigation assistance technologies, such as the interactive display function of augmented reality, can enhance the perspective perception of surgeons combining virtuality and reality and make up for the lack of 3D imaging in the surgical field.[27] In addition, the robot-assisted surgical technology also has a strong application prospect in facial contouring surgery, providing a new solution to the problem that the surgical guide is easy to slide and difficult to place during surgery.[28]

With the development of modern plastic surgery, the multidisciplinary application of fat graft, dermal fills, facelift procedures, and energy-based equipment makes facial bone contouring proceeds a more minimally invasive, effective, and comprehensive treatment.

SUMMARY

The widespread and acceptance of facial contour surgery in Asia have been made in recent decades. Through the standardized perioperative procedures, in our experience, the incidence of severe complications has been reduced. The application of 3D printing technology contributes to the standardization and improvement of safety and accurate of facial bone contouring surgery. With the comprehensive development of minimally invasive medical cosmetology in the world, the combination of soft tissue contour surgery and minimally invasive procedures for facial bony contouring will make the facial bone contouring surgery safer and more effective.

CLINICS CARE POINTS

- Preoperative three-dimensional (3D) digital design based on Asian ethnic features helps to communicate surgical plans.
- The use of personalized 3D-printed osteotomy template can improve surgical safety, and those procedures should be performed by fellowship-trained plastic surgeons.
- Anatomy-based facial bone osteotomy with intraoperative hemostasis and postoperative pressure bandage dressing are crucial to prevent sever complications such as hematoma.

DISCLOSURE

This work was supported by the project of Science and Technology Commission of Shanghai Municipality (Nos. 19441912300); Clinical Research Plan of SHDC (No. SHDC2020CR3070B); The project of Shanghai Jiao Tong University School of Medicine Two-hundred Talent (No. 20161420); The project of Shanghai Municipal Key Clinical Specialty (shslczdzk00901) and the project of Clinical Research Program of 9th People's Hospital affiliated to Shanghai Jiao Tong University School of Medicine (JYLJ202108).

SUPPLEMENTARY DATA

Supplementary data related to this article can be found online at https://doi.org/10.1016/j.cps.2022.08.002.

REFERENCES

1. Yang J, Xu H, Yang X, et al. The emergence of craniofacial surgery in China. J Craniofac Surg 2014;25(1):6–8.
2. Wu G, Xie Z, Shangguan W, et al. The accuracy of a patient-specific three-dimensional digital ostectomy template for mandibular angle ostectomy. Aesthet Surg J 2022;42(5):447–57.
3. Lin L, Shi Y, Tan A, et al. Mandibular angle split osteotomy based on a novel augmented reality navigation using specialized robot-assisted arms–A feasibility study. J Craniomaxillofac Surg 2016;44(2):215–23.
4. Tan A, Chai Y, Mooi W, et al. Computer-assisted surgery in therapeutic strategy distraction osteogenesis of hemifacial microsomia: accuracy and predictability. J Craniomaxillofac Surg 2019;47(2):204–18.
5. Liew S, Wu WT, Chan HH, et al. Consensus on changing trends, attitudes, and concepts of asian beauty. Aesthetic Plast Surg 2016;40(2):193–201.
6. Liew S, Wu WTL, Chan HH, et al. Consensus on changing trends, attitudes, and concepts of asian beauty. Aesthetic Plast Surg 2020;44(4):1186–94.
7. Li D, Xu H, Xu L, et al. The aesthetic proportion index of facial contour surgery. J Craniofac Surg 2015;26(2):586–9.
8. Whitaker LA, Pertschuk M. Facial skeletal contouring for aesthetic purposes. Plast Reconstr Surg 1982;69(2):245–53.
9. Yang DB, Park CG. Infracture technique for the zygomatic body and arch reduction. Aesthetic Plast Surg 1992;16(4):355–63.
10. Kim YH, Seul JH. Reduction malarplasty through an intraoral incision: a new method. Plast Reconstr Surg 2000;106(7):1514–9.
11. Cho BC. Clinical notes - reduction malarplasty using osteotomy and repositioning of the malar complex: clinical review and comparison of two techniques. J Craniofac Surg 2003;14(3):383–92.
12. Kook MS, Jung S, Park HJ, et al. Reduction malarplasty using modified I-shaped osteotomy. J Oral Maxillofac Surg 2012;70(1):E87–91.
13. Hong SE, Liu SY, Kim JT, et al. Intraoral zygoma reduction using I-shaped osteotomy. J Craniofac Surg 2014;25(3):758–61.
14. Mu X. Experience in East Asian facial recontouring: reduction malarplasty and mandibular reshaping. Arch Facial Plast Surg 2010;12(4):222–9.
15. Baek SM, Kim SS, Bindiger A. The prominent mandibular angle: preoperative management, operative technique, and results in 42 patients. Plast Reconstr Surg 1989;83(2):272–80.
16. Yang DB, Park CG. Mandibular contouring surgery for purely aesthetic reasons. Aesthetic Plast Surg 1991;15(1):53–60.
17. Yang J, Wang L, Xu H, et al. Mandibular oblique ostectomy: an alternative procedure to reduce the width of the lower face. J Craniofac Surg 2009;20(Suppl 2):1822–6.
18. Cui H, Zhao H, Xu H, et al. An innovative approach for facial rejuvenation and contouring injections in asian patients. Aesthet Surg J Open Forum 2021;3(2):ojaa053.

19. Adams WM. Bilateral hypertrophy of the masseter muscle; an operation for correction; case report. Br J Plast Surg 1949;2(2):78–81.

20. Deguchi M, Iio Y, Kobayashi K, et al. Angle-splitting ostectomy for reducing the width of the lower face. Plast Reconstr Surg 1997;99(7):1831–9.

21. Han K, Kim J. Reduction mandibuloplasty: ostectomy of the lateral cortex around the mandibular angle. J Craniofac Surg 2001;12(4):314–25.

22. Hwang K, Lee DK, Lee WJ, et al. A split ostectomy of mandibular body and angle reduction. J Craniofac Surg 2004;15(2):341–6.

23. Lee TS. Standardization of surgical techniques used in facial bone contouring. J Plast Reconstr Aes 2015;68(12):1694–700.

24. Li J, Hsu Y, Khadka A, et al. Surgical designs and techniques for mandibular contouring based on categorisation of square face with low gonial angle in orientals. J Plast Reconstr Aesthet Surg 2012; 65(1):e1–8.

25. Xu HS, Zhang C, Shim YH, et al. Combined use of rapid-prototyping model and surgical guide in correction of mandibular asymmetry malformation patients with normal occlusal relationship. J Craniofac Surg 2015;26(2):418–21.

26. Baek SM, Chung YD, Kim SS. Reduction malarplasty. Plast Reconstr Surg 1991;88(1):53–61.

27. Lin L, Xu C, Shi Y, et al. Preliminary clinical experience of robot-assisted surgery in treatment with genioplasty. Scientific Rep 2021;11(1):6365.

28. Lin L, Sun M, Xu C, et al. The prospective, single-center, randomized controlled trial: assessment of robot-assisted mandibular contouring surgery in comparison with traditional surgery. Aesthet Surg J 2022;42(6):567–79.

Orthognathic Surgery to Enhance the Smile

Alan Yan, MD, Yu-Ray Chen, MD*

KEYWORDS

- Smile • Orthognathic surgery • Surgery-first • LeFort I • Bilateral split sagittal osteotomy
- Genioplasty • Dentofacial deformity

KEY POINTS

- A detailed facial and smile analysis, as well as careful patient selection, are essential in achieving a favorable surgical outcome.
- Orthognathic surgery improves a person's smile by correcting malocclusion, treating excessive or insufficient incisal display, altering the lip line, improving smile arc, correcting asymmetry, and adjusting tooth inclination.
- In the surgery-first approach, orthodontic treatment is undertaken after orthognathic surgery.
- The postsurgical rapid orthodontic tooth movement after maxillary and mandibular osteotomies allows for a shorter course of orthodontic treatment.
- Meticulous surgical techniques and thorough understanding of the facial anatomy are paramount to minimize the risk of avoidable complications such as unexpected fracture of the mandibular ramus or the pterygoid plates.

INTRODUCTION

A smile is an integral component of our social interaction with others. As Dale Carnegie once wrote, a smile "creates happiness in the home, fosters goodwill in a business, and is the countersign of friends."[1] It is the universal language that helps make a good first impression. Studies have shown that those who are happy are more productive in the workplace.[2] A smile encourages trust and makes a person appear more attractive. Improvement of the smile can be achieved by surgery, orthodontics, cosmetic dentistry, or a combination of the aforementioned. In this review, we focus on how orthognathic surgery can be utilized as a treatment modality to create an esthetic smile.

INDICATIONS AND CONTRAINDICATIONS TO ORTHOGNATHIC SURGERY

Orthognathic surgery is indicated for those with dentofacial deformity accompanied by malocclusion. At our institution, the majority of our patients are females (67%) between the ages of 20 to 29 years (65%). Mandibular prognathism is the most prevalent indication (68%), followed by bimaxillary protrusion (21%), and facial asymmetry (11%) (see the section titled, "Case Demonstrations").[3] More recently, people with normal occlusion also seek orthognathic surgical treatment to improve their smile. Orthognathic surgery is contraindicated for those who are medically not healthy enough for surgery or those with body dysmorphic disorder.

Orthognathic surgery is an effective modality to improve smile by treating the following:

- Correct malocclusion
- Treat excessive or insufficient incisal display
- Altered lip line (treat gummy smile)
- Improve smile line by rotation of the maxillomandibular complex
- Correct asymmetry (row, yaw)
- Assist in correcting teeth inclination

Department of Plastic & Reconstructive Surgery, The Craniofacial Center, Chang Gung Memorial Hospital, 5 Fushing Street, Gueishan Shiang, Taoyuan, Taiwan R.O.C. 333
* Corresponding author.
E-mail address: uraychen@cgmh.org.tw

Clin Plastic Surg 50 (2023) 81–89
https://doi.org/10.1016/j.cps.2022.07.001
0094-1298/23/© 2022 Elsevier Inc. All rights reserved.

PREOPERATIVE EVALUATION AND SPECIAL CONSIDERATIONS

Preoperative evaluation of the patient serves a twofold purpose. Firstly, the patient's esthetic and surgical goals are addressed, which will be incorporated into a suitable and realistic surgical plan. Secondly, the initial consultation will allow the surgeon to perform a thorough facial and smile analysis, during which the patient's facial morphology, skeletal, dental, and soft tissue features will be elucidated. Radiographic studies (cephalometric, panoramic radiograph, and facial bone computer tomography) are useful in identifying skeletal and dental relationships; the status of the temporomandibular joint; and the presence of pathologic lesions. Appropriate photographic documentation of the patient smiling and in repose should be recorded. With the advent of virtual surgical planning, three-dimensional (3D) photography of the patient, in addition to facial bone computer tomography, has become an essential preoperative study.

Preoperative analysis should include a facial skeletal evaluation as well as a smile analysis.[4] In short, the skeletal evaluation should include a description of the overall symmetry of the patient's face (chin point deviations from the midline, discrepancy between the vertical position of the inferior border of the mandible between the left and right, and occlusal canting). The vertical proportionality of the face is elucidated by comparing the height of the lower face from the menton to the subnasale relative to the midface from the subnasale to the glabella.

From the lateral view, the sagittal positions of the maxillary and mandibular skeletal bases are compared. Overall facial convexity or concavity is established by connecting a line from the glabella to the subnasale to the pogonion. Patients with mandibular prognathism (Class III malocclusion) typically present with an overall concave facial profile with a divergent chin point, whereas patients with bimaxillary protrusion often have an overall convex profile with chin retrusion.

Smile analysis begins with the identification of the occlusion type as well as an assessment of the dental alignment, arch coordination, dental midline, and incisor inclination. The amount of upper incisor and gingival display while smiling and in repose should be noted. The lip line, defined as the inferior border of the upper lip as it relates to the teeth and gingiva when smiling, should expose the maxillary teeth and only the interdental papillae during a smile. A high lip line, or a gummy smile, can be due to periodontal causes (such as a shortened incisor height), which can be treated with crown-lengthening procedures. Another cause is vertical maxillary excess, as usually seen in bimaxillary protrusion (**Fig. 1**). It is treated by orthognathic surgery to impact the maxilla, as seen later in clinical examples.

The smile arc, an imaginary line along the incisal edges of the maxillary incisors and canines, is another important component of an esthetic smile (**Fig. 2**).[5] The ideal or consonant smile arc should coincide with or follow the curvature of the lower lip when smiling. A flat or reverse smile arc can often be improved by performing posterior impaction of the maxilla and clockwise rotation of the maxillomandibular complex.

The microesthetic features of the smile, such as papillary contours, gingival contours, relative proportions of the maxillary incisors and canines, and tooth inclination, should also be assessed and documented during preoperative evaluation (**Table 1**).[4,6]

Finally, facial soft tissue attributes, such as the nasolabial angle, mentolabial angle, interlabial gap, and presence of mentalis strain, should be assessed in both static and dynamic poses. Adequate skeletal support of the soft tissue is important, and it allows the surgeon to anticipate soft tissue response after skeletal alteration. As soft tissue does not always respond to intended skeletal displacements, patients should be informed of potential soft tissue changes, such as lengthening of the upper lip, deepening of the nasolabial fold, and widening of the nasal base that may result from orthognathic surgery.

SURGICAL PLANNING/TECHNIQUE

The traditional treatment sequence for orthognathic surgery begins with presurgical orthodontics to obtain optimal dental alignment before surgery itself. Our institution has championed the

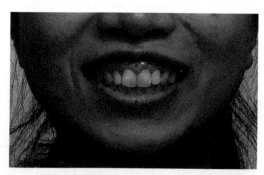

Fig. 1. A high lip line, or gummy smile, can be due to vertical maxillary excess, as seen in bimaxillary protrusion. Surgical treatment includes LeFort I osteotomy with intrusion (impaction) of the anterior maxilla.

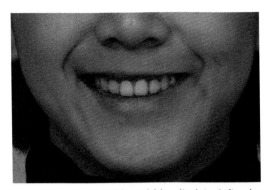

Fig. 2. The smile arc (*dotted blue line*) is defined as the line along the incisal edges of the maxillary incisors and canines. The ideal or consonant smile arc should coincide with or follow the curvature of the lower lip when smiling.

Table 1 Microesthetic features of smile	
Components	**Esthetic Features**
Midline	Perpendicular to the incisal plane; parallel/coincident to the midline of the face
Buccal corridor	Full and symmetric, but not completely eliminated
Papillary contour	Pointed and fill the interdental spaces to the contact point
Gingival margin of maxillary incisors & canines	Along a horizontal line with lateral incisors slightly lower than the line
Gingival zenith point	Maxillary central incisors & canines: distal to the long axis Maxillary lateral incisors: coincident with the long axis
Apparent widths of maxillary incisors & canines	Central incisor: lateral incisor: canine = 1.6:1: 0.6 (golden ratio)
Teeth inclination	More pronounced axial inclination from central incisors to canines
Incisal embrasure	Progressive increase in depth from central incisors to canines

surgery-first orthognathic surgical approach, where the majority of orthodontic adjustment is undertaken after completion of surgery. The surgery-first approach utilizes the greater potential for rapid tooth movement after maxillary and mandibular osteotomies, thereby shortening the time required for orthodontic treatment.[7–12] Our surgical technique, which has been detailed previously, is summarized here.[13]

Bilateral Sagittal Split Osteotomy

Our preferred technique for performing a bilateral sagittal split osteotomy (BSSO) of the mandible is the modified Hunsuck technique (**Fig. 3**).[14] The mandible is incised via a vestibular incision. Subperiosteal dissection of the medial aspect of the ascending ramus is then performed to expose the lingula and the inferior alveolar neurovascular bundle, which is retracted and protected. A horizontal corticotomy of the medial aspect of the ascending ramus is performed just superior to the mandibular foramen.

The sagittal osteotomy of the mandibular body with a reciprocating saw follows the anterior oblique line up to the level of the first molar, where it is joined by the vertical osteotomy of the buccal cortex of the mandibular body. A similar procedure is completed on the contralateral side before actual splitting is performed.

Splitting of the proximal and distal mandibular segments is accomplished by a series of osteotomies. Osteotomy of the medial cortex of the mandibular angle, which remains with the proximal segment, is performed to ensure long-term stability after repositioning the mandible as muscular forces are no longer restricting its excursion. Mandibular angle contouring can be performed concurrently, and the resected medial cortex of the angle can be used as a bone graft if necessary.

The mobile distal segment of the mandible is now guided into its new position with the occlusal splint, and intermaxillary fixation (IMF) is accomplished. Bony adjustments are made as necessary to provide optimal contact between the segments. The condyle should be in a relaxed position within the glenoid fossa. Osteosynthesis is achieved with two 2.0 millimeters titanium plates secured with monocortical screws along the body of the mandible. The IMF is released to verify the occlusion. The wound is closed in layers with absorbable sutures.

LeFort I Osteotomy

An intraoral labial-buccal incision is made, preserving an adequate cuff of mucosa to facilitate final closure (**Fig. 4**). Subperiosteal dissection then

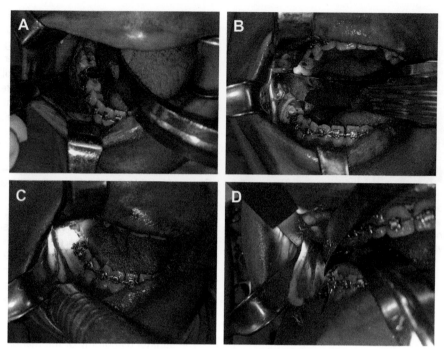

Fig. 3. BSSO. (*A*) A buccal vestibular incision begins at the anterior border of the ramus and extends anteriorly along the mandibular body up to the second premolar. The incision is then taken onto the bone, and subperiosteal dissection is performed. to expose the lateral aspect of the mandible. (*B*) Subperiosteal dissection of the medial aspect of the ascending ramus is then performed to expose the lingual; the inferior alveolar neurovascular bundle is identified and protected. Horizontal corticotomy of the medial ascending ramus is performed just superior to the mandibular foramen. (*C*) The sagittal split osteotomy of the mandibular ramus is performed based on the technique described by Hunsuck. (*D*) The pterygomasseteric muscle sling is detached, and the medial surface of the mandible can be used as an alternative source of bone grafts if needed.

exposes the anterior maxillary wall, infraorbital foramen, lateral zygomaticomaxillary buttress, and pterygomaxillary junction. The nasal mucosa is elevated off the nasal piriform, and intranasal dissection extends onto the nasal floor and the lateral nasal wall, and medially onto the septum and vomer. The nasal septum is separated from the maxillary crest. The planned osteotomy is then marked out, maintaining a distance of at least 5 millimeters above the tooth root apices. Horizontal osteotomy is performed from the posterior-lateral maxillary wall, across the anterior maxillary wall, and onto the lateral nasal wall. Pterygomaxillary disjunction begins with the use of a right-angled oscillating saw and is completed with a curved osteotome. A posterior maxillary wall osteotomy is performed through gentle tapping with a thin osteotome. Once the osteotomies are complete, the maxilla can be down fractured with digital pressure without excessive force.

With the maxilla fully mobilized, it is guided into the occlusal splint either as a single piece or in multiple segments and stabilized with the IMF. If a BSSO is performed concurrently, the maxillomandibular complex is placed in the desired position sequentially by intermediate and final occlusal splints, as directed by virtual surgical planning. Areas of bony interference are removed, as in cases of maxillary impaction or setback. The nasal septum may need to be partially resected to prevent septal buckling. If there is significant inferior maxillary extrusion, interpositional grafts can be used. The final position of the maxilla is secured with titanium plates and screws at the medial and lateral buttresses. The IMF is released to verify the occlusion. An alar cinch suture is placed to control the width of the alar base, and the intraoral incision is closed in layers with absorbable sutures.

POSTOPERATIVE CARE AND EXPECTED OUTCOME

The IMF is routinely removed before the patient is extubated. For multiple-segment osteotomies of the maxilla or mandible, a dental splint is applied for 2 weeks to provide additional stability if needed. Patients are instructed to use chlorhexidine solution for oral rinsing. A liquid diet is initiated as soon as possible after surgery and a soft diet is gradually advanced within 2 weeks.

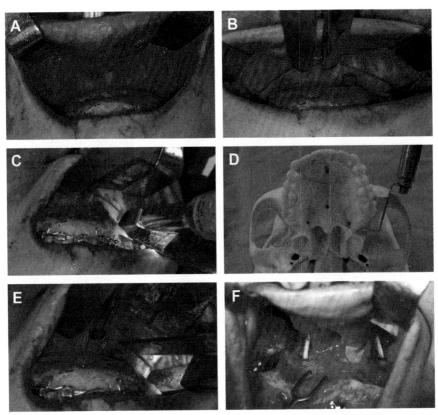

Fig. 4. LeFort I osteotomy. (*A*) After making an intraoral labial-buccal incision, subperiosteal dissection is performed to expose the anterior maxillary wall, infraorbital foramen, lateral zygomaticomaxillary buttress, pterygomaxillary junction, and nasal piriform. The nasal septum is separated from the maxillary crest. (*B*) The planned osteotomy is marked 5 mm above the canine root apices. (*C, D*) The pterygomaxillary osteotomy is performed with a right-angled oscillating saw followed by a curved thin-blade osteotome for completion. (*E*) Posterior maxillary wall osteotomy is performed under gentle tapping with a thin osteotome. (*F*) Downfracturing of the maxilla is performed with digital pressure after completion of all osteotomies, with preservation of the descending palatine vessels (shown next to *arrow*).

Nonsteroidal anti-inflammatory drugs are routinely prescribed for pain relief. Broad-spectrum parenteral antibiotics are given after the operation and then converted to an oral form for 1 week. To reduce the discomfort from soft tissue swelling, patients are advised to routinely apply ice packs and elevate their heads, and nasal decongestants are used for the first few days after surgery. Most patients are discharged 2 days after the surgery once their oral intake is adequate and they are able to ambulate. They are followed up at 1 week, 1 month, 4 months, and 1 year after surgery. Postoperative orthodontic treatment is initiated 4 weeks after surgery.

In the surgery-first orthognathic approach, orthodontic treatment is initiated postoperatively and continues monthly to align the dental arches and fine-tune the smile profile. At our institution, the mean treatment time from orthognathic surgery to bracket debonding lasts about 9 months.[15]

MANAGEMENT OF COMPLICATIONS

Inferior alveolar nerve injury remains the most common complication after orthognathic surgery. While 90% of patients experience transient sensory disturbance of the lower lip immediately after surgery, only 10% of patients experience symptoms lasting longer than 6 months.[16]

An unexpected fracture of the mandibular ramus occurred in 1% to 3% of the patients. This often occurs as a result of the surgeon's attempt to prevent an inferior alveolar nerve injury, thereby making the mandibular ramus too thin. Most unexpected fractures are incomplete and can be identified intraoperatively before the ramus has been split completely. For inadvertent complete

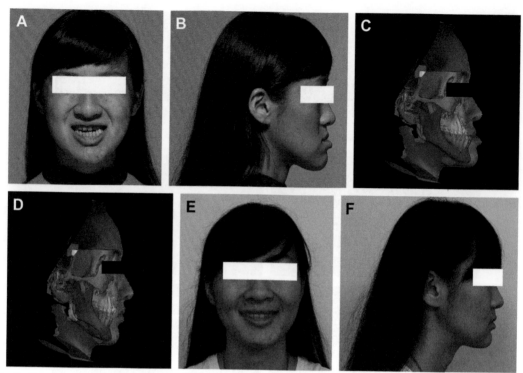

Fig. 5. Class III malocclusion (mandibular prognathism). Preoperative frontal (*A*) and profile (*B*) views reveal a flat smile arc, anterior open bite, and a concave profile on sagittal view. Virtual surgical planning (*C, D*) of LeFort I osteotomy and BSSO includes mandibular setback, as well as clockwise rotation of the maxillomandibular complex to improve the smile arc. Postoperative frontal (*E*) and profile (*F*) views.

ramus fractures, rigid fixation with miniplates is necessary.

Injury to the descending palatine artery is not uncommon when performing LeFort I osteotomies. Bleeding is controlled with cauterization to prevent postoperative hematoma. Injury to the facial artery is uncommon. If it does occur, we recommend ligation of the vessel to prevent the development of a late pseudoaneurysm.

REVISION AND SUBSEQUENT PROCEDURES

A small percentage of patients will require revision or secondary orthognathic surgery,[17] which is usually done at least 1 year after the initial surgery to allow for consolidated skeletal structures and stabilized soft tissues.[18] The four main indications for revision orthognathic surgery are unexpected postsurgical skeletal growth, dental relapse, skeletal relapse, and unsatisfactory esthetic results.[17] To improve the esthetic result, facial bone contouring as well as facial lipofilling can be performed concomitantly[19] or as secondary procedures.

CASE DEMONSTRATIONS

These concepts are illustrated in the following clinical examples.

Case 1: Class III Malocclusion with Mandibular Prognathism

This 23-year-old woman presented with class III malocclusion with mandibular prognathism (**Fig. 5**). Her preoperative facial and smile analysis is characterized by an anterior open bite, a flat smile arc, and a concave profile in sagittal view. To treat the dentofacial deformity and improve her smile, the surgical plan includes a LeFort I osteotomy and BSSO to set back the mandible, as well as clockwise rotation of the maxillomandibular complex to improve the smile arc.

Case 2: Class II Malocclusion with Bimaxillary Protrusion

This 24-year-old woman presented with class II malocclusion with bimaxillary protrusion (**Fig. 6**). She also exhibited a gummy smile due to maxillary excess. To treat the dentofacial deformity and improve her smile, the surgical plan includes a LeFort I osteotomy with an anterior segmental osteotomy (Wassmund), together with a BSSO with an anterior segmental osteotomy (Kole), to intrude the maxilla and improve the proclination of her incisors.

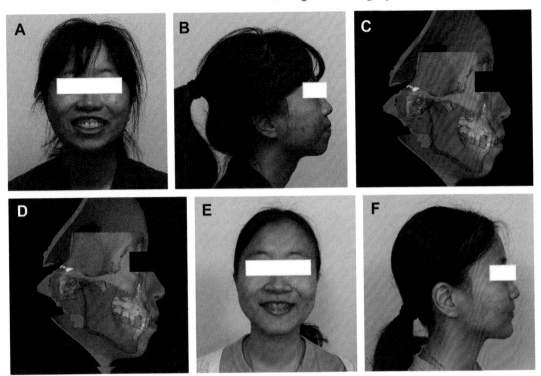

Fig. 6. Bimaxillary protrusion. Preoperative frontal (*A*) and profile (*B*) views reveal a gummy smile and a convex profile on sagittal view. Virtual surgical planning (*C, D*) includes a LeFort I osteotomy with an anterior segmental osteotomy (Wassmund), together with a BSSO with an anterior segmental osteotomy (Kole), to intrude the maxilla and improve the proclination of her incisors. Postoperative frontal (*E*) and profile (*F*) views.

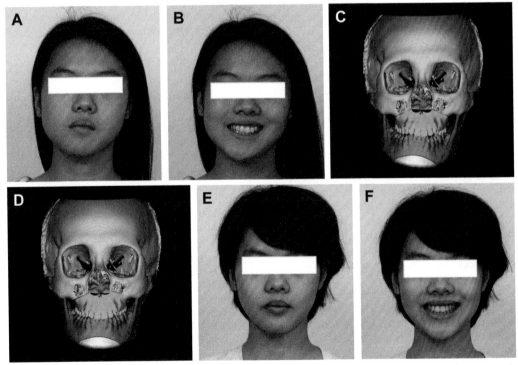

Fig. 7. Facial asymmetry. Preoperative frontal views (*A, B*) reveal occlusal canting as well as deviation of the dental midline and chin point. Virtual surgical planning (*C, D*) includes LeFort I osteotomy to intrude the left maxilla and extrude the right maxilla, BSSO, and an osseous genioplasty to correct the chin point deviation. Postoperative frontal views (*E, F*).

Case 3: Facial Asymmetry

This 20-year-old woman presented with facial asymmetry, characterized by deviation of the dental midline, chin point, and occlusal canting (**Fig. 7**). To treat the dentofacial deformity and to improve her smile, the surgical plan includes a LeFort I osteotomy to intrude the left maxilla and extrude the right maxilla, a BSSO, and an osseous genioplasty to correct the chin point deviation.

DISCUSSION

A successful surgical outcome is comprised of thorough preoperative evaluation followed by careful surgical planning and precise execution of each surgical step. Equally important but often overlooked is the understanding and management of the patient's surgical goals and expectations. A surgery that is well planned and perfectly carried out can still result in a dissatisfied patient if there is a disconnect between patient expectations and the limitations of surgery. Management of patients with unrealistic expectations has become more and more important, as more and more people are seeking orthognathic surgery for esthetic rather than functional purposes. Elderly patients with bimaxillary protrusion, for instance, are at the highest risk of developing an aged appearance after surgery as a result of attenuated midfacial soft tissue support after setback and/or intrusion of the maxilla. They should therefore be forewarned and prepared to accept this likely consequence. At our institution, all patients were instructed to maintain good sleep and exercise regularly before undergoing orthognathic surgery. From the senior author's experience, this preoperative preparation of the mind and body positively impacts patient recovery.

Surgical planning for orthognathic surgery has come a long way, from the classic 2D planning with mounted plaster models and cephalograms, to virtual simulated planning in 3D using computer software, cone beam computer tomography, 3D photographs, and digital dental casts. Since 2017, our institution has adopted the two-splint technique together with 3D planning.[20] This provides the surgeon with "infinite" opportunities to perform the surgery virtually until all the desired surgical results are achieved. It also provides the patients a glimpse of the postsurgical appearance, and final last-minute changes can be made to meet their goals. However, even a perfectly executed surgery that follows the virtual simulated plans precisely may not yield an esthetic result if there is an error in the surgical plan itself. And when it happens, the surgeon must be decisive to discard the virtual surgical plan and convert the surgery to the one-splint technique, using the intraoperative checkpoints to control facial symmetry and guide the final result.[21]

To achieve a stable surgical result with minimal relapse and complications, osteotomies should be performed safely while rigid fixation is placed after assuring maximal bony contact without interference and liberal use of bone grafts. Finally, effective collaboration between the surgeon and orthodontist is essential to obtain a balanced outcome that incorporates both facial and dental ideals.[13]

SUMMARY

The design of an esthetic smile consists of a detailed analysis of the facial skeleton as well as the tooth, lips, gingival tissues, and their collective appearance. Symmetry and balance of the dentofacial features are paramount, with the maxillary incisors and canines serving a vital role in smile analysis. Orthognathic surgery serves as a powerful tool in improving the smile. It is important to keep in mind that the concept of a beautiful smile is often influenced by a person's cultural, ethnic, and racial backgrounds. Moreover, the most natural and beautiful smiles are often not perfect by any scientific standard; an esthetic smile is often achieved not by perfection but rather through the subtlety of imperfection.

CLINICS CARE POINTS

- To minimize intraoperative blood loss, the mean blood pressure is maintained at around 60 mm Hg with the aid of hypotensive agents.

- During LeFort I osteotomy, pterygomaxillary disjunction is performed with the use of a right-angled oscillating saw followed by a curved osteotome. Excessive force during downfracture should be avoided to prevent unfavorable fractures.

- If the mandibular ramus is split too thin (in an attempt to avoid inferior alveolar nerve injury) during bilateral sagittal split osteotomy, unexpected ramus fracture can occur. The fracture is usually incomplete and can be identified and treated intraoperatively.

- Stability of LeFort I and bilateral sagittal split osteotomy is achieved by rigid fixation with plates and screws, removal of areas of bony interference, maximal contact between bony segments to be fixated, and liberal use of bone grafts when necessary. Intermaxillary fixation is usually removed at the end of surgery.

- Meticulous layered closure of soft tissue eliminates the need for drain placement, which improves patient comfort postoperatively.

DISCLOSURE

The authors have nothing to disclose.

REFERENCES

1. Carnegie D. How to win friends & influence people. New York City, USA: The World's Work (1913) Ltd; 1953. p. 310, viii.
2. Oswald AJ, Proto E, Sgroi D, University of Warwick. Department of E. Happiness and productivity. Warwick economic research papers no 882. Department of Economics, University of Warwick; 2008:42 p. : ill.
3. Chou PY, Denadai R, Yao CF, et al. History and evolution of orthognathic surgery at chang gung craniofacial center: lessons learned from 35-year experience. Ann Plast Surg 2020;84(1S Suppl 1): S60–8.
4. Sarver D, Jacobson RS. The aesthetic dentofacial analysis. Clin Plast Surg 2007;34(3):369–94.
5. Sarver DM. The importance of incisor positioning in the esthetic smile: the smile arc. Am J Orthod Dentofacial Orthop 2001;120(2):98–111.
6. Davis NC. Smile design. Dent Clin North Am 2007; 51(2):299–318, vii.
7. Ko EW, Hsu SS, Hsieh HY, et al. Comparison of progressive cephalometric changes and postsurgical stability of skeletal Class III correction with and without presurgical orthodontic treatment. J Oral Maxillofac Surg 2011;69(5):1469–77.
8. Liao YF, Chiu YT, Huang CS, et al. Presurgical orthodontics versus no presurgical orthodontics: treatment outcome of surgical-orthodontic correction for skeletal class III open bite. Plast Reconstr Surg 2010;126(6):2074–83.
9. Liou EJ, Chen PH, Wang YC, et al. Surgery-first accelerated orthognathic surgery: orthodontic guidelines and setup for model surgery. J Oral Maxillofac Surg 2011;69(3):771–80.
10. Liou EJ, Chen PH, Wang YC, et al. Surgery-first accelerated orthognathic surgery: postoperative rapid orthodontic tooth movement. J Oral Maxillofac Surg 2011;69(3):781–5.
11. Wang YC, Ko EW, Huang CS, et al. Comparison of transverse dimensional changes in surgical skeletal Class III patients with and without presurgical orthodontics. J Oral Maxillofac Surg 2010;68(8):1807–12.
12. Yu CC, Chen PH, Liou EJ, et al. A Surgery-first approach in surgical-orthodontic treatment of mandibular prognathism–a case report. Chang Gung Med J 2010;33(6):699–705.
13. Pu LLQ. Aesthetic plastic surgery in Asians: principles & techniques. USA: CRC Press/Taylor & Francis; 2015. 2 volumes (xxxiv, 1138 pages).
14. Hunsuck EE. A modified intraoral sagittal splitting technic for correction of mandibular prognathism. J Oral Surg 1968;26(4):250–3.
15. Huang CS, Chen YR. Orthodontic principles and guidelines for the surgery-first approach to orthognathic surgery. Int J Oral Maxillofac Surg 2015; 44(12):1457–62.
16. Yoshioka I, Tanaka T, Khanal A, et al. Relationship between inferior alveolar nerve canal position at mandibular second molar in patients with prognathism and possible occurrence of neurosensory disturbance after sagittal split ramus osteotomy. J Oral Maxillofac Surg 2010;68(12):3022–7.
17. Reyneke JP. Reoperative orthognathic surgery. Oral Maxillofacial Surg Clin N Am 2011;23(1):73–92, vi.
18. Raffaini M, Pisani C, Conti M. Orthognathic surgery "again" to correct aesthetic failure of primary surgery: report on outcomes and patient satisfaction in 70 consecutive cases. J Craniomaxillofac Surg 2018;46(7):1069–78.
19. Wang YC, Wallace CG, Pai BC, et al. Orthognathic surgery with simultaneous autologous fat transfer for correction of facial asymmetry. Plast Reconstr Surg 2017;139(3):693–700.
20. Ng JH, Chen YA, Hsieh YJ, et al. One-splint versus two-splint technique in orthognathic surgery for class III asymmetry: comparison of patient-centred outcomes. Clin Oral Investig 2021;25(12):6799–811.
21. Yu CC, Bergeron L, Lin CH, et al. Single-splint technique in orthognathic surgery: intraoperative checkpoints to control facial symmetry. Plast Reconstr Surg 2009;124(3):879–86.

Periorbital Rejuvenation for Asians

Yun-Nan Lin, MD[a], Yi-Chia Wu, MD, PhD[a,b], Shu-Hung Huang, MD, PhD[a,b,c,d], Chih-Kang Chou, MD, MS[e], Hidenobu Takahashi, MD[f], Tsai-Ming Lin, MD, PhD[e],*

KEYWORDS

• Periorbita • Periorbital rejuvenation • Fat grafting • Microautologous fat transplantation

KEY POINTS

- Several problems with Asian periorbita necessitate effective and long-term treatment.
- We have categorized periorbital rejuvenation in Asians into 6 main issues.
- We provide several promising and straightforward strategies for these problems utilizing autologous fat grafting and innovative instrumentation.
- Comprehensive illustrations and satisfactory long-term results demonstrate the feasibility and indispensability of microautologous fat transplantation for periorbital rejuvenation in Asian patients.

 Video content accompanies this article at http://www.plasticsurgery.theclinics.com.

INTRODUCTION

"The eye is the window to the soul." In pursuing aesthetic beauty, the eyes are the central draw of the face and may be the point of focus for human appearance. In Asians, the established ideal is fullness of the upper eyelids with a natural eyelid crease, few wrinkles around the eyelids, a lack of baggy appearance in the lower eyelid, and no depressions over the tear trough (nasojugal groove) or lid–cheek junction (palpebromalar junction). The periorbital areas are mainly the main areas of focus for facial rejuvenation, either for women or men. Lower blepharoplasty (transcutaneous or transconjunctival), botulinum toxin A, fillers, and laser treatment have offered solutions historically. Microautologous fat transplantation (MAFT) has been postulated by Lin and colleagues,[1] and its efficacy has been illustrated by using the innovative instrument, MAFT-GUN,[2] to demonstrate its feasibility in facial rejuvenation.[3–11] In this article, we explore the MAFT technique combined with other modalities, provide detailed descriptions of the technique, and illustrate its long-term results for periorbital rejuvenation in Asians.

Authorship: Y.-N. Lin: First author with the contribution to surgical operation, data analysis, and interpretation. T.-M. Lin: The corresponding author contributes to the surgical procedure, data analysis, and interpretation. Y.-C. Wu, S.-H. Huang, C.-K. Chou: Contributed to the data interpretation and analysis. H. Takahashi: Contributed to surgical operation, compiled the DVD, and created the animation.

[a] Division of Plastic Surgery, Department of Surgery, Kaohsiung Medical University Hospital, No. 100, Tzyou 1st Road, Kaohsiung City 807, Taiwan; [b] Department of Surgery, School of Medicine, College of Medicine, Kaohsiung Medical University, Tzyou 1st Road, Kaohsiung City 807, Taiwan; [c] Hyperbaric Oxygen Therapy Room, Kaohsiung Medical University Hospital, No. 100, Tzyou 1st Road, Kaohsiung City, Taiwan; [d] Graduate Institute of Medicine, College of Medicine, Kaohsiung Medical University, No. 100, Tzyou 1st Road, Kaohsiung City, Taiwan; [e] Charming Institute of Aesthetic and Regenerative Surgery (CIARS), 2F.-1, No. 172, Ziqiang 2nd Road, Qianjin District, Kaohsiung City 801, Taiwan; [f] Department of Surgery, Kaohsiung Medical University Hospital, No. 100, Tzyou 1st Road, Kaohsiung City 807, Taiwan
* Corresponding author.
E-mail address: k79157@gmail.com
Twitter: @TsaiMingLinMD (T.-M.L.)

Clin Plastic Surg 50 (2023) 91–100
https://doi.org/10.1016/j.cps.2022.07.009

INDICATIONS AND CONTRAINDICATIONS

Based on the goal of harmonious tissue recontouring and skin texture improvement, we will illustrate 6 strategies for 6 problems in Asian periorbita in this article. The issues include sunken upper eyelids, sunken upper eyelids with multiple folds, crow's feet (fine wrinkles over the lateral orbital area), baggy eyes with skin redundancy, baggy eyes without skin redundancy, and moderate baggy eyes with deformities of tear trough/lid–cheek junction or an infraorbital dark circle (IODC) (**Fig. 1**). The individual strategy for each of these problems is as follows (**Fig. 2**).

Preoperative Evaluation and Special Considerations

The authors evaluate Asian periorbital rejuvenation according to the following key points:

Sunken upper eyelids

Sunken upper eyelids are a problem that bothers patients who may feel tired, exhausted, or sick-looking. They often request consult for depression recontouring as fullness over the upper eyelids. Unfortunately, in situ, dermal/dermo-fat sheet grafting does not show positive results in long-term follow-up. Filler injection is also not suggested or favored, given the potential risks such as nodulation due to thin skin and potential vascular insults in this location. However, Lin has illustrated the application of MAFT and showed a promising result by fat grafting.[2] Its indispensability in fewer morbidities and favorable long-term outcomes has been demonstrated in approximately 100 cases.

Sunken upper eyelids with multiple folds

In Asians, a double eyelid crease is desired, although only approximately 50% of the population are born with this presentation.[12] Therefore, double-eyelid blepharoplasty is the most frequently performed aesthetic surgery in the Asian population. However, in a delicate but not uncommon scenario, sunken upper eyelids combined with multiple folds present the complexity

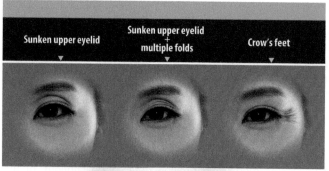

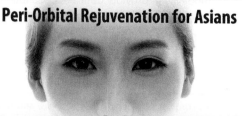

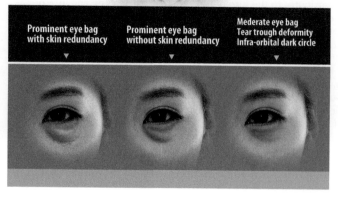

Fig. 1. There are 6 issues in Asian periorbital rejuvenation; include sunken upper eyelids, sunken upper eyelids with multiple folds, crow's feet (fine wrinkles over the lateral orbital area), baggy eyes with skin redundancy, baggy eyes without skin redundancy, and moderate baggy eyes with deformities of tear trough/lid–cheek junction or an infraorbital dark circle (IODC).

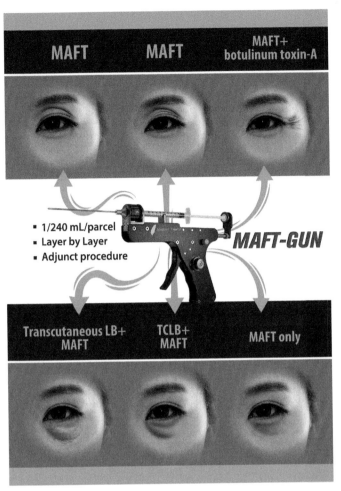

Fig. 2. The corresponding strategy for each of the 6 issues for peri-orbital rejuvenation relies on the primary strategy, MAFT technique, and other adjunctive procedures. The purified fat is transferred to a 1-mL syringe and loaded with a MAFT-GUN (Dermato Plastica Beauty Co., Ltd., Kaohsiung, Taiwan). In peri-orbital rejuvenation, a single delivered fat parcel volume is predetermined at 1/240 mL (0.0042 mL) by turning the 6-graded volume dial to 240.

in the face of adopting a promising surgical intervention. Studies showing successful treatment of sunken upper eyelids and recreation of the desired curvature of the double eyelid simultaneously are limited in the literature, although surgeons have proposed several modalities.[13–15] In the authors' previous publication,[2,3] a unique strategy was demonstrated for managing these 2 problems in one procedure; the technical details and results are highlighted in this article.

Crow's feet (fine wrinkles over lateral orbital areas)

Wrinkles over the periorbital areas are often and favorably selected to be treated by botulinum toxin A (BTX) injection to achieve a satisfactory result.[16] However, crow's feet (or wrinkles over the bilateral orbital areas) necessitate repeated injection to maintain the effect, and the deepening static wrinkles are always refractory to BTX. Therefore, to achieve a long-lasting treatment outcome, an increase in dermal thickness and the amount of extracellular matrix (such as collagen or elastin

fiber) is warranted. The MAFT technique can provide sustainable improvements in crow's feet and dermis thickening over this area.

Baggy eyes with skin redundancy

Lower blepharoplasty can rejuvenate the lower eyelids and necessitates various modifications to treat the associated deformities, such as the tear trough/lid–cheek junction depression. The authors have advocated a strategy of 3 simple steps for refining transcutaneous lower blepharoplasty for aging eyelids with promising results. This technique includes step 1, subciliary transcutaneous lower blepharoplasty to remove redundant skin only (or combine limited resection of a strip of orbicularis oculi muscle); step 2, conservative removal of 3 orbital fat compartments; and step 3, the MAFT technique for recontouring the deformities of tear trough/lid–cheek junction.[11]

Baggy eyes without skin redundancy

For those who request to improve the appearance of moderate to severe baggy eyelids

Table 1
Five determinant scenarios in Asian periorbital rejuvenation and the corresponding strategies

	Characteristics	Strategies	Author's Comment
A. Sunken appearance of the upper eyelid	Hollowness in the upper eyelid area	Fat Grafting	• Using the MAFT technique and delivering fat grafting at 1/240 mL per parcel • 0.5~1.5 mL/side by MAFT-GUN • Zone I, total layers; Zone II, superficial layer only; and Zone III, no-touch area
B. Multiple folds over the upper eyelid	Multiple parallel shallow folds, sometimes with a dominant fold	Fat grafting	• Please ensure that the desired main crease height (the lowest of the folds or 6~8 mm from the ciliary margin) is the lower margin of Zone II • Same technique as mentioned above
C. Crow's feet in the lateral orbital area	Dynamic or static radial wrinkles of lateral canthal ligament	Fat grafting	• Fan-shaped total layers of fat grafting • MAFT technique with MAFT-GUN • 1/240 mL per parcel, 1~2 mL/side • Botulinum toxin A might be adjunct
D. Degree of lower eye bag	Mild baggy eye (some moderate candidates) Moderate ~ severe baggy referred to as E strategy	Fat grafting	• MAFT only if the baggy eye appearance is acceptable. 1.0 ~3.0 mL/side. MAFT technique with MAFT-GUN • Lower blepharoplasty is mandatory in moderate to severe baggy eyes (see E).
E. Redundancy of lower eyelid skin	Moderated ~severe baggy eyes Prominent skin redundancy or not	Redundancy: Transcutaneous LB; No redundancy: transconjunctival LB	• In the authors' series for Asians, transcutaneous LB for those aged >50 years and transconjunctival LB for those aged <40 years • For those aged 40~50 years, redundancy is the determinant factor for choosing the method of LB

MAFT, microautologous fat transplantation; MAFT-GUN, is a patented instrument for fat grafting produced by Dermato Plastica Beauty Co., Ltd., Kaohsiung, Taiwan; LB, lower blepharoplasty.

without skin redundancy over the lower eyelid area, transconjunctival lower blepharoplasty is the most appropriate option. As in the strategy mentioned above, a direct approach through the conjunctiva to remove orbital fat, followed by the MAFT procedure in the tear trough/lid–cheek junction areas, is highly preferred.

Table 2
Surgical procedures for periorbital rejuvenation in Asian patients

	Main Strategies	Technique/Instrument/ Adjunct	Anatomic Considerations	Authors' Comment
A. Sunken appearance of the upper eyelid	Fat grafting	MAFT (1/240 mL per parcel)/ MAFT-GUN	Three layers are deep, supraperiosteal; middle, between deep and orbicularis oculi muscle; and superficial, between orbicularis oculi muscle and skin dermis. Zone I (total layers) and Zone II (superficial) Zone III, No-touch area	Zone I 0.5~1.0 mL, Zone II 0.2~0.5 mL Fig. 2
B. Multiple folds over the upper eyelid	Fat grafting	MAFT (1/240 mL per parcel)/ MAFT-GUN	As A The designed double eyelid crease will be preferably set along the lower margin of Zone II, which clinically may be the lowest fold or 6~8 mm from the ciliary margin.	Similar to A Fig. 2
C. Crow's feet in the lateral orbital area	Fat grafting	MAFT (1/240 mL per parcel)/ MAFT-GUN Botulinum toxin A	Total layers (deep, supraligament of lateral canthus; middle, between deep and orbicularis oculi muscle; superficial, between middle and skin dermis)	Fan-shaped area transplantation 1~2 mL/side Botulinum toxin A may be necessary
D. Degree of lower eye bag	Fat grafting	MAFT (1/240 mL per parcel)/ MAFT-GUN	Total layers (deep, supraperiosteum; middle, between deep and orbicularis oculi muscle: superficial, between mid and eyelid dermis) in the deformities of tear trough/lid-cheek junction	2.5~3.0 mL/side, deep: 25%, middle: 50%, and superficial: 25% The amount may increase once the midcheek furrow necessitates contouring. Fig. 2
E. Redundancy of the lower eyelid skin	Fat grafting	MAFT (1/240 mL per parcel)/ MAFT-GUN/ Lower blepharoplasty	Redundancy of skin: transcutaneous LB; no redundancy: transconjunctival LB (TCLB) Conservative orbital fat removal without extensive dissection or other procedure MAFT as D	The three simple steps, combining MAFT and transcutaneous lower blepharoplasty, comprise the preferable procedure for skin redundancy. If there is no redundancy, then TCLB is an optional choice. The delivered fat amount is similar to that noted for D. Fig. 2

MAFT, microautologous fat transplantation; MAFT-GUN, is a patented instrument for fat grafting produced by Dermato Plastica Beauty Co., Ltd., Kaohsiung, Taiwan; LB, lower blepharoplasty.

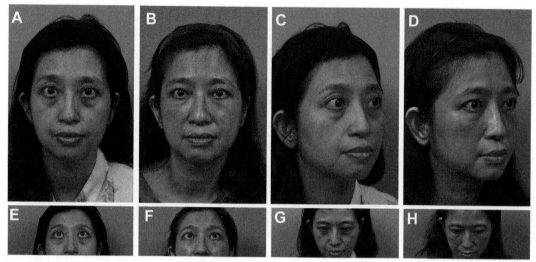

Fig. 3. A 40-year-old female presented for her sunken upper eyelid, tear trough deformity (depression), moderate eye bag, and infraorbital dark circle (IODC) for microautologous fat transplantation (MAFT) (*A, C, E, G*). MAFT was performed to deliver a 2.0/2.0-mL (left/right) for the sunken upper eyelid and 2.5/2.5-mL (left/right) for the tear trough/lid–cheek junction. Five years and nine months after a single MAFT session (*B, D, F, H*), the fullness of her upper eyelid was well maintained with a nice curvature of the double eyelid crease. The improvement of IODC and nice recontouring of the deformities of tear trough and lid/cheek junction further demonstrated the effects of the MAFT technique.

Moderate baggy eyes with tear trough/lid–cheek junction deformities or combined with the infraorbital dark circle

Younger Asians may request a consultation to evaluate a moderate or minimal baggy eye appearance. Occasionally, conjunct problems such as deformities over tear trough/lid–cheek junction or IODC necessitate treatment with the same procedure. The authors have experienced more than 200 cases in this category with good long-term follow-up.

Table 1 illustrates the symptoms and signs of each scenario and its corresponding strategy.

Surgical Procedures

All patients received total intravenous anesthesia during fat grafting. Appropriate local anesthesia was applied at donor and recipient inserting sites with 0.3 to 0.5 mL of 2% lidocaine HCl with epinephrine (1:50,000). Lipoaspirates were harvested from the lower abdomen or inner thigh. The donor site was infiltrated with a tumescent solution (10 mL of 2% lidocaine [20 mg/mL]: 30 mL of Ringer lactate solution: 0.2 mL of epinephrine [1:1000]). Approximately 10 to 15 minutes after infiltration, fat was harvested from the donor site with a blunt-tip cannula (diameter, 2.5 or 3.0 mm; 1 side-hole sized 1 mm 2 mm). The lipoaspirate volume was approximately equal to the volume of the tumescent solution to ensure

that fat constituted a major proportion of the lipoaspirate. To minimize damage to the lipoaspirate, the plunger of a 10-mL syringe connected to a liposuction cannula was withdrawn to approximately 2 to 3 mL to maintain a negative pressure of 270 to 330 mm Hg.[3–11,17] Lipoaspirates were processed and purified by centrifugation at 3000 rpm (approximately 1200 g) for 3 minutes. This procedure minimized graft contamination due to environmental exposure and manual manipulation. Centrifugation facilitated the separation of the lipoaspirate into layers. The top layer contained oil from ruptured fat cells; the middle layer contained purified fat; and the bottom layer contained blood, cellular debris, and fluid. The purified fat was carefully transferred into a 1-mL Luer-slip syringe using a transducer. The syringe containing purified fat was loaded into a MAFT-GUN (see **Fig. 2**) and connected to an 18-gauge, blunt-tip cannula. The device was set by adjusting a dial to deliver fat parcels to 0.0042 mL (i.e., 1/240 mL) with each trigger deployment (see **Fig. 2** and **Table 2**). A puncture incision was made on the midcheek (tear trough/lid–cheek junction, and crow's feet) or later upper eyelid (for sunken upper eyelid) with fat parcels delivered from deep, middle, and superficial layers according (see **Table 2**).[3–5,11] More surgical details for these scenarios are demonstrated in and Video 1–5 and **Table 2**.

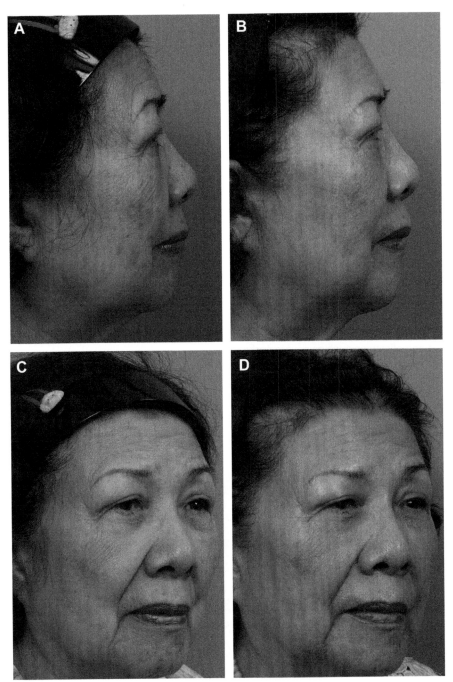

Fig. 4. A 79-year-old lady wished for facial rejuvenation of her crow's, skin texture, fine wrinkles, and aging spots over the cheek (*A, C*). The rejuvenating effect of fat grafting was demonstrated with the MAFT technique. One session of the MAFT technique was performed over the crow's feet (1.5/1.5-mL, left/right) and cheek areas (3.5/3.5-mL, left/right). Five months after the MAFT session, the crow's feet and the wrinkles, aging spots, and skin texture over the lower eyelid and cheek areas were improved (*B, D*).

Postoperative Care and Expected Outcome

We apply flesh-colored article tape to all MAFT areas and remove them two days after surgery. Then, patients self-administer nonsteroidal anti-inflammatory drugs for a few days when necessary, and although mild to moderate swelling/ecchymosis occurs, it usually subsides gradually within 7–10 days. After fat grafting, hyperbaric oxygen therapy (HBOT) is optional suggested management. The authors have deployed a single-chamber HBOT routinely postoperatively for one week (1.4 ATM, 60–90 minutes/day) (CA200-OX II, Kuang Tai Metal Industrial Co., Ltd., Taiwan) since 2020 with improved recovery from swelling on both recipients and donor sites. Patients are also encouraged to receive a lymphatic massage to facilitate the subsiding of the swelling. Donor-site care followed a postliposuction routine, and patients wore a pressure garment at the donor site for three months. The recipients' appearance was noted to be "natural" one month after MAFT and showed favorable rejuvenation effects at three months. The results of fat grafting were long-term, as shown in **Figs. 3–6**.

Management of Complications/Revision or Subsequent Procedures

For the past decade, authors have dealt with more than 1500 cases of periorbital rejuvenation without any significant complications such as severe nodulation/fibrosis, vascular insults/blindness, or cerebral infarction. Among these, touchup was required in less than 1% of cases, and most of them were requests for increased fullness instead of responses to complications or under-correction.

The MAFT technique for facial rejuvenation recontouring has demonstrated favorable long-term effects. However, in Asians, for periorbital rejuvenation to address the problems mentioned above, a touchup procedure may still be occasionally required. For sunken eyelids, an initial session of MAFT did not offer satisfactory results in severe sunken eyes, and a touchup procedure was indicated 4–6 months after the initial process. Meanwhile, a similar situation may necessitate a touchup for the recontouring of tear troughs in the lower eyelid areas, although the average fat survival/retention rate is estimated to be 60–70%. There is no over-correction concept using the MAFT technique; therefore, over-grafting should not be a problem.

Case Demonstrations

Four cases represent the long-term follow-up effects of periorbital rejuvenation using the MAFT technique combined with other procedures, lower blepharoplasty, rigottomy,[18] or botulinum toxin A (see **Figs. 3–6**).

DISCUSSION

Good craftsmanship depends on the use of the appropriate tool. For the past few decades, the evolution progression necessitates a new technique and device/instrument for improving facial aesthetics. This article described the MAFT technique and advocated the clinical application of

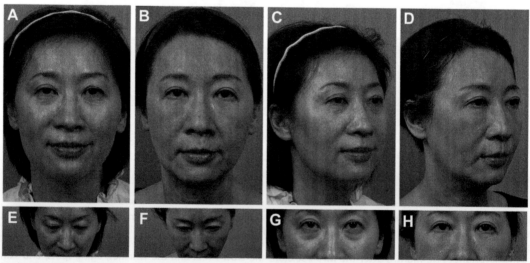

Fig. 5. This 55-year-old woman requested rejuvenation of her aging lower eyelid (*A, C, E, G*). A transcutaneous lower blepharoplasty was performed in conjunction with MAFT to remove right and left orbital fat (0.41 g and 0.42 g, respectively) that was then transplanted in the right and left tear troughs and lid–cheek junctions (3.5 mL and 4.0 mL, respectively). At 6 years after surgery, retention of the fat volume in her tear trough and lid–cheek junction areas was well maintained. After long-term follow-up, the AP (*B*) and oblique (*D*) views show good recontouring in the tear troughs and lid–cheek junctions. A downward view (*H*) demonstrates the eliminated infraorbital fine wrinkles and the rejuvenation with appropriate volume restoration. The fine wrinkles and skin texture over the lower eyelid areas were improved and maintained (*F*).

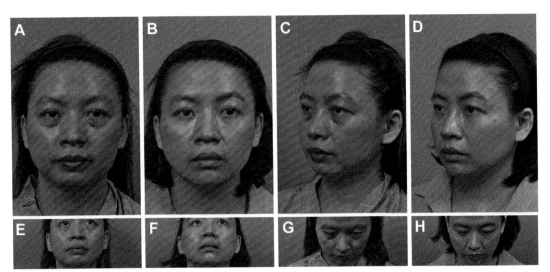

Fig. 6. This 38-year-old woman was consulted for fat grafting to improve her lower eyelid, including moderate baggy eye, depression of teary trough/lid–cheek junction, and infraorbital dark circle (IODC) (*A, C, E, G*). A transconjunctival lower blepharoplasty (TCLB) with MAFT for recontouring the tear trough deformity/lid–cheek junction was performed in terms of no skin redundancy noted. The total fat volumes of 3.5/3.0-mL (left/right) were placed after removing orbital fat volumes of 0.30/0.32 gram by TCLB. Two years and five months after the operation, the improved appearance of her lower eyelid was maintained (*B, D*). The recontoured tear trough and the lid–cheek junction with an improved appearance of the baggy lower eyelid are shown in the upward-looking (*F*) and downward-looking view (*H*), further indicating the skin rejuvenation effects with diminished IODC.

MAFT-GUN in fat grafting procedures. Fat grafting provides volumetric restoration and skin rejuvenation for periorbital rejuvenation concerns, necessitating an innovative, anticipated technique. Reliable and long-term results, as shown in **Figs. 3–6**, illustrate the novelty and indispensability of the MAFT technique.

The deficiency of soft tissue, baggy eyelid due to protruded orbital fat, ongoing aging skin redundancy, and wrinkles, deformities of the tear trough, and lid–cheek junction depression altogether are the key issues of periorbital aging in Asians. Clinically, we apply the lower blepharoplasty to remove the orbital fat for improving the baggy appearance and eliminating redundant skin, if ever. Moreover, we meticulously perform the MAFT technique to recontour the ongoing soft tissue deficiency, regenerate the aging skin problems (wrinkles or thinning skin), and rejuvenate the periorbital area. The advantage of the MAFT technique is that it is a simple and reliable procedure for surgeons with low morbidity and high long-term satisfaction. The limitation of this technique is that it is an instrument, MAFT-GUN dependent, and the short learning curve is fast might be individual variables.

In general, Caucasians and Asians share the basic periorbital anatomy in common. However, Caucasians have thinner skin and more skeletonization while aging than Asians. Moreover, the cultural aspect (the Asians disfavor sunken upper eyelids) might influence the request from the patient's point of view for the management of periorbital aging. The preoperative consultation for individualized surgical planning is necessary for every case in Asian periorbital rejuvenation according to the abovementioned six key points.

SUMMARY/CONCLUSION

For periorbital rejuvenation in Asians, we offer the MAFT technique as the primary strategy and combine it with other modalities such as transcutaneous/transconjunctival lower blepharoplasty and botulinum toxin A. Long-term results show the reliability and indispensability of fat grafting for periorbital rejuvenation. The sustainable volumetric restoration and rejuvenating effects further demonstrate the desirability of the MAFT technique and the reliable, innovative instrument MAFT-GUN.

CLINICS CARE POINTS

- The periorbital areas where patients ask for rejuvenation should be evaluated, followed by a proposal of the necessary strategies.
- Surgical intervention can be performed effectively based on the microautologous fat transplantation (MAFT) technique with adjunctive procedures.

- Good postoperative care is mandatory.
- Promising rejuvenation effects appear one month following MAFT and persist for years.

ETHICS STATEMENT

There is no ethical concern in this study.

ACKNOWLEDGMENTS

The authors would like to thank Mr. Chia-Hsiu Chien for his preparation of **Figs. 1** and **2** and the animations in the videos.

DISCLOSURE

Dr T.-M. Lin owns the patent rights to the MAFT-GUN and is a scientific adviser for Dermato Plastica Beauty Co. Ltd., the manufacturer of the MAFT-GUN device. None of the other authors have any financial disclosures or conflicts of interest.

SUPPLEMENTARY DATA

Supplementary data related to this article can be found online at https://doi.org/10.1016/j.cps.2022.07.009.

REFERENCES

1. Lin TM, Lin SD, Lai CS. The treatment of nasolabial fold with free fat graft: preliminary concept of Micro-Autologous Fat Transplantation (MAFT). Paper presented at: The 2nd Academic Congress of Taiwan Cosmetic Association Taipei. Taiwan, May 7, 2007.
2. United States Patent, Patent No.: US 7,632,251 B2. 2009.
3. Lin TM, Lin TY, Chou CK, et al. Application of microautologous fat transplantation in the correction of sunken upper eyelid. Plast Reconstr Surg Glob Open 2014;2(11):e259.
4. Lin TM, Lin TY, Huang YH, et al. Fat grafting for recontouring sunken upper eyelids with multiple folds in Asians-novel mechanism for neoformation of double eyelid crease. Ann Plast Surg 2016;76(4):371–5.
5. Lin TM. Total facial rejuvenation with microautologous fat transplantation (MAFT). In: Pu LLQ, Chen YR, Li QF, et al, editors. Aesthetic plastic surgery in Asians: principles and techniques. 1st edition. St. Louis (MO): CRC Press; 2015. p. 127–46.
6. Kao WP, Lin YN, Lin TY, et al. Microautologous fat transplantation for primary augmentation rhinoplasty: long-term monitoring of 198 Asian patients. Aesthe Surg J 2016;36(6):648–56.
7. Lee SS, Huang YH, Lin TY, et al. Long-term outcome of microautologous fat transplantation to correct temporal depression. J Craniofac Surg 2017;28(3):629–34.
8. Chou CK, Lee SS, Lin TY, et al. Micro-autologous fat transplantation (MAFT) for forehead volumizing and contouring. Aesthetic Plast Surg 2017;41(4):845–55.
9. Lin YN, Huang SH, Lin TY, et al. Micro-autologous fat transplantation for rejuvenation of the dorsal surface of the aging hand. J Plast Reconstr Aesthet Surg 2018;71(4):573–84.
10. Huang SH, Huang YH, Lin YN, et al. Micro-autologous fat transplantation for treating a gummy smile. Aesthet Surg J 2018;38(9):925–37.
11. Huang SH, Lin YN, Lee SS, et al. Three simple steps for refining transcutaneous lower blepharoplasty for aging eyelids: the indispensability of microautologous fat transplantation. Aesthet Surg J 2019;39(11):1163–77.
12. Harry S, Hwang 1, Spiegel Jeffrey H. Aesthet Surg J the effect of "single" vs "double" eyelids on the perceived attractiveness of Chinese women. Aesthet Surg J 2014;34(3):374–82.
13. Chen CC, Chen SN, Huang CL. Correction of sunken upper-eyelid deformity in young asians by minimally-invasive double-eyelid procedure and simultaneous orbital fat pad repositioning: a one-year follow-up study of 250 cases. Aesthet Surg J 2015;35(4):359–66.
14. Lee W, Kwon SB, Oh SK, et al. Correction of sunken upper eyelid with orbital fat transposition flap and dermofat graft. J Plast Reconstr Aesthet Surg 2017;70(12):1768–75.
15. Jiang L, Li H, Yin N, et al. Free orbital fat grafting during upper blepharoplasty in asians to prevent multiple upper eyelid folds and sunken upper eyelids. J Craniofac Surg 2020;31(3):685–8.
16. Ballard TNS, Vorisek MK, Few JW. Impact of botulinum toxin type a treatment of the glabella and crow's feet on static forehead rhytides. Dermatol Surg 2019;45(1):167–9.
17. Chou CK, Lin TM, Chiu CH, et al. Influential factors in autologous fat transplantation - focusing on the lumen size of injection needle and the injecting volume. J IPRAS 2013;9:25–7.
18. Roger KK, Rigotti G, Cardoso E, et al. Megavolume autologous fat transfer: part II. Practice and techniques. Plast Reconstr Surg 2014;133(6):1369–77.

Asian Upper Blepharoplasty
A Comprehensive Approach

Chunmei Wang, MD, PhD[a], Lee L.Q. Pu, MD, PhD[b],*

KEYWORDS

• Asians • Upper blepharoplasty • Double eyelid • Cosmetic surgery • Comprehensive approach

KEY POINTS

- Both height and length of the new upper skin crease should be properly determined.
- More "ideal" anatomy of the upper eyelid can be created by removing excess tissues of the upper eyelid.
- The desirable anatomic structure of the upper eyelid should be reconstructed.
- If indicated, a medial epicanthoplasty can be added to enhance cosmetic result.

 Video content accompanies this article at http://www.plasticsurgery.theclinics.com.

INTRODUCTION

Asian upper blepharoplasty is commonly referred to as a "double eyelid" surgery and is the most common cosmetic surgical procedure performed in East Asian countries, especially for women, as about 50% of Asian women have a single fold of their upper eyelid.[1,2] The primary goal of Asian upper blepharoplasty is to create a well-defined supratarsal skin crease so that the eye looks more open and more aesthetically pleasing. Most Asian women desire more a "natural look" of their eyes that still respects their identity other than being more westernized look.[2] For years, Asian upper blepharoplasty has been considered as a relatively simple procedure as long as a suprastarsal skin crease for each upper eyelid is symmetrically created after surgery.[3,4]

Because there are several differences of the upper eyelid anatomy between Caucasians and Asians, the surgeon who performs an Asian upper blepharoplasty should also address several other anatomic features of an Asian upper eyelid such as epicanthal fold, ptosis or pseudoptosis, eyelash inversion, and excess fat of the upper eyelid in addition to scar formation after the surgery.[5–7] Most experts in the field believe that Asian upper blepharoplasty requires finesse, precision, and clear understanding of the eyelid anatomy in addition to the patient's expectation and unique culture sensitivity.[1–9]

Several techniques for Asian upper blepharoplasty have been reported in the literature, some seem to be simple and some seem to be somehow complicated and difficult to learn.[3,4,6,7,10,11] There is lack of a standardized technique that is relatively easy to follow but comprehensive enough that addresses all relevant structures of Asian upper eyelid so that more natural look and aesthetically pleasing result can be achieved. Over the last decade, the authors have developed a comprehensive approach that could address all anatomic features or structures of the Asian upper eyelid for Asian upper blepharoplasty. With this approach, patients may come close to have a more natural and beautiful look of their eyelids without a visible

a Department of Plastic and Aesthetic Surgery, Institute of Dermatology, Southern Medical University, 2 Lujing Road, Yuexiu District, Guangzhou, P.R. China 510030; b Division of Plastic Surgery, University of California Davis Medical Center, 2335 Stockton Boulevard, Suite 6008, Sacramento, CA 95817, USA
* Corresponding author.
E-mail address: llpu@ucdavis.edu

Clin Plastic Surg 50 (2023) 101–109
https://doi.org/10.1016/j.cps.2022.07.006

scar when they close eyes but aesthetically attractive when they open eyes. In this article, we describe our comprehensive approach for Asian upper blepharoplasty. Our preferred preoperative design and step-by-step surgical technique for Asian upper blepharoplasty are also described in detail.

Special Considerations of Upper Eyelid Anatomy in Asians

Asian upper eyelid, especially Mongolian type, has significant differences of the anatomy compared with one of Caucasians: absent supratarsal skin crease, low tarsal height, abundant preseptal fat, eyelash ptosis, and presence of medial epicanthal fold. The preseptal fat may often prolapse into pretarsal area. The insertion of the levator is usually beneath the upper tarsal edge or at the tarsal edge[12](**Fig. 1**). Therefore, Asians often have droopy eyelid, bloated eye, invisible eyelid skin fold or single eyelid, or even epicanthus. Although the primary goal of Asian upper blepharoplasty is to create a supratarsal skin crease, all other anatomic structures should also be alternated so that more natural look and aesthetically pleasing result can be achieved in either statistical or dynamical expression after such a procedure.[13,14]

Indications and Contraindications

As the ultimate goal for Asian upper blepharoplasty is to create natural looking double eyelid, the procedure itself can be indicated for all ages of patients, women or men (**Fig. 2A**). It can also be indicated for patients with less noticeable supratarsal fold or even less desirable shape of the fold (**Fig. 2B**). There is no absolute contraindication for the procedure as long as patients have good motivation and realistic expectation for the

procedure. Patients with a history of hypertrophic scar or keloid formation might be relatively contraindicated for the procedure.

Our standardized informed consent includes noticeable scar formation, asymmetry, less desirable cosmetic outcome, and future revision, if indicated. All procedures are performed under local anesthesia in our outpatient operating rooms.

Preoperative Design and Marking

Based on our understanding of the applied anatomy of an Asian upper eyelid as well as the sense of beauty and desirable outcome for Asian patients, the authors have developed a comprehensive approach for Asian upper blepharoplasty. The standard measurement of a beautiful eye for Far East Asian women has been described and should be considered as a reference for every single patient (**Fig. 3**). With use of a small forceps or a special double eyelid designer to mimicking the effect of fan-shaped, crescent-shaped, or parallel double eyelid, the preferred shape of new double eyelid is confirmed with the patient.

The height of the upper eyelid skin crease is marked from the edge of the eyelid in a supine position when the eye is closed. In general, the optimal height for Asian women is 6 to 8 mm (for Asian men 4–6 mm) above the eyelid margin in the center of the upper eyelid. The new height of the upper eyelid skin crease can be adjusted according to the patient's desired result and the distance from the eyebrow to the eyelid margin. The length of the upper eyelid crease can be determined based on 1:3 or 1:4 ratio between the height and length of the upper eyelid skin crease. Once the central height of the upper eyelid skin crease is determined, a skin pitch test is done to determine the amount of the upper eyelid skin that can be removed. In general, a maximal 3 to

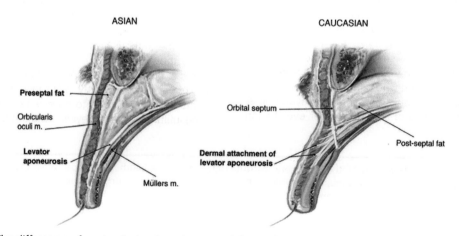

ASIAN   CAUCASIAN

Preseptal fat

Orbicularis oculi m.

Levator aponeurosis

Müllers m.

Orbital septum

Post-septal fat

Dermal attachment of levator aponeurosis

Fig. 1. The differences of anatomic structures between Asian and Caucasian upper eyelids.

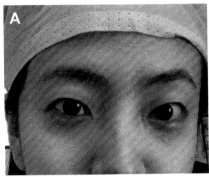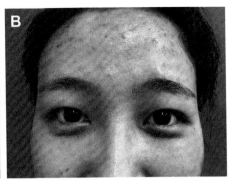

Fig. 2. (*A*) A typical Asian woman with "single eyelid" who desires upper blepharoplasty to "create double" eyelid; (*B*) a typical Asian woman with less noticeable supratarsal fold who desires upper blepharoplasty to create more obvious supratarsal fold.

5 mm skin resection is needed in order to produce the effect of eyelashes' elevation but without causing eyelid ectropion. A skin incision marking can then be finalized. If medial canthoplasty is indicated, the medial upper eyelid incision is extended to a Z-plasty or V-to-Y fashion in the medial canthal area (**Fig. 4**A, B).

SURGICAL PROCEDURES
Creating More Ideal Anatomy of the Upper Eyelid

All upper blepharoplasty procedures are performed under local anesthesia. A total of 5 cc 1% lidocaine with 1:100,000 epinephrine is precisely infiltrated into each upper eyelid skin incisions from skin to tarsus. It takes at least 3 minutes to have full aesthetic and vasoconstrictive effects.

The upper eyelid skin incision is made with a knife through the subcutaneous tissue down to the orbicularis ocular muscle. A strip of the excess upper eyelid skin (usually 3–5 mm) is excised (**Fig. 5**). With a scissor's dissection, the underlying orbicularis ocular muscle is excised to explore the septum. The lower part of the eyelid skin in front of

the orbicularis oculi muscle and tarsus are dissected free. The thinning of this part of the eyelid is performed by removing the upper two-thirds of the orbicularis oculi muscle in front of the tarsus but preserving the full layer of the orbicularis oculi muscle in the lower one-third in front of the tarsus (**Fig. 6**); this is followed by excision of preseptal fat and an appropriate amount of the central fat pad once the septum is opened (**Fig. 7**). In this way, an "ideal anatomy" of the upper eyelid in Asians can be created by removing all above "excess" tissues.

Reconstructing the Desirable Anatomic Structure of the Upper Eyelid Skin Crease

After above tissue removal, the levator aponeurosis is then identified and its function is evaluated intraoperatively. If the upper eyelid margin needs to be raised, its proper position can be adjusted with plication of the levator aponeurosis above the upper edge of the tarsus with 7-0 nylon interrupted sutures. This procedure may be common for relatively older patients or patients with preexisting eyelid ptosis or pseudoptosis. The degree of the levator aponeurosis suspension can be

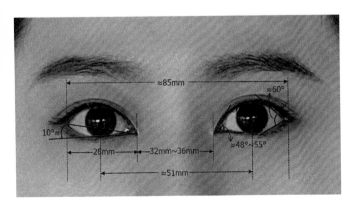

Fig. 3. Ideal and standard measurements of Asian periorbital anesthetics.

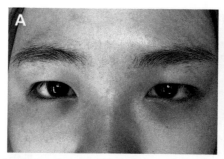
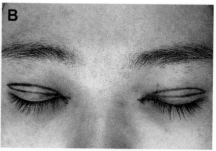

Fig. 4. An intraoperative view shows before (*A*) and after marking of each eyelid skin incision and its extended medial epicanthoplasty incision (*B*).

determined intraoperatively by the range of movement for the created upper eyelid skin crease and controlled by allowing for the upper eyelid margin to rest at the superior limbus by covering 0.5 to 1.0 mm of the upper cornea. The eyelashes can also be raised after this maneuver (**Fig. 8**). In this way, the desirable anatomic position of the tarsus in an upper eyelid can be created. The upper eyelid skin incision is then closed precisely through the septum and the mobile portion of the levator aponeurosis 3 to 5 mm above the upper edge of the tarsus with 7-0 nylon suture in an interrupted fashion once the proper shape of the incision closure and the proper degree of eye lashes' elevation are determined to be optimal (**Fig. 9**). The symmetry and shape for each incision closure can be adjusted by removing more eyelid skin as indicated.

Medial Epicanthoplasty as Needed

Because of the unique anatomy of upper eyelid in Asians, medial epicanthoplasty is often needed to enhance cosmetic result for Asian upper blepharoplasty. In the investigators' practice, about 50% of patients would need medial epicanthoplasty in

conjunction with their upper blepharoplasty. The skin incision can be designed in either Z-plasty or Y-to-V fashion. The ectopic superficial orbicularis oculi muscle and the fibers of the superficial medial ligament fibers are transected to form a double opposite triangular skin cross flaps or a Y-to-V advancement flap. Attention should be made to ensure that the skin closure after medial epicanthoplasty can match the skin closure after upper blepharoplasty skin incision (**Fig. 10**). A video is included to show our preoperative design, marking, and operative technique (Video 1).

POSTOPERATIVE CARE AND EXPECTED OUTCOME

The incision is covered with a small Vaseline gauze and a light pressure dressing. Immediate postoperatively, the patient is asked to have head elevation and to use an ice pack for the incision site during the first night. Oral antibiotics is given for the first 3 days. The suture is usually removed about 1 week postoperatively (**Fig. 11**). Each patient is followed-up for up to 1 year after surgery and as needed after 1 year.

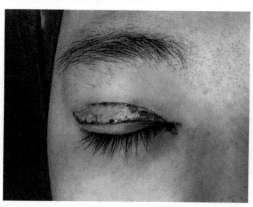

Fig. 5. An intraoperative view shows the extent of the eyelid skin excision.

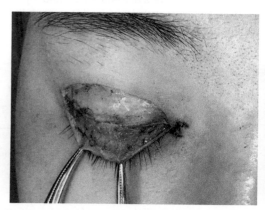

Fig. 6. An intraoperative view shows the excision of the orbicularis ocular muscle within the extend of the skin resection and in front of the tarsal plate.

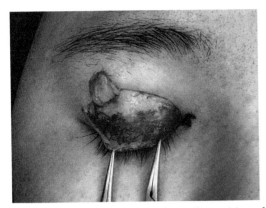

Fig. 7. An intraoperative view shows the excision of the septal fat.

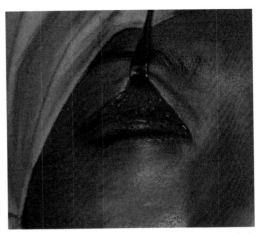

Fig. 9. An intraoperative view shows closure of the skin incision. Please note that the suture is through the septum and the mobile portion of the levator aponeurosis.

More than 800 patients with various ages underwent upper blepharoplasty for creation of double eyelid as a primary procedure or conversion from less visible to more optimal double eyelid as a secondary procedure by the authors with this comprehensive approach. An average length for bilateral upper blepharoplasty in the authors' practice is 1.5 hours. The surgical outcomes, including patient satisfaction and postoperative complications, were retrospectively reviewed by clinical documentation and postoperative photography for each patient. Minimum follow-up time was 1 year, ranging from 1 to 7 years postoperatively. Photos were taken at the follow-up visit. Each patient was asked whether she felt satisfactory about the aesthetic outcome after upper blepharoplasty for creation of double eyelids.

MANAGEMENT OF COMPLICATIONS OR REVISIONS

No surgical complications that required reoperation was observed in the investigators' practice during the follow-up period. Less than 2% of our patients required surgical revision for asymmetry or less optimal shape of the upper eyelid. However, after a minor revision surgery, again it was performed under local anesthesia as an office procedure; all those patients were eventually satisfactory for their final outcome.

Case Demonstrations

Case 1: see **Fig. 12A–C.**
Case 2: see **Fig. 13A–C.**
Case 3: see **Fig. 14A–C.**
Case 4: see **Fig. 15A–C.**

DISCUSSION

Asian upper blepharoplasty is often referred to as a "double eyelid surgery" by creating a supratarsal skin crease in the upper eyelid. The aesthetic

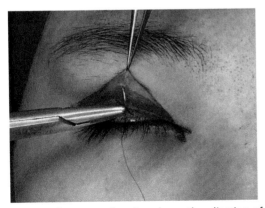

Fig. 8. An intraoperative view shows the plication of the levator aponeurosis.

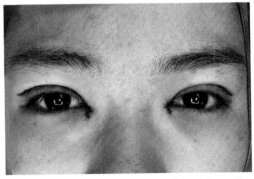

Fig. 10. An intraoperative view shows immediate result after upper blepharoplasty and medial epicanthoplasty.

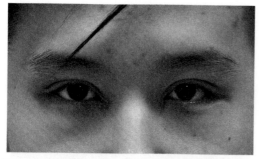

Fig. 11. A 21-year-old Asian man with no natural supratarsal eyelid crease had Asian upper blepharoplasty for creation of a nature "double eyelid." At 1-week postoperative follow-up, he had a minimal swelling and ecchymosis, and the scar of his newly created supratarsal fold was less noticeable.

outcome after such a procedure is often dramatic and can change the look of one's periorbital region or even some features of the face. It is the most common cosmetic procedure for Asians especially for young women.[8,15] However, Asian upper blepharoplasty is not a simple operation as it sounds.[7,8] Less satisfactory results are still relatively common based on the reports from previous publications and the investigators' observation.[4,6,8,16] For example, the supratarsal skin crease is unnaturally too high or too deeper, and the scar of the new supratarsal skin crease is too prominent. Therefore, most experts in Asian upper blepharoplasty believe that a thorough understanding of the Asian eyelid anatomy and the patient's expectation, accurate preoperative

planning to address anatomic features of the Asian eyelid, and precise execution of the surgical procedure are all necessary steps for an optimal outcome.[2,6,7,9]

Asian upper blepharoplasty is not just for creation of a double eyelid. Based on a good understanding of the differences of upper eyelid anatomy between Caucasians and Asians, there are several "other issues" in an Asian upper eyelid that also need to be addressed when planning an Asian upper blepharoplasty. In addition to creating a reliable dermal attachment to the levator aponeurosis through an open technique, excess skin, preseptal or septal fat, and orbicularis ocular muscle should also be removed.[9,10,13,16] In this way, an "ideal anatomy" of the upper eyelid in Asians, which is more mimic to a Caucasian one, can be created by removing all above "excess" tissues. Such a newly created Asian upper eyelid can look thinner and less full after the procedure. Because many Asian upper eyelids have a droopy look, a typical feature of upper eyelid psudoptosis,[6,7] such a condition can be corrected by proper tightening of the levator aponeurosis via plication. In this way, a desirable anatomic position of the tarsus in an upper eyelid can be created. The proper position of the tarsus often results in an overall more dynamic expression of the upper eyelid and dramatically change the eye's expression from a dull to an attractive look, one of the most important aesthetic features that are well liked by many Asian patients especially women. Furthermore, medial epicanthal fold, if present, should also be corrected properly by a medial

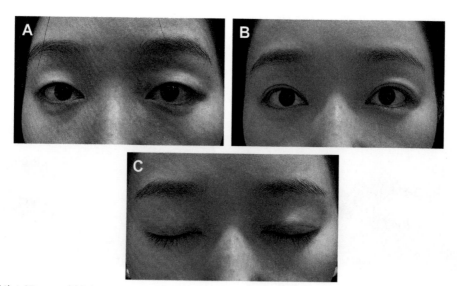

Fig. 12. (*A*) A 27-year-old Asian woman with no natural supratarsal eyelid crease. (*B*) The result at 6 months after Asian upper blepharoplasty for creation of a nature "double eyelid." (*C*) The scar of her new supratarsal fold was almost invisible.

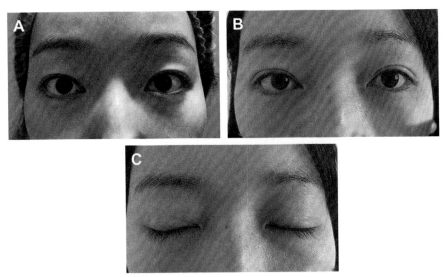

Fig. 13. (*A*) Another 27-year-old Asian woman with less noticeable supratarsal eyelid crease. (*B*) The result at 12 months after Asian upper blepharoplasty for creation of a more pleasing "double eyelid." (*C*) The scar of her new supratarsal fold was almost invisible.

epicanthoplasty that can be incorporated with the medial upper blepharoplasty incision.[14]

Although several procedures for Asian upper blepharoplasty are described in the literature, there is lack of a standardized approach that is comprehensive and can result in a consistent but optimal result for most of the patients.[6,8,9,11,16] Some techniques seem to be less reliable such as a closed technique, and many others may fail to address all anatomic problems of the Asian upper eyelid. For example, an open technique can create a dermal attachment to the levator aponeurosis by a scar formation but does not remove excess skin, orbicularis ocular muscle, and preseptal or septal fat. In addition, a simple open approach, commonly performed by others, may not correct pseudoptosis of the upper eyelid by repositioning the tarsus in the upper eyelid. The

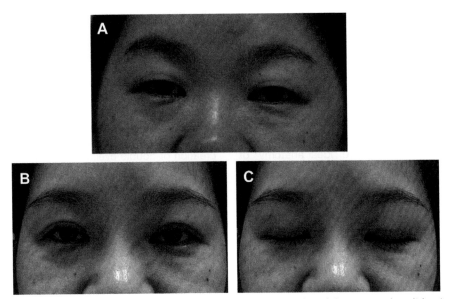

Fig. 14. (*A*) A 37-year-old Asian woman with less noticeable supratarsal eyelid crease and eyelid aging. (*B*) The result at 4 months after Asian upper blepharoplasty for creation of a more pleasing "double eyelid." In this case, a significant amount of the orbital fat was removed. In addition, more upper eyelid skin was also removed. (*C*) The scar of her new supratarsal fold was almost invisible.

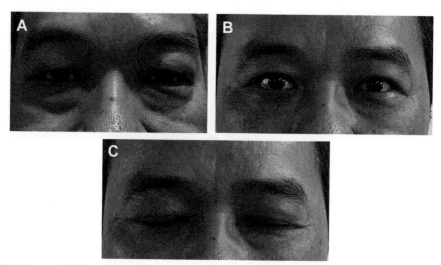

Fig. 15. (*A*) A 46-year-old Asian man with no nature supratarsal eyelid crease and eyelid aging. (*B*) The result at 14 months after Asian upper blepharoplasty for creation of a more pleasing "double eyelid." In this case, a significant amount of the orbital fat was removed including transconjunctival lower blepharoplasty for fat removal. In addition, more upper eyelid skin was also removed. (*C*) The scar of his new supratarsal fold was almost invisible.

Hinge technique, the use of a vascularized orbital septum as a flap to create a fibrous extension from the levator aponeurosis to the dermis at the location of eyelid crease, may be another versatile technique to reconstruct the anatomic and physiologic architecture of the natural Asian "double eyelid."[17] It becomes obvious, however, that a more comprehensive approach is needed for Asian upper blepharoplasty that can clearly address all anatomic problems of the Asian upper eyelid.

We believe our comprehensive approach for Asian upper blepharoplasty may achieve a higher satisfactory outcome but a very low revisional rate. In our approach, each anatomic problem of the Asian upper eyelid is addressed through an open technique. In that way, a dermal attachment of levator aponeurosis can securely be established. The upper eyelid skin, orbicularis oculi muscle, and preseptal or septal fat are appropriately excised to form a more "ideal anatomy" of the Asian upper eyelid. Once the eyelid becomes thinner, the fullness of the upper eyelid can be corrected or minimized so that the cosmetic result can be enhanced. For each patient, any excess skin above the new upper eyelid skin crease can be removed as much as possible so that the eyelashes can also be raised. This step may enhance the cosmetic result after Asian upper blepharoplasty and may also prevent future upper eyelid from aging. Partial removal of the orbicularis ocular muscle in front of the tarsus may further make the upper eyelid thinner, avoid the formation of "a sausage eye," and reduce restrains on an eye

opening so that the eye fissure becomes larger and the eye opening can be accelerated; this is one of the key components of our procedure that may improve the dynamic beauty of the eye after Asian upper blepharoplasty. Appropriate plication of the levator aponeurosis can correct pseudoptosis of eyelid, increase corneal exposure, and improve attractive look of the eye. The upper eyelid skin incision is closed with an interrupted suture through the septum and the mobile part of the levator aponeurosis 3 to 5 mm above the upper edge of the tarsal plate, and this can form a "sandwich" type adhesion that makes opening of eyes more pleasing and closed without a visible scar. In addition, medical epicanthoplasty is added and incorporated with the upper blepharoplasty incision to correct medial epicanthal fold so that the cosmetic result can be enhanced. Our approach indicates that Asian upper blepharoplasty is no longer a simple procedure for just a creation of double eyelid and requires a comprehensive approach for an optimal outcome.

SUMMARY

A high satisfactory outcome of Asian upper blepharoplasty can be achieved with this comprehensive approach. Our approach addresses each anatomic problem of an Asian upper eyelid and can create more ideal anatomy and a proper position of an Asian upper eyelid. With incorporation of needed medical epicanthoplasty, a more natural and aesthetically pleasing result can be accomplished. Our approach may be considered as a standardized technique for Asian upper blepharoplasty that ensures good to excellent outcome but with very low revisional rates.

CLINICS CARE POINTS

- Proper preoperative evaluation and operative design for the procedure can be critical for Asian upper blepharoplasty.
- Effective communication with patients and understanding their desire for the outcome may be another important step for happy patients.
- Meticulous surgical techniques and precise execution of surgical procedures can ensure an optimal outcome for Asian upper blepharoplasty.

DISCLOSURE

The authors have no financial interest to declare in relation to the drugs, devices, and products mentioned in this article.

SUPPLEMENTARY DATA

Supplementary data related to this article can be found online at https://doi.org/10.1016/j.cps.2022.07.006.

REFERENCES

1. Weng CJ. Oriental upper blepharoplasty. Semin Plast Surg 2009;23:5–15.
2. Fakhro A, Yim HW, Kim YK, et al. The evolution of looks and expectations of Asian eyelid and eye appearance. Semin Plast Surg 2015;29:135–44.
3. Takayanagi S. Asian upper blepharoplasty double-fold procedure. Aesthet Surg J 2007;27:656–63.
4. Ma GFY, Cheng MS. Mini-incision double Eyelid-plasty. Aesthet Surg J 2010;30:329–34.
5. Chee E, Choo CT. Asian blepharoplasty- an overview. Orbit 2011;30:58–61.
6. Yoon KC, Park SH. Systematic approach and selective tissue removal in blepharoplasty for your Asians. Plast Reconstr Surg 1998;102:502–8.
7. Lee CK, Ahn ST. Asian upper lid blepharoplasty. Clin Plast Surg 2013;40:167–78.
8. Kruavit A. Asian blepharoplasty: an 18-year experience in 6215 patients. Aesthet Surg J 2009;29:272–83.
9. Chen WPD. Techniques, principles and benchmarks in Asian blepharoplasty. Plast Reconstr Surg Glob Open 2017;7:e2271.
10. Chen WPD. Asian upper blepharoplasty. JAMA Facial Plast Surg 2018;20:249–50.
11. Park KS, Park DDH. Objective outcome measurement after upper blepharoplasty: an analysis of different operative techniques. Aesthetic Plast Surg 2017;41:64–72.
12. Wang CM, Mei XX, Pu LLQ. Asian upper blepharoplasty in women: a comprehensive approach for a natural and aesthetically pleasing outcome. Aesthet Surg J 2021;41:1346–55.
13. Sun L, Chen X, Liu G, et al. Subcutaneous fat in the upper eyelids of Asians: Application to blepharoplasty. Clin Anat 2020;33:338–42.
14. Saononan P. The new focus on epicanthoplasty for Asian eyelids. Curr Opin Ophthalmol 2016;27:457–64.
15. Lee H, Shin HH, Park MS, et al. Comparison of surgical techniques and results of upper blepharoplasty between Asian males and females. Ann Plast Surg 2013;70:6–9.
16. Sun WY, Wang YQ, Song T, et al. Orbicularis-tarsus fixation approach in double-eyelid blepharoplasty: a modification of Park's technique. Aesth Plast Surg 2018;42:1582–90.
17. Wong CH, Hsieh MKH, Wei FC. Asian upper blepharoplasty with the Hinge technique. Aesth Plast Surg 2022. in press.

Revision of Asian Upper Blepharoplasty

Chang-Chien Yang, MD

KEYWORDS

- Revision upper blepharoplasty • Fixation of the pretarsal flap • Blepharoptosis • Scar • Double fold
- Puffy fold • Pretarsal swelling • The height of double fold

KEY POINTS

- Rediscover the key components of upper blepharoplasty: lifting power of the eyelid, iso-tension fixation of the pretarsal flap, and natural distribution of desired skin tension.
- Understand the determining variables of double-fold height through a linear geometric model.
- Understand the pathogenesis of complications of upper blepharoplasty and plan revision surgery accordingly.

INTRODUCTION

Upper blepharoplasty is the most popular esthetic surgery in east Asian countries. However, revision of upper blepharoplasty is also the most executed revision surgery for esthetic purposes in these countries. As the eye contact is probably the most evaluated individual identity, together with the intrinsic delicacy of double-fold formation, and strong demand for symmetry and naturally beautiful fold. All these make upper blepharoplasty surgery to become one of the most challenging esthetic surgeries in the modern era.

KEY COMPONENTS OF UPPER BLEPHAROPLASTY

The majority of suboptimal results of upper blepharoplasty arise from misunderstanding or negligence of the key components of blepharoplasty surgery. Thorough understanding of the key components of blepharoplasty is essential for the revision of upper blepharoplasty. The three key components of upper blepharoplasty are as follows:

1. To ensure that there is enough lifting power for eyelid uprising:

   The eyelid skin has good plication for double fold only if the eyelid is lifted well.[1] Patients with undetected blepharoptosis tend to have unexpected fold formation after upper blepharoplasty as the surgery itself can bring a subtle change in the balance between lifting power and weight-bearing for the eyelid. The prevalence of subclinical blepharoptosis is also high in east Asian countries. Many upper blepharoplasty surgeries are performed with negligence of existing blepharoptosis and as a result, suboptimal result occurs.

2. Iso-tension fixation of the pretarsal flap:

   Although not every upper blepharoplasty is performed with fixation of the pretarsal flap, it is essential for surgeons to ensure that there is a secure iso-tension fixation of the pretarsal flap to achieve the good formation of the double fold. Non-iso-tension fixation of the pretarsal flap almost always results in the suboptimal formation of the double fold, no matter whether it is high-tension or low-tension fixation.

3. Natural distribution of desired skin tension:

   Many surgeons consider trimming redundant skin as one of the key components in upper blepharoplasty. Well, it is not wrong but it is not solid enough. It is better to think all the procedures including the excision of skin are to achieve the natural distribution of the new skin tension, which

Artwood Plastic Surgery Clinic, 4F-2, No.309, Sec. 3, Roosevelt Road, Taipei City 10647, Taiwan
E-mail address: doctor@artwood.com.tw

Clin Plastic Surg 50 (2023) 111–120
https://doi.org/10.1016/j.cps.2022.08.007
0094-1298/23/© 2022 Elsevier Inc. All rights reserved.

are truly desired for. Without natural distribution of skin tension, patients will look "operated." This thinking of skin tension is more important in the revision of upper blepharoplasty as almost all cases are altered in skin condition, and sometimes it is too complicated to determine the exact amount of "redundant" skin.

SPECIAL CONSIDERATIONS IN ASIAN REVISION UPPER BLEPHAROPLASTY
Linear geometric model for fold formation in the upper lid

Surgeons must be capable to evaluate and find a way to meet the demand of the patients who ask for revision of upper blepharoplasty. In the real world, patients who ask for revision surgery tend to be pickier than those who do not. A simplified linear geometric model (**Fig. 1**) can help surgeons to determine how the fold can be changed. In this linear model, there are two basic presumptions: the thickness of the skin and tissue is ignored; and the skin tension is distributed evenly throughout the brow to the eyelashes.

In revision upper blepharoplasty, it is very useful to combine correction of blepharoptosis if there is any subclinical ptosis, especially when there is tight skin and high fold, which is very common in revision surgery.

Fixation of the Pretarsal Flap

Fixation of the pretarsal flap is one of the most important components of upper blepharoplasty.[1] It plays a decisive role in defining the double fold (**Fig. 2**).

CLASSIFICATION OF SUBOPTIMAL UPPER BLEPHAROPLASTY RESULTS AND THEIR MANAGEMENT

Clinically patients ask for revision surgery because they subjectively feel symptoms. It is practical to classify the suboptimal results according to the complaints. The pathophysiology and resolution will be addressed accordingly.

Prominent scar

The most common prominent scar is a depressive scar, which most commonly is resulted from high-tension fixation of the pretarsal flap. It is seen with a typical stepping scar. The other reasons for prominent scar are as follows: over-excision of the orbicularis oculi muscle (OOM); poor incision design to cross Langer's line, which often occurs at lateral or medial canthal areas; and poor suture technique with focal hypertensive closure.

Solution
If the residual skin is ample, redesign with excision of the old scar and try to hide the scar along the natural crease or at least follow the Langer's line. Save OOM and close the OOM gap by suturing the stumps if it is over-excised. High-tension fixation must be divided and redo the fixation as iso-tension (**Fig. 3**).

Depth of fold: shallow fold/deep fold/loss of fold

The depth of the fold is a more subjective issue. The variation of individual preference can be widely different in habitant areas, ethnic groups, occupations, and so on. However, the depth of the fold is relative to the tension of fixation of the pretarsal flap. A fixation with higher tension tends to result in a deeper fold and vice versa. Strong high-tension fixation creates a typical triad of the deep fold, puffy fold, and eversion of eyelashes (see **Figs.** 2C and 3A).

Strong deep folds do not look natural and may also have a dragging effect to exacerbate blepharoptosis. A fixation that connects the dermis directly to the posterior lamella tends to be strong but it is also a high-tension fixation; as a result, it forms a deeper fold.

If the connection between the posterior lamella and anterior lamella is weak due to a loose fixation, the fold becomes shallower or even disappears (see **Fig. 2D**). High folds tend to be deeper than low folds even if the fixations are similar iso-tensive ones (see **Fig. 2E**).

Solution
Respect patients' preferences and provide your advice. Adjust the tension of fixation of the pretarsal flap to achieve a proper tension in the pretarsal skin. If the pretarsal flap is tensely fixed, it is necessary to dissect the pretarsal flap caudally to release the tension.[2] If the tension remains high, the eyelash is going to evert immediately when the fixation suture is completed. On the contrary, with low-tension fixation the pretarsal skin is going to be slack. Avoid direct dermis to tarsal plate fixation for it creates both deep fold and stepping scar.[1]

Low fold/high fold

As the linear geometric model described, the height of the fold is relative to the level of fixation of the pretarsal flap, the amount of the tissue volume and the skin, and the amount of eyelid opening (see **Fig 1**). In daily practice, the level of fixation is the primary factor that determines the height of the fold. A low fixation level will create a low fold. On the contrary, a high level of fixation creates a

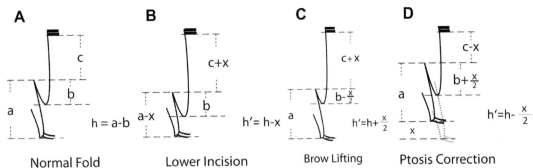

Normal Fold   Lower Incision   Brow Lifting   Ptosis Correction

Fig. 1. (*A*) a= pretarsal flap height, b= skin length of overlap, and c= the vertical distance of brow to the fold line fixation point. In this linear model, the height of double fold equals (a-b). The total length of skin from brow to eyelash equals to (a+2b+c). (*B*) With lower incision /fixation level, the new fold height will have 1:1 amount of reduction as incision /fixation level. Note that the total skin amount in this figure still equals to (a+2b+c). (*C*) In case of brow lifting, in this model lifting the brow has the same effect as skin excision. The reduction of new fold height equals to half of the amount of skin excision or brow lifting. In this figure the skin amount still equals to (a+2b+c) because the brow is stretched up instead of skin excision. (*D*) In case of correction of blepharoptosis, the reduction of new fold height equals half the amount of eyelid lifting. This is important in revision surgery because correction of blepharoptosis can help to reduce the height of fold even under tight skin condition. In this figure the total skin amount is still equals to (a+2b+c).

high fold (see **Fig. 2**E). With redundant overlapping skin, the height of the fold is low. With tighter skin, the fold tends to be higher. Ptotic eyelid has a higher fold.[1] Clinically high folds are also commonly seen in the triad of high-tension fixation because high-tension fixation also tends to create higher folds (see **Figs. 2**C and **3**).

Solution for high folds

1. If the skin is ample enough, it is better to excise the old skin scar to reduce the folding tendency at the old scar site. Do not excise OOM or "scar-like" tissue, it can be sutured to pile up, increasing the resistance of folding at the old fold level.[1]

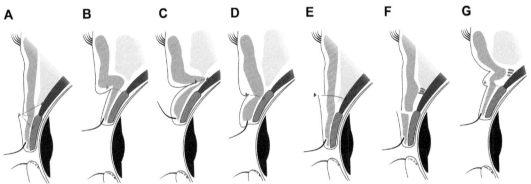

Fig. 2. (*A*) fixation of the pretarsal flap. The green line indicates the natural iso-tension fixation, which is ideally perpendicular to the longitudinal axis of the pretarsal flap. The red line is kind of high-tension fixation. The blue line indicates low-tension fixation. The non-iso-tension fixations tend to have inferior esthetic results. (*B*) iso-tension fixation indicated as green line. The fold forms normally. (*C*) High-tension fixation indicated as red line. It forms a typical triad of deep fold, puffy fold, and eversion of the eyelashes. The scar in this figure will show typical stepping. (*D*) Low-tension fixation (*blue line*) creates shallow fold. Sometimes shallow fold can also look slightly puffy as this figure shows. More anterior lamella tissue is confined to a smaller posterior base. This will also create puffy look. The eyelashes are shaded by the lengthy hanging skin. (*E*) High fixation creates high fold. High fold tends to be puffier than lower fold because there is more anterior lamella tissue included in the fold. Green line indicates iso-tension fixation. Compare with **Fig. 2**A. (*F*) Inadvertent adhesion between anterior and posterior lamella indicated as blue marks. There is trace or no dimpling at all while the eye is closed. (*G*) When the eye is opened, triple fold forms. The higher triple fold can be more dominant and the designated fold becomes shallow even with iso-tension fixation (indicated as *green line*). Very high triple fold is usually classified as sunken eye.

2. Divide the high fixation. Set the new fixation at the proper level and make iso-tension fixation.
3. The height of the fold can be further reduced if more skin is preserved.
4. Dissect the pretarsal flap caudally if the flap is tensely fixed[2] (see **Fig. 3**; **Fig. 4**).

Solution for low folds

1. Low fold with redundant skin can be treated by mere skin excision. If the fixation is slack, redo the fixation as proper tension can further increase the height.
2. Low fold with very low incision scar: although high-tension fixation creates a higher fold but it also creates an unnatural deep and puffy fold. Non-incision buried suture double-fold surgery can help to reset a higher height of the fold in a limited range. If the patient accepts two scars, a new higher incision at the proper level is another solution to achieve a higher height of the fold.[1]

Puffy eyelid/prolonged swelling/congestion of pretarsal flap

High-tension fixation of the pretarsal flap creates all these three symptoms together as one of the triad complications. The flap is so stretched that the small vessels in the pretarsal flap are dilated and congested. It usually takes months to subside as the skin is eventually expanded. However, the puffiness remains for decades as too much soft tissue is included and confined in the flap by the high-tension low–high fixation (see **Fig. 2**C).

High fold tends to be puffier than folds with normal heights because a higher fold enrolls more tissue in the pretarsal flap.

Solution

1. If the pretarsal flap itself is fixed in stretched status, do a dissection of the pretarsal flap caudally to relieve the tension.
2. Redo fixation as iso-tension.
3. It is not necessary to excise pretarsal orbicularis muscle in most circumstances. However, if a long pretarsal orbicularis muscle stump is left on site, the excessive muscle stump can be trimmed off to avoid puffiness.

Eversion of the eyelashes

There is three pathogenesis of the eversion of the eyelashes:

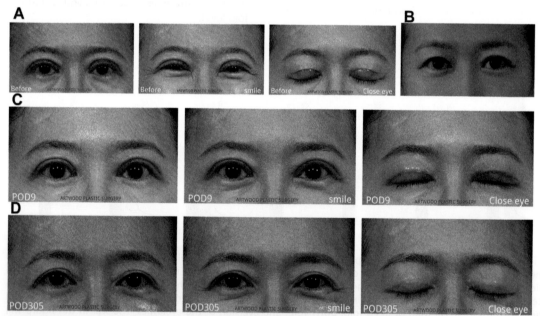

Fig. 3. (A) A case of typical triad of high-tension fixation presented 2 months after her primary upper blepharoplasty. The fold is deep and puffy, the eyelashes are much everted. The pretarsal skin is tensely fixed with a stepping scar. Patient also reports difficulty to open eyes. (B) Photograph of the same patient taken 2 years ago shows no belpharoptosis. High-tension fixation may drag the levator movement and injure the levator complex. It is not rare to see blepharoptosis as a complication of blepharoplasty. (C) 9 days after revision surgery. The tension of the pretarsal flap is relieved instantly when the high-tension fixation is divided and refix at iso-tension position. The injured aponeurosis is repaired and advanced slightly. The stepping scar is removed. The skin tension is now distributed evenly. Left side has undergone a minor revision at day 6. (D) 10 months after revision surgery. The scar is barely noticeable.

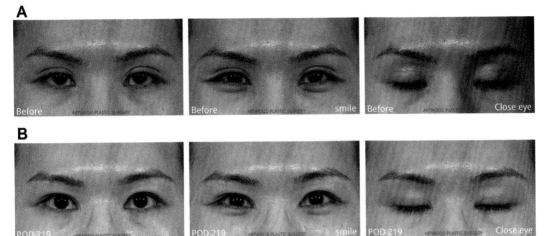

Fig. 4. (*A*) A case with high fold and multiple scars after two times of blepharoplasty with epicanthoplasty. The newer high incision and fixation defines the dominant high folds. Note even under iso-tension fixation, the folds still look puffy in high folds. In the close-eye view, the flash light is dimmed to show the two scars more clearly. (*B*) Seven months after revision surgery. Skin amount is barely enough for excision of old scars. The old scar and the skin between two scars are removed during the revision surgery. Subclinical blepharoptosis is corrected to further shorten the height of the fold. Revision of epicanthoplasty is also performed to reduce the visible depressive epicanthal scar.

1. The eyelashes will evert whenever the pretarsal skin is stretched.[1] That is the reason why eversion of the eyelashes is one of the typical triad symptoms of high-tension fixation of the pretarsal flap (see **Figs.** 2C and 3A). It is the most common pathogenesis of everted eyelashes.

2. In some badly or multiply operated cases, the anterior lamella becomes too short to match with the posterior lamella length. In this circumstance after skin closure, the eyelashes become everted.[1]

3. Sometimes the surgeon did the correction of ptotic eyelid and advanced the levator complex with sutures bite at lower tarsal plate. The tarsal plate is then elevated and rotated externally to create eversion.

Solution

1. Redo the fixation as iso-tension. Dissect the pretarsal flap to relieve the tension and stretching, as the solution of puffy fold solution (see **Fig.** 3).

2. In case of a mismatch of anterior and posterior lamella length, the lower pretarsal skin can be fixed to the tarsal plate and reduce the stretching of lower pretarsal skin.[1,3]

3. Shorten the posterior lamella by wedge resection of the tarsal plate on the posterior surface with a small stripe of the conjunctiva.

4. Check the advancing sutures in ptosis surgery. A bite within 2 mm distal to the cephalic end of tarsal plate is not likely to rotate the tarsal plate externally.

Triple fold/multiple folds

When the anterior lamella is inadvertently adhered to the posterior lamella at a position higher than the designated fixation level, an unwanted fold occurs as triple fold (see **Fig.** 2F, G). If there are multiple sites of adherence, multiple folds occur. This complication is commonly seen in cases whose orbital fat was removed roughly or excessively with or without the preseptal connective tissue. Excise OOM above fixation level can leave a gap in OOM which induces adhesion. If the retro-orbicularis oculi fat (ROOF) is trimmed off completely, the risk of adhesion will be increased.[1] During the correction of high folds, if the old scar is preserved, it is a potential folding site. As a rule, the triple fold is not visible while the eye is closed or in downgaze (see **Fig.** 2F). The triple fold can be more dominant, and the designated fold becomes shallower (see **Fig.** 2G; **Fig.** 5A).

Solution

1. Try to redrape the residual orbital fat or septum to separate the adhered sites of anterior and posterior lamella. Fix the orbital fat/septum remnant to the distal aponeurosis if necessary.

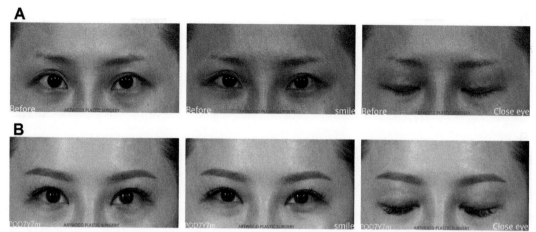

Fig. 5. (*A*) This patient has triple fold after several revision blepharoplasty surgeries. The left eye is also slightly ptotic at medial one-third. The triple fold is more dominant and the designated fold is shallower. The surgical plan is to divide the adhesion and re-drape the residual orbital fat to prevent re-adhesion. Correction of subclinical ptosis is also helpful to diminish the triple fold as this triple fold is close to the designated fold. Revision of epicanthoplasty is also included for patient's preference. (*B*) More than seven years after revision surgery. Patient is happy for the natural, brighter and brilliant effect of the ptosis correction.

2. Fill the OOM gap by suturing the OOM stumps.
3. Ptosis correction can help to narrow down the discrepancy gap between the designated fold and triple fold. If the gap is small, it may become unnoticed after ptosis correction (**Fig. 5**).
4. ROOF flap can be dissected and transposed to separate the adhered sites if no residual fat or septum can be used.
5. Trim off the old high fold scar if possible. Increase the resistance of folding as the solution of the high fold.
6. Free fat graft has a very low successful rate to really separate the adhered sites, it tends to create supra-tarsal roughness instead (**Fig. 6**A). However, desperate patients may rather accept rough supra-tarsal puffiness than a triple fold. If the triple fold is concealed by mere excessive fat graft, a drawback is that the eyelid looks puffy in downgaze, especially downgaze in three-quarters view. Traditional presentations that do not include this view or not even a close-eye view provide insufficient information about this drawback (**Fig. 6**B). This is why iatrogenic supra-tarsal puffiness/roughness is so prevalent.

Supra-tarsal puffiness

The most common cause of supra-tarsal puffiness is unprocessed thick ROOF. The second common cause is iatrogenic fat graft excessively (see **Fig. 6**A, B). It is not rare for previous surgeons to choose to do excessive free fat graft to alleviate triple fold as described in the triple fold section.

Solution

1. Trim off ROOF properly in the revision surgery. Leave at least a thin layer of ROOF with the membranous connective tissue to prevent triple fold.
2. For iatrogenic puffiness, trim off the excessive fat graft and make a smooth transition. Surgeons may have to solve the triple-fold problem after the removal of the excessive fat graft (**Fig. 6**C, D).

Sunken eye

Although the sunken eye is traditionally considered as a senile change, it is very commonly seen in patients with blepharoptosis disregarding patients' age. It is well known that correction of blepharoptosis helps to improve the sunken eye.[4] In fact, even in senile patients with primary sunken eyes, many of them also have attenuated and dislocated levator aponeurosis. Iatrogenic dislocation of levator aponeurosis is a common cause of sunken eyes after upper blepharoplasty. The dislocated aponeurosis exerts a pulling force at a much higher level to form a sunken eye when the eye is opened. Similar to triple folds, most sunken eyes are not obvious while the eye is closed (**Fig. 7**A).

Solution

1. Check first if there is blepharoptosis. Almost all sunken eyes in revision cases have a minor degree of ptosis at least. Look for dislocated aponeurosis during surgery, make anatomical reduction/repair of the dislocated aponeurosis.

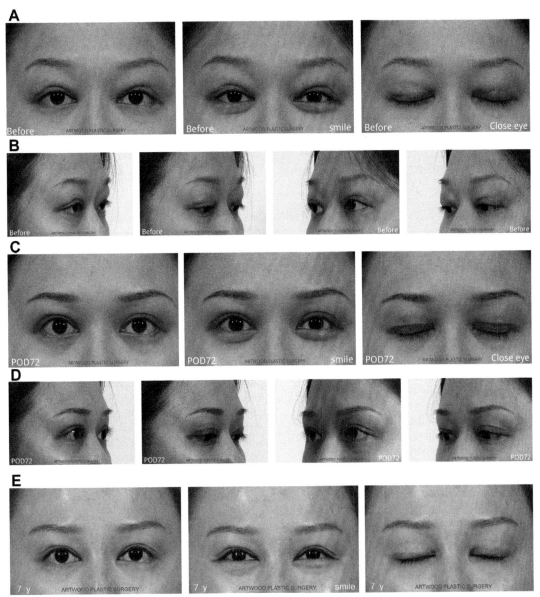

Fig. 6. (*A*) This patient had triple fold after her primary blepharoplasty and received succeeding free fat graft for reduction of the triple fold. In the frontal views under normal flash light setting, the supratarsal puffiness may not be well seen. (*B*) In three-quarters views especially downgaze, the drawback of mere fat graft for triple fold is clear. Iatrogenic supratarsal puffiness with roughness is evident in downgaze three-quarters views. (*C*) She underwent revision surgery including scar excision, correction of blepharoptosis, correction of high fold, and careful trimming off the excessive fat graft. The original triple fold was prevented with re-draping of the residual orbital fat. (*D*) Supratarsal bulkiness and roughness is significantly reduced after surgery. (*E*) 7 years after revision surgery.

2. Do not excise OOM. Excessive OOM can be rolled up to enhance volume.
3. Relocate the orbital fat as a fat flap and fix it to the distal aponeurosis.
4. Usually 1,2,3 will be enough to correct sunken eyes (**Fig. 7**). If the fat graft is still needed, do either a dermal fat graft or micro fat graft in the ROOF layer at the same time or succeeding surgery.[5]

Blepharoptosis

Blepharoptosis is quite prevalent in general population of east Asian countries.[6] When regular blepharoplasty is performed on patients with neglected subclinical ptosis, apparent blepharoptosis can occur due to the dragging effect of high-tension fixation. High fixation with high tension

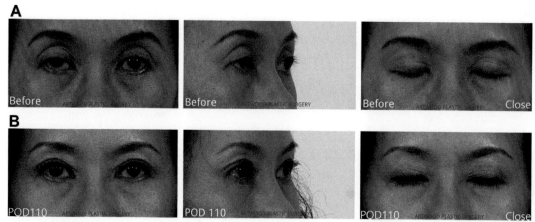

Fig. 7. (*A*) Typical sunken eyes. Patient underwent a correction surgery for blepharoptosis years ago but seemingly the surgery is not successful. She has very profound sunken eyes while the eyes are opened. Note in the close-eye view the sunken eye is unnoticeable. (*B*) After advancing and reattaching the dislocated levator aponeurosis, blepharoptosis and sunken eye are mostly corrected. No fat graft is needed. Note the close-eye view is almost the same as preop.

does not only drag the levator movement but may also attenuate the levator aponeurosis. The attenuated aponeurosis may be further injured inadvertently during surgery. This is why blepharoptosis is commonly seen in cases with a typical high-tension fixation triad (see **Fig. 3**A).

Patients who developed blepharoptosis after primary upper blepharoplasty have the strongest motivation to seek secondary revision help. It is obviously one of the reasons why the correction of blepharoptosis plays very important role in the revision of upper blepharoplasty.

Solution

Correction of blepharoptosis is discussed in another article. It is impossible to over-emphasize the importance of correction of blepharoptosis in revision upper blepharoplasty (see **Figs. 3–7**). As mentioned, correction of blepharoptosis helps to reduce fold height, alleviate deep fold, triple fold, and sunken eyes.

Asymmetry

Any symptoms mentioned above can result as asymmetry if they are not happening symmetrically in both eyes. Treat every individual complication accordingly. However, the right and left hemifaces are never symmetry. As a rule, left eye slants more than right eye. The left periorbital tissue is less abundant as the right side.

The brows can be asymmetry. It is well known that higher brow results in higher fold.[1] But first of all, check if asymmetric blepharoptosis exists before jumping into conclusions of asymmetry brows. In fact, in patients with asymmetric brows,

most of them have blepharoptosis with asymmetric compensation of brow-raising movement.

Frowning/Heavy sensation to open eyes

This is a pure subjective symptom different from all other objective complications mentioned above. Patients complain unpleasant heavy sensation when opening eyes. Many of them frown automatically to alleviate the unpleasant annoying sensation without self-aware. Adhesion between posterior and anterior lamella at high level is believed to be the culprit of this rarely known symptom. The adhesion site is usually over medial or medio-central portion of levator complex at a high level near to the Whitnall's ligament. This adhesion exerts dragging when patients open eyes and triggers a reflex to raise brows just like ptotic patients do. But raising brows this time pulls the anterior lamella with the adhered posterior lamella outward against the natural inward movement of posterior lamella due to the high-level adhesion. The conflict of movement is so unpleasant that patient automatically frown to reduce the outward pull and the annoying heavy sensation.

Clinically a *brow fixation test* is very useful to detect this kind of high-level adhesion. If patients feel significant relief of heavy sensation when opening eyes with brow fixed by doctor's thumb, it is a positive result. A positive brow fixation test is highly correlated with adhesion at high level.

Solution

As the frowning/heavy sensation on opening eye is essentially adhesion between anterior and posterior lamella at high level, it is also commonly seen simultaneously with other adhesion related complications such as triple fold, very high and deep fold. The treatment is similar to triple fold but usually requires more extensive dissection to re-mobilize the fixed adhesion sites. Prevention of re-adhesion like triple fold solution is more important because at this high level the adhesion is apt to recur.

CLINICAL CASES DEMONSTRATIONS

Case 1 (see **Fig. 3**A–D).
   Case 2 (**Fig. 4**A, B).
   Case 3 (see **Fig. 5**A, B).
   Case 4 (see **Fig. 6**A–E).
   Case 5 (see **Fig. 7**A, B).

DISCUSSION

There are several valuable surgical pearls of revision upper blepharoplasty which are very helpful for clinical practice. Surgeons can assess the skin redundancy by checking skin tension at siting position with patients' eyes closed. Raise patient's brow slowly with your thumb and observe the tension change of the eyelid skin until the eyelashes begin to evert. The travel distance of brow represents the maximum of skin affordable for excision or scar removal. The remaining tissue and skin resources can be estimated with this maneuver in a precise way. Surgeons should now be able to match the practical surgical plan with the patient's expectation.

It is better to excise only the full thickness of skin with scar at the beginning of surgery if this is affordable for patients' limited resources. It should be emphasized that do not excise so called "scar tissue". This maneuver is not helpful for preventing re-adhesion. In the contrary, gaping of tissues may occur and triple fold or depressive scar arises instead. After careful dissection the faulty fixation should be divided and the pretarsal flap can be dissected caudally in case the pretarsal flap was fixed tensely.

The fold height can be readjusted during surgery. Excise more skin will increase the fold height. Reduction of supratarsal tissue volume will also increase the fold height (see **Fig. 1**). But be aware that commonly it is not good to increase the fold height by intentionally fixing the pretarsal flap deeper or tenser. That kind of maneuver is apt to create unnatural deep and puffy fold. During dissection, always look for the residual orbital fat or stump of septum, use them to separate anterior and posterior lamella. This is the most effective way to prevent re-adhesion or unwanted adhesion. Attenuated levator aponeurosis may split and retract quite cephalically. Failure to repair such aponeurotic retraction can be devastating to the surgical result by formation of triple fold or asymmetric blepharoptosis.

It cannot be over-emphasized that correction of blepharoptosis is very helpful not only to alleviate other complications of upper blepharoplasty but also earns more satisfaction of patient (see **Fig. 5**).

The optimal timing for revision upper blepharoplasty should be addressed here. If the skin resource is ample enough, ideally the old scar should be removed for esthetic purpose. In noncomplicated cases with ample skin, timing of surgery is not related to the surgical result, providing the surgeon knows what to do. It is surprisingly easy to do revision surgery within 2 weeks after the first surgery because the original wound can be split open and the neovascularization and adhesion is not bothering yet (see **Fig. 3**C). For those patients with shortage of skin, it is better to wait for 6 months or longer to have the scar matured. In complicated cases such as cases with multiple ptosis correction surgeries, it is better to wait for 6 months or longer to have the injured levator complex healed; otherwise, the injured levator complex may be retarded to response to any advancement or shortening.

SUMMARY

The difference between optimal and complicated Asian upper blepharoplasty can be merely scanty because of the mobile and delicate nature of eyelid. Surgeons do upper blepharoplasty as daily practice should also be capable to do revision upper blepharoplasty. Follow the systemic approach method in this article with accumulation of experiences, which can be accelerated by observation of properly performed procedures, it is possible to resolve almost all kinds of complications of upper blepharoplasty.

CLINICS CARE POINTS

- The majority of complicated Asian upper blepharoplasty comes with under-estimated or under-corrected blepharoptosis.
- It is wise to always note patients' levator function before performing any upper blepharoplasty.
- Surgeons who wish to master revision of Asian upper blepharoplasty should also be very familiar to do correction of belpharoptosis.

DISCLOSURE

The author declares no competing interests.

REFERENCES

1. Cho IC. The art of blepharoplasty. Republic of Korea: Koonja Publishing, Inc.; 2017. ISBN: 979-11-5955-234-2.
2. Kim KK, Kim WS, Oh SK, et al. High double eyelid fold correction using wide dual-plane dissection. Ann Plast Surg 2017;78(4):365–70.
3. Cho IC, Kim BJ, You HJ, et al. Surgical correction of upper eyelid ectropion presenting dry eye symptoms. Aesthet Surg J 2021;41(1):NP1–9.
4. Mawatari Y, Fukushima M, Kawaji T. Changes in sunken eyes combined with blepharoptosis after levator resection. Plast Reconstr Surg Glob Open 2017;5(12):e1616.
5. Lee W, Kwon SB, Oh SK, et al. Correction of sunken upper eyelid with orbital fat transposition flap and dermofat graft. J Plast Reconstr Aesthet Surg 2017; 70(12):1768–75.
6. Paik JS, Han K, Yang SW, et al. Blepharoptosis among Korean adults: age-related prevalence and threshold age for evaluation. BMC Ophthalmol 2020; 20(1):99.

Advanced Approach to Asian Lower Blepharoplasty

Chin-Ho Wong, MBBS (Singapore), MRCS(Ed), MMed (Surg), FAMS (Plast Surg)

KEYWORDS

- Low lid • Eye bags • Asian • Oriental • Modern • Blepharoplasty • Mid cheek • Rejuvenation

KEY POINTS

- Understanding the surgical anatomy of the lower eyelid and mid cheek is key to safe and atraumatic dissection via the lower eyelid.
- The key concept for safety is dissecting in the ideal plane of the facial soft tissue spaces with precise release of the retaining ligaments that separate these spaces.
- Either the transconjunctival or subciliary approach may be used depending on patients' requirements and desired outcomes.
- The transconjunctival approach is safe and effective for patients with prominent eye bags, tear trough deformity, and lid–cheek junction with minimal skin excess.
- The subciliary approach has the main advantage of allowing a concomitant cheek lift to be incorporated into the procedure.

 Video content accompanies this article at http://www.plasticsurgery.theclinics.com.

INTRODUCTION

Patients presenting for lower eyelid surgery usually complain of "looking tired" and often attributes this to the presence of their eye bags. They come in requesting for their eye bags to be removed; hence, colloquially lower blepharoplasty has been called eye bag removal surgery. For many years, this was taken as the essence of lower blepharoplasty, and the surgical techniques were accordingly focused solely on elimination of the eye bags. However, modern lower blepharoplasty is so much more than just simplistic eye bag removal. It is important to appreciate that patients presenting for lower blepharoplasty are actually looking for rejuvenation of the mid cheek and to *look more youthful* and not merely for removal of the eye bags. The eye bags—bulging of the

preseptal segment of the lower lid—are perhaps one of the most obvious change of the aging mid cheek, accordingly the patients may attribute their aging appearance solely to this aspect of their aging mid cheek. However, it is not the sole physical change responsible for the features of the aging mid cheek.[1] *Collectively*, these changes result in the "tired" look, accordingly to effectively address this "tired" look, all these aspects of the aging mid cheek need to be addressed

To understand the esthetic goals of lower eyelid surgery, one has to appreciate that the lower eyelid is an integral part of the mid cheek and to optimize outcomes of lower eyelid surgery, the lower eyelid cannot be treated in isolation. This is this paradigm shift in modern lower eyelid surgery. Although the procedure is called lower blepharoplasty, as the access is through the lower eyelid,

The authors declare no conflict of interest in this present work. None of the authors has a financial interest in any of the products, devices, or drugs mentioned in this article.
W Aesthetic Plastic Surgery, Mount Elizabeth Novena Specialist Center, #06 – 28/29, 38 Irrawaddy Road, Singapore 329563, Singapore
E-mail address: drwong@waesthetics.com

aging changes of the entire mid cheek have to be treated as a whole to achieve optimal esthetic results. Accordingly, removal of the eye bags alone, without concomitantly addressing other aspects of the aging mid cheek, will lead to suboptimal outcomes and disappointment for the patient and the surgeon. To effectively rejuvenate the mid cheek, each component that changes with aging has to be addressed. The technique selection depends on the specific aging changes need to be addressed for the individual patient. Understanding the surgical anatomy is the key to the development of anatomically sound surgical approaches that are effective while minimizing trauma from the surgery and thereby reducing downtime and complications.

THE YOUTHFUL MID CHEEK AND CHANGES OF THE MID CHEEK WITH AGING

The youthful mid cheek is full with smooth contours, without surface grooves or bulges.[1,2] With aging, changes occur at the two fundamental levels: the mid cheek *skeleton* and the overlying *soft tissues*.[3–7] The mid cheek skeleton, especially the maxilla medially, retrudes significantly with aging. The resultant loss of projection and support for the overlying soft tissues predisposes to sagging of the tissue, which gives the visual impression of loss of soft tissue volume. Where the soft tissues overlie retaining ligaments, the skin remains firmly attached to the underlying skeleton and manifests as surface grooves, given different names at different locations on the face. These include the nasojugal groove, so-called tear trough deformity, medially, and mid cheek furrow more laterally, whereas over the facial soft tissue spaces laxity in the roof of the space manifests as a surface bulge. In the lower eyelid, bulging over the preseptal space results in the development of eye bags. Laxity over the roof of the prezygomatic space is the anatomical basis for malar mounds or bags. This combination of relatively strong fixation in areas directly overlying retaining ligaments contrasted with laxity of tissue in the roof of adjacent soft tissue spaces results in segmentation of the mid cheek into three segments: the lid–cheek, malar, and nasolabial segments (**Fig. 1**).

SURGICAL ANATOMY OF THE MID CHEEK AND DISSECTION PLANES

To produce natural results and minimize downtime associated with surgical dissection, the key is to use the mid cheek facial soft tissue spaces, which are preexisting gliding planes that are avascular with no vital structures traversing within (**Fig. 2**).[4]

To access these spaces, the retaining ligaments in the boundary of the spaces must be sharply released. Once released, the surgeon will note the profound mobility of the roof with traction. This approach may be summarized as "through the facial soft tissues spaces with precise release of intervening retaining ligaments."[8,9] In terms of dissection plane, this is a sub- superficial musculoaponeurotic system (sub-SMAS) dissection. This concept will be detailed in the surgical techniques below. Aging of the facial skeleton may be addressed by skeletal augmentation, using either structural fat grafting, facial fillers, or even hydroxyapatite bone substitute.

PATIENT SELECTION FOR SURGICAL TECHNIQUE

Patient selection is a key to ensure optimal outcomes. Two surgical approaches are available for lower blepharoplasty: the transconjunctival or subciliary (transcutaneous) approaches. Each approach has its pros and cons and depending on the specific anatomy, requests, and expectations of the patient, one or the other may be preferred. The transconjunctival approach is advantageous for being safe and effective with a quicker recovery and is the method of choice for patients with early aging changes with little or no skin excess or laxity. For patients with more significant aging changes and requesting for a more significant improvement, a more aggressive approach incorporating some form of mid cheek tightening is required to deliver a more profound rejuvenation. In this group of patients, therefore, the subciliary approach is preferred because the required mid cheek lift may be incorporated into the procedure.

TRANSCONJUNCTIVAL APPROACH: THE EXTENDED TRANSCONJUNCTIVAL LOWER EYELID BLEPHAROPLASTY

The transconjunctival lower eyelid blepharoplasty offers an advantageous access to the lower eyelid and mid cheek because of its safety (by avoiding trauma to the anterior lamella of the lower eyelid) and its quick recovery.[10–13] The transconjunctival fat removal only type of procedures is very popular, effective for patients with true lower eyelid fat pad excesses, and is easy to perform. The benefit of the procedure is limited to the lid–cheek segment of the mid cheek, however, due to the limited nature of the dissection. However, for more profound rejuvenation via the transconjunctival approach, it is necessary to take the dissection significantly caudal to the orbital rim.[11,12] This type

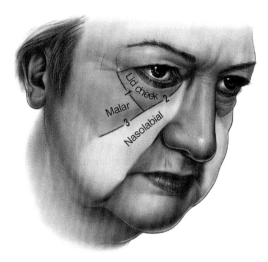

Fig. 1. In youth, the spaces are tight, being more potential than real. The retaining ligaments are stout and the *transitions between spaces* are not discernible. With aging, the spaces expand to a greater extent than the laxity that develops in the ligaments within their boundaries, resulting in bulges between areas of relative fixation. This results in the "segmentation" of the mid cheek into three characteristic segments: the lid–cheek, malar, and nasolabial segments. (*Courtesy of* Levent Efe, MD, Melbourne, AU.)

of procedure, called the extended transconjunctival lower blepharoplasty, as described below, is more versatile and powerful to address aging changes of the mid cheek. This approach is

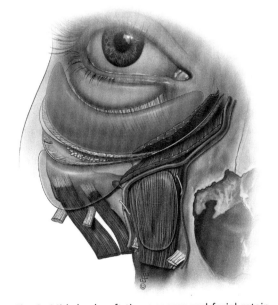

Fig. 2. Mid cheek soft tissue spaces and facial retaining ligaments of the mid cheek. (*Courtesy of* Levent Efe, MD, Melbourne, AU.)

good for patients with prominent eye bags, with tear trough deformity with minimal laxity of the mid cheek soft tissues. In patients with mid cheek loss of projection, structural fat grafting may be performed at the same time.

Markings and Preparation

Preoperatively, with the patient upright, the location and amount of fat pads to be removed are determined and marked. A mental image of the expected fat to be excised should be visualized as the key component to good results is precise removal of fat. The mid cheek groove, anatomically formed by the tear trough ligament and orbicularis retaining ligament (ORL), that needs to be released is also marked. The procedure can be performed either under local or general anesthesia. The cornea is anesthetized with two drops of Alcaine 0.5% eye drops (Alcon-Couvreur, Belgium). The cornea is lubricated with some Duratears (Alcon-Couvreur) and protective corneal eye shield placed. The conjunctiva, lower eyelid, and mid cheek are anesthetized with a mixture of 10 mL of 1% ropivacaine, 10 mL 1% lidocaine, and 0.25 mL of 1:1000 adrenaline. The lower lid, mid cheek, and lateral orbital rim are infiltrated with a total of 3 mL of the local anesthetic mixture each side.

Surgical Technique

See Video 1 for demonstration of the author's surgical technique.[14] With two fine skin hooks applying gentle upward traction on the lower eyelids, an approximately 15-mm transconjunctival incision is made about 2 mm inferior to the lower edge of the tarsus using a sharp point diathermy, incising through the conjunctival and lower eyelid retractors. The skin hooks are replaced by a small, insulated Desmarres retractor. The preseptal space is bluntly entered with a tenotomy scissors. The orbital septum is then opened directly over the areas where the fat pads would be removed. The orbital fat pads are excised as indicated and meticulous hemostasis performed.

The Desmarres is replaced with the blunt end of a cat's paw retractor and the preseptal space then bluntly developed to its boundaries with a gentle sweeping motion with a cotton bud, carefully looking for the white line that defines the location of the arcus marginalis. A key landmark, the origin of the palpebral part of the orbicularis oculi is located slightly caudal to the arcus marginalis. With the assistant holding the retractor upward and the surgeon pushing the orbital septum down with the cotton bud, the orbicularis oculi is sharply released with cutting cautery at its bony origin. The palpebral part of the orbicularis oculi, tear trough ligament, and the orbital part of the orbicularis oculi are sequentially released, taking care that the dissection stays close to the anterior maxilla. The end point of the release is the visualization of muscular fibers of the levator labii superioris (LLS). This heralds the entrance into the premaxillary space and, accordingly, the complete release of the tear trough ligament (**Fig. 3**). More laterally, the medial part of the ORL is also released. The excised fat is then placed under the tear trough ligament as free fat grafts and secured with Vicryl 6-0 percutaneous sutures. These are secured with Steristrips. The conjunctival incision is closed with two or three buried 6-0 plain catgut sutures. Mid cheek structural fat grafting, if indicated, is then performed using the Coleman technique.

SUBCILIARY APPROACH: THE MID CHEEK LIFT VIA THE FACIAL SOFT TISSUE SPACES

In patients with more advanced aging changes, with sagging of the mid cheek, malar bags, and prominent nasolabial folds, it is important to incorporate tightening of the mid cheek soft tissue into the surgical procedure.[15,16] The subciliary approach is indicated for patients with cheek laxity, sagging, malar bags, and heavy nasolabial folds, whereas any skin excess may be addressed at the same time.

Preoperative Markings

The areas of fat excess and the extent of the tear trough to be corrected are marked. The mental quantitation of fat redistribution and/or removal is made. The precise planning of this aspect is crucial for effective blending of the lid–cheek junction. The procedure can be performed under local or general anesthesia. The lower eyelid, mid cheek, and lateral orbital rim are anesthetized with 4 to 5 mL of the previously described local anesthetic mixture each side.

Surgical Technique

Our surgical technique is demonstrated in Video 2.[17,18] A subciliary incision is made. The skin is raised off the orbicularis oculi. A blunt tenotomy scissor is then introduced into the suborbicularis plane and the preseptal space opened with gentle spreading of the blades. The orbicularis oculi is then cut with cautery to approximately the level of the medial corneoscleral limbus, ensuring preservation of about 5 to 7 mm of pretarsal orbicularis oculi. The preseptal space is a bloodless plane that can be fully opened bluntly using a cotton tip to its boundary, which is the

orbicularis oculi origin medially and the ORL laterally. Medially, over the maxilla, the origin of the orbicularis oculi (the palpebral and orbital parts of the orbicularis oculi), and the tear trough ligament located between them are sharply released with cutting cautery. Complete release then brings the dissection into the premaxillary space, heralded by the visualization of the suborbicularis oculi fat adherent to the underside of the orbicularis oculi muscle fascia in the roof and the LLS muscle in the floor (**Fig. 4**). More laterally, the ORL is released with cutting cautery in the preperiosteal plane. A complete release of the ORL, over the body of the zygoma, takes the dissection into the prezygomatic space. The zygomaticofacial nerve (and its associated vessels), emerge from a foramen in the body of the zygoma, closely associated with the inferior lamella of the ORL. Accordingly, visualizing this nerve heralds the entrance into the prezygomatic space and the complete release of the ORL. More laterally, the ORL continues as the lateral orbital thickening (LOT), the inferior part of which needs to be released, up to the level of the lateral canthus, to allow free elevation of the mid cheek. With this release (surgically connecting the three facial soft tissue spaces of the mid cheek, the preseptal, premaxillary, and prezygomatic), upward traction on the orbicularis oculi allows free and unhindered elevation of the entire mid cheek. This is the end point for the surgical release.

To address the eye bags and tear trough deformity, depending on the patient's anatomy, one of two maneuvers may be selected. In patients with a tear trough deformity without a significant palpebromalar groove, transposition of the medial and middle fat pads over the medial orbital rim, onto the anterior maxilla is performed. The orbital septum is opened and the fat pads transposed over the rim and secured with Vicryl 6-0 sutures. In patients presenting with more advanced aging changes with a deep lid–cheek junction, a septal reset is done. Fat removal is done conservatively, only in patients with a true excess of retro-orbital fat, usually from the lateral compartment. A canthopexy is routinely performed with a 5-0 Ethilon suture secured to the periosteum of the orbital rim at a location vertically above the lateral canthus. If an upper blepharoplasty is not performed concomitantly, this canthopexy suture may be placed via a small 8 mm upper eyelid crease incision.

The mid cheek lift is achieved by orbicularis suspension. This is performed in a superolateral vector with Vicryl 3-0 sutures secured to the lateral orbit periosteum, ensuring that the malar eminence and the upper nasolabial fold lifts sufficiently with tightening of the sutures. Two of these

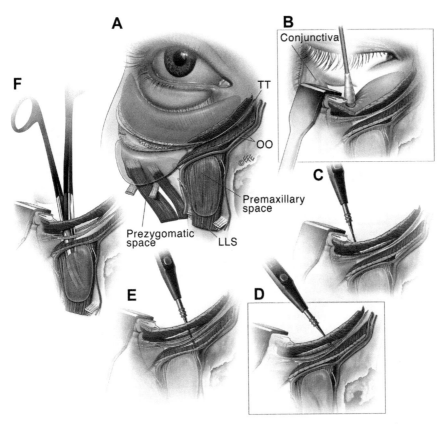

Fig. 3. The anatomy of the tear trough ligament. (*A*) Facial soft tissue spaces and retaining ligaments of the mid cheek. (*B*) Bluntly opening the preseptal space. Sharp release of the palpebral part of the orbicularis oculi (*C*), tear trough ligament (*D*), and the orbital part of the orbicularis oculi (*E*). (*F*) Bluntly opening the premaxillary space with tenotomy scissors. This is the concept of atraumatic dissection by dissecting in the facial soft tissue spaces and precisely releasing the retaining ligaments that separate the spaces. (*Courtesy of* Levent Efe, MD, Melbourne, AU.)

cheek-lift fixation sutures are placed. Excess orbicularis is trimmed laterally. Bunching of the skin below the lateral canthus is usually observed with this maneuver, and addressed by further mobilizing the skin off the orbicularis and redraping the skin in a more vertical direction. The excess skin is then conservatively trimmed and the incision closed. Mid cheek fat grafting is then performed using the Coleman technique in selected patients to correct deflation of the mid cheek. The fat is placed in tiny aliquots in a multiplanar manner. The volume of fat injected ranges from 1.5 to 4.0 mL per side depending on the degree of deflation present.

POSTOPERATIVE CARE AND EXPECTED OUTCOME

The benefit of the transconjunctival approach is its relative safety.[10–14] By avoiding trauma to the middle lamella of the lower lid, the risk of middle lamella contracture that may result in lower eyelid

malposition, scleral show, and ectropion is minimized. The surgical trauma associated with the surgical access is minimized by using this "through the spaces approach" as detailed above; this would minimize downtime of the procedure (**Fig. 5**A, B). **Figs. 6** and **7** show the long-term result of this technique. This technique has consistently been effective in eliminating the tired look, with long-term effective correction of the tear trough deformity and in rejuvenating the mid cheek. The long-term safety and efficacy of release of the tear trough ligament and its associated release of the orbicularis oculi origins has been documented.[19] The lower eyelid remains stable with no increased incidence of scleral show or ectropion.

Commitment to meticulous postoperative care is crucial in subciliary techniques. The mid cheek is taped with Steristrips for 5 days and sutures removed after about 6 days. Lower eyelid massaging is started 2 weeks after the operation. This is done by gently pushing the lower lid supero-medially against the globe and holding it

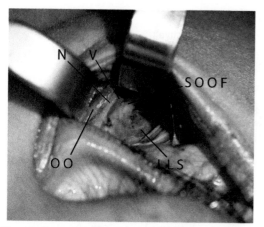

Fig. 4. Entrance into the premaxillary space is achieved by complete release of the orbicularis origin (OO) (with concomitant release of the tear trough ligament). This is confirmed by the visualization of the levator labii superioris (LLS) in the floor and the suborbicularis oculi fat (SOOF) in the roof. Note the close association of the angular vein (V) and terminal branches of the zygomatic nerve (N) with the orbicularis oculi muscle medially. Injury to these structures is avoided during the preperiosteal release of the muscle by staying close to the bone.

in position for 1 minute, for up to five times a day. This is generally continued for about 1 month. Patients are seen weekly in the initial postoperative period to check on the lower eyelid position and healing in general. The long-term results of the mid cheek lift are shown in **Fig. 8A, B.**

MANAGEMENT OF COMPLICATIONS

Complications for the transconjunctival approach are relatively minor and infrequent. These include inadequate fat pad removal requiring revision in less than 5%, significant bruising specifically from injury to the angular vein, lumpiness of the grafted fat, prolonged swelling in some patients, and transient chemosis usually lasting less than a few days.[13] Chemosis is rare with the transconjunctival approach. More serious complications reported in the literature include corneal abrasions, lid retraction, diplopia from injury to the inferior oblique muscle, and dreaded retrobulbar bleed. Of note, these are rare when the technique is done correctly and is the reason for the preference of many surgeons for this technique, for its safety and quicker recovery.

The subciliary approach delivers profound results but has a relatively higher potential risks of complications compared with the transconjunctival approach. Reported complications include prolonged swelling, mid cheek edema, and prolonged chemosis. Prolonged chemosis (more than 1 month) is one of the more problematic and common complications with more aggressive subciliary surgery. Chemosis reported to occur in up to 10% to 15% and is due to disruption of the lymphatic of the lower eyelid in *anatomically predisposed patient*. Chemosis usually resolves with conservative treatment of eye lubrication and lower eyelid massaging. In very symptomatic patients, a temporary tarsorrhaphy to relieve symptoms and promote resolution of the chemosis should be considered.[20] As a technical pearl, consider doing a tarsorrhaphy if chemosis is noted at the end of the surgery and keep the suture for several days. One of the feared complications of the subciliary approach is lower eyelid positional issues. These include scleral show, lid retraction, and ectropion. Patients with certain anatomy such as a negative vector orbit, preexisting scleral show (the so-called "polar bear syndrome") with laxity and poor recoil of the lower eyelids, are at greater risk of these complications. To support the lower eyelid in the early recovery period, canthopexies were routinely done for all patients undergoing the subciliary approach.[17,18] These problems may arise anytime between immediate postoperation to 6 weeks after the surgery. Accordingly, it is important to follow patients closely in the early postoperative period. Even a hint of lower eyelid malposition demands an immediate proactive approach. Rigorous lower eyelid massaging as described above should be started. Early scarring in the middle lamella may benefit from injections of small amounts of a mixture of triamcinolone and 5-fluorouracil into the orbital septum, which is effective to prevent and reduce early scar formation and should be repeated judiciously to resolve the situation. In refractory cases, it would be advisable to wait for at least 4 (preferably 6) months before attempting correction. Techniques to correct scleral show include tarsal strip canthoplasty and dermal pennant flap. Correction of ectropion is more complicated, depending on the severity and location of the contracture, in addition to canthoplasty or tarsal strip, a posterior lamella spacer graft (for posterior lamella shortage), and a mid cheek lift (for anterior lamella shortage) may be needed. If the lower eyelid is stiffened and is unable to elevate freely, reconstruction of the posterior lamella spacer would be needed. Material used may be autologous tissue (hard palate or ear cartilage) or acellular dermal matrix.

DISCUSSION

With current understanding, mid cheek aging may be conceptualized as several components:

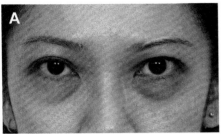 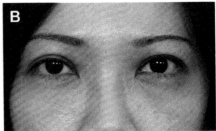

Fig. 5. (A) and (B) A 40-year-old woman presented with a very tired look. She underwent transconjunctival lower blepharoplasty with tear tough ligament release and fat redistribution. Shown here 7 days postsurgery.

retrusion of the facial skeleton, predisposing to loss of support of soft tissues resulting in laxity or sagging, primarily over the roof of facial soft tissue spaces in contrast to the tethering of the retaining ligaments resulting in surface grooves.[3–7] To effectively rejuvenate patients with significant mid cheek aging, three aspects of the aging mid cheek need to be addressed: first, the prominent eye bags, second the sagging and laxity of the cheeks, and finally, the deflation or volume loss that occurs with aging. Depending on the pathology present, these individual aspects need to be specifically targeted to achieve natural and harmonious rejuvenation of the mid cheek. Depending on the individual anatomy and requests, these objectives may be achieved either via transconjunctival or subciliary approaches.

Release of the tear trough ligament is a key maneuver in rejuvenation of the mid cheek.[8] To prevent reattachment of the ligament to the anterior maxilla and to correct retrusion of the maxilla here, interpositional fat is needed, either transposed as a flap or as free fat grafts of the excised orbital fat. The importance of this maneuver can be clearly demonstrated in patients whose appearance becomes "less attractive" when they smile.[14,19] These are typically patients with hypertrophic orbicularis oculi, small eye bags at rest, and maxillary retrusion. With animation, strong contraction of the periorbital muscles squeezes the retro-orbital fat pads forward and medially against the tightly fixed tear trough ligament, increasing the bulging of the eye bags and prominence of the tear trough deformity. Removal of the eye bags alone, which has the effect of reducing the bulge, provides only a partial solution. With release of the tear trough ligament and orbicularis origins (OOs), the tethering effect is eliminated and the *dynamics* of the smile changed. This change in *vectoring* of the action of the orbicularis oculi gives a more relaxed and beautiful smile (**Figs. 9** and **10**).

A recent long-term study on the effect of release of the tear trough ligament and associated origins of the orbicularis documented the safety of this maneuver in the long term as well as noted the esthetic benefits of this release.[19] With release of the ligament, the following long-term changes were evident. First, the tethering with smiling was eliminated. Second, the vector of contraction of the orbicularis oculi changed to a more upward and outward direction. In combination with the elimination of the blocking effect of the tear trough ligament on elevation of cheek soft tissues with smiling, these effects incombination result in the elevation of the visual location of the lid–cheek

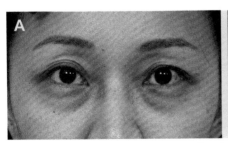 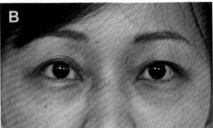

Fig. 6. (A) and (B) A 34-year-old woman presented with eye bags and a "tired look." She underwent transconjunctival lower blepharoplasty with tear tough ligament release and fat redistribution; also, fat grafting of the mid cheek and upper eyelid. Sharp needle intradermal fat grafting was also performed. Shown 1-year post-operation. Note the improvement of the tear trough deformity with elimination of the lid–cheek junction and also the improvement of the dark eye circles, giving a fresher and more youthful appearance.

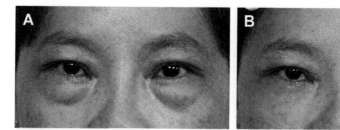

Fig. 7. (A) and (B) A 51-year old woman presented with large eye bags and prominent lid cheek junction. An extended transconjunctival eye bag removal was performed. No fat grafting was performed for her. Here, she is shown at 1-year postsurgery. The eye bags have been effectively eliminated and the tear trough deformity and prominent lid cheek junction effaced giving a more youthful and vibrant appearance.

junction when the patient smiles, giving the impression of a more youthful and pleasant smile (see **Fig. 9**). Third, with release of the OOs, the muscle contraction becomes less efficient. This has two potential benefits on the esthetics of the smile. For patients who have a prominent pretarsal bulge due to orbicularis hypertrophy, the bulge on smiling becomes less prominent postoperatively, resulting in a more esthetic appearance. The reduced efficiency of contraction also resulted in slightly fewer crow's feet with smiling (see **Fig. 10**).

The mid cheek is an area of compaction of structures. Safe dissection may be done with

good technique. This may be achieved with the application of retraction to move vital structures out of the dissection. From the lower eyelid, the preseptal space is opened, with traction on the origins of the orbicularis oculi under tension, and the muscle (and the closely associated tear trough ligament) is released, staying close to the anterior maxilla while applying upward retraction on the tear trough ligament. This is important as the blood vessels (the angular vein and artery) are located in close relation, on the underside of the orbital part of the orbicularis oculi close to its origin, and therefore need to be lifted out of the way of the

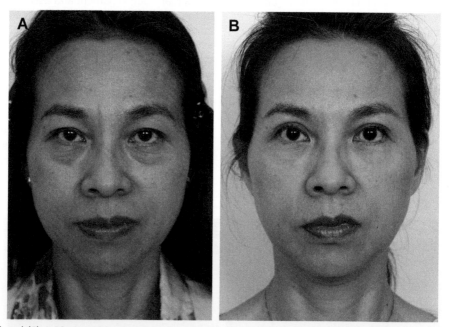

Fig. 8. (A) and (B) A 53-year-old woman presented with the complaints of looking tired and difficulty opening her upper eyelids. Specifically, she complained of cheek sagging and prominence of her upper nasolabial folds. A lower blepharoplasty with mid cheek lift was performed for her to concomitantly tighten the cheek and improve the nasolabial folds. The medial and central fat pads were transposed over the orbital rim and the lateral fat pad excess conservatively excised. Mid cheek fat grafting was also performed. Bilateral upper eyelid ptosis correction with levator advancement as previously described[22,23] was performed at the same time. She is shown here at 1-year postsurgery.

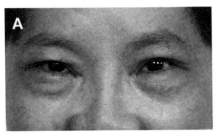 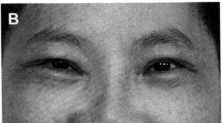

Fig. 9. (*A*) and (*B*) This long-term result demonstrates the benefits of the release of the tear trough ligament and origins of the orbicularis oculi on the esthetics of the patient's smile. The lid–cheek junction was eliminated and "elevation" of the lid–cheek junction with smiling gives a more pleasant and youthful smile.

dissection (Fig. 65.14).[14,17] The extent of the release is determined preoperatively, by marking the indent of tear trough deformity and its lateral extension as the palpebromalar groove. With the right eye as reference, this release usually extends from the 4 o'clock to the 7 o'clock positions. Medially, the release should not extend medial to the 4 o'clock position, as in this area the angular nerve (which innervates the inner canthal orbicularis, glabella, and procerus) and the angular artery and vein become very closely associated with the tear trough ligament and are at risk of injury.[21]

Laterally, the release may be done as needed depending on the preoperative plan. For a lift of the mid cheek, the ORL and the inferior part of the LOT need to be released to mobilize the mid cheek (**Fig. 11**).

When considering mid cheek lifts via the lower eyelid, two planes of dissections are used, the subperiosteal and the preperiosteal planes. The subperiosteal plane is popular for its simplicity and when properly applied is effective in lifting the mid cheek. However, the subperiosteal plane has the problem of prolonged swelling and has significant potential

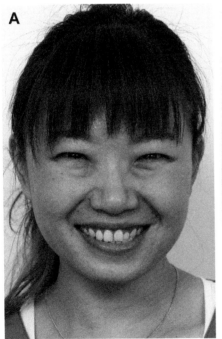 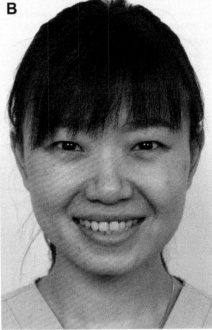

Fig. 10. (*A*) and (*B*) 33-year-old woman presented with the primary concern of prominent eye bags when smiling. An extended transconjunctival lower eyelid blepharoplasty was performed. (*B*) At 6 months postsurgery, note the elimination of the eye bags and augmentation of the anterior maxilla with good survival of the free fat grafts. The benefit of releasing the tear trough ligament is evident when the patient smiles. Elimination of the tethering and scrunching centered at the tear trough ligament results in a more relaxed and beautiful smile.

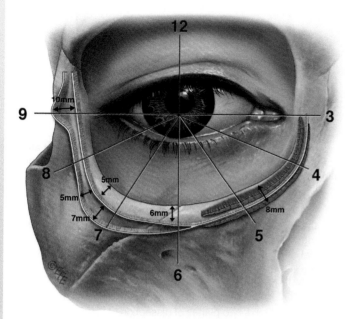

Fig. 11. Extent of the release of the tear trough–orbicularis retaining ligament complex generally extends from the 4 o'clock to the - 7 o'clock position for treatment of the tear trough deformity and from 4 o'clock to 9 o'clock for mid cheek lift. (*Courtesy of* Levent Efe, MD, Melbourne, AU.)

complications. The preperiosteal approach has been used by several authors, but the anatomy is complicated and not well described, hence the exact dissection approach was poorly understood. With recent advances in the understanding of the mid cheek anatomy, particularly the anatomy medially, that of the tear trough ligament and the premaxillary space,[8,9] we can now harness this knowledge in safely and effectively mobilizing the mid cheek. The preperiosteal plane offers some advantages over the subperiosteal technique in that, first, division of the ligament at the preperiosteal level allows the entire superficial fascia (composing the composite of skin, subcutaneous tissue, and orbicularis oculi) to redrape and lift more effectively to tighten the superficial fascia. Second, recurrence is less likely, as the release permanently separates the superficial fascia from the deep fascia (in contrast to the subperiosteal dissection which, in essence, leaves the tear trough–ORL complex, intact). Finally, swelling and bruising are much less than with the subperiosteal dissection.[17,18]

SUMMARY

Using the mid cheek facial soft tissue spaces to release the tear trough ligament and mobilize the mid cheek is a safe and effective technique. As the spaces are anatomical glide planes, dissection is easy, atraumatic, and bloodless. The key is the precise release of the retaining ligaments that separate the spaces. Using this anatomy, recovery is quick and the results lasting, with low complication rates.

CLINICS CARE POINTS

- To deliver optimal results with lower blepharoplasty, aging changes of not just the lower eyelid, but the entire mid cheek should be addressed.

- Understanding the surgical anatomy of the mid cheek is crucial in designing effective and safe surgical approaches in lower eyelid blepharoplasty.

- Patient selection for either using the transconjunctival or subciliary approach depends on patient anatomy and requests.

- For patients with early aging changes, prominent eye bags and tear trough deformity, minimal sagging of the cheeks or skin excess, and the extended transconjunctival lower eyelid blepharoplasty with or without concomitant fat grafting is the procedure of choice.

- For patients with more advanced aging changes, sagging of the cheeks, festoons and for patients specifically seeking a cheek lift to improve their nasolabial folds, the mid cheek lift via the facial soft tissue spaces would be the preferred approach.

- Achieving atraumatic dissection by using the concept of dissecting through the facial soft tissue spaces with precise sharp release of the retaining ligaments that separate the spaces is crucial in lower eyelid surgery to minimize complications and hasten recovery.

SUPPLEMENTARY DATA

Supplementary data related to this article can be found online at https://doi.org/10.1016/j.cps.2022.07.010.

REFERENCES

1. Mendelson BC, Jacobson SR. Surgical anatomy of the midcheek: facial layers, spaces, and the midcheek segments. Clin Plast Surg 2008;35:395–404 [discussion: 393].
2. Wong CH, Mendelson B. Newer understanding of specific anatomic targets in the aging face as applied to injectables: aging changes in the craniofacial skeleton and facial ligaments. Plast Reconstr. Surg 2015;136(5 Suppl):44S–8S.
3. Mendelson B, Wong CH. Changes in the facial skeleton with aging: implications and clinical applications in facial rejuvenation. Aesthetic. Plast Surg 2012;36(4):753–60.
4. Mendelson BC, Wong CH. Anatomy of the aging face. In: Neligan PC, Warren RJ, editors. Plast Surg. Aesthetic, 2, 3rd ed. Elsevier; 2012. p. 78–92.
5. Mendelson BC. Facelift anatomy, SMAS, retaining ligaments and facial spaces. In: Aston SJ, Steinbrech DS, Walden JL, editors. Aesthetic plastic surgery. London: Saunders; 2009. Section 3.
6. Mendelson BC, Muzaffar AR, Adams WP Jr. Surgical anatomy of the midcheek and malar mounds. Plast Reconstr Surg 2002;110(3):885–96 [discussion: 897–911].
7. Muzaffar AR, Mendelson BC, Adams WP. Surgical anatomy of the ligamentous attachments of the lower lid and lateral canthus. J Plast Reconstr Surg 2002;110(3):873–84 [discussion: 897–911].
8. Wong CH, Hsieh MK, Mendelson B. The tear trough ligament: anatomical basis for the tear trough deformity. Plast Reconstr. Surg 2012;129(6):1392–402.
9. Wong CH, Mendelson B. Facial soft-tissue spaces and retaining ligaments of the midcheek: defining the premaxillary space. Plast Reconstr Surg 2013; 132(1):49–56.
10. Jelks GW, Jelks EB. The "no touch" lower blepharoplasty. Can J Plast Surg 2009;17:102–3.
11. Sullivan PK, Drolet BC. Extended lower lid blepharoplasty for eyelid and midface rejuvenation. Plast Reconstr Surg 2013;132:1093–101.
12. Goldberg RA. Transconjunctival orbital fat repositioning: transposition of orbital fat pedicles into a subperiosteal pocket. Plast Reconstr Surg 2000; 105:743.
13. Hidalgo DA. An integrated approach to lower blepharoplasty. Plast Reconstr Surg 2011;127(1):386–95.
14. Wong CH, Mendelson B. Extended transconjunctival lower eyelid blepharoplasty with release of the tear trough ligament and fat redistribution. Plast Reconstr Surg 2017;140(2):273–82.
15. Codner MA, Wolfli JN, Anzarut A. Primary transcutaneous lower blepharoplasty with routine lateral canthal support: a comprehensive 10-year review. Plast Reconstr Surg 2008;121:241–50.
16. Schiller Jeffrey D. Lysis of the Orbicularis retaining ligament and orbicularis oculi insertion: a powerful modality for lower eyelid and cheek rejuvenation. Plast Reconstr Surg 2012;129(4):692e–700e.
17. Wong CH, Mendelson B. Midcheek lift using facial soft-tissue spaces of the midcheek. Plast Reconstr. Surg 2015;136(6):1155–65.
18. Wong CH, Hsieh MK, Mendelson B. Mid cheek lift via the facial soft tissue spaces. Plast Reconstr Surg 2022. In press.
19. Wong CH, Mendelson B. Long-term static and dynamic effects of the release of the tear trough ligament and origins of the orbicularis oculi in lower eyelid blepharoplastry. Plast Reconstr Surg 2019; 144(3):583–91.
20. Weinfeld AB, Burke R, Codner MA. The comprehensive management of chemosis following cosmetic lower blepharoplasty. Plast Reconstr Surg 2008; 122(2):579–86.
21. Caminer DM, Newman MI, Boyd JB. Angular nerve: new insights on innervation of the corrugator supercilii and procerus muscles. J Plast Reconstr Aesthet Surg 2006;59(4):366–72.
22. Wong CH, Hsieh MKH, Mendelson B. Upper eyelid ptosis correction with levator advancement in asian patients using the musculoaponeurotic junction of the levator as the key reference point. Plast Reconstr Surg 2020;146(6):1268–73.
23. Wong CH, Hsieh MKH, Mendelson B. A comprehensive approach to asian upper eyelid ptosis correction: the levator musculo-aponeurotic junction formula. Aesthet Surg J 2021;41(10): 1120–9.

Primary Rhinoplasty Combined with Pyriform Aperture Augmentation in Asians

Zhao Jianfang, MD, PhD[a,b], An Yang, MD[a,*], Li Dong, MD[a,*]

KEYWORDS

- Comprehensive rhinoplasty • Pyriform aperture augmentation • Mid-face concavity • Nasal base
- Alar base • Columella base

KEY POINTS

- Asians commonly have unpleasant facial profiles of mid-face concavity.
- Pyriform aperture augmentation includes nasal alar base augmentation and nasal columella base augmentation.
- Pyriform aperture augmentation greatly improves mid-face concavity and increases the visual effect of nasal projection.
- This technique would especially be suitable for rhinoplasty with mid-face concavity in indicated Asian patients.

INTRODUCTION

In recent 20 years, comprehensive rhinoplasty has developed rapidly in Asia because it meets the needs of augmentation and extension of the external nose for Asians. However, for those who have a small nose with insufficient skin, there may be insufficient external nose protrusion after the operation even when the extension and elevation of the external nose is enough during the surgery. Likewise, excessive extension and elevation of the external nose may also lead to many complications.

To find a more reliable surgical strategy, our group conducted a three-dimensional (3D) research on the nasal-facial relationship of 250 Chinese volunteers. The results showed that the mid-face concavity had a severe impact on the nasomental angle (protrusion of the external nose), columella-labial angle, and nasofrontal angle, whereas the mid-face concavity was uncommon in beautiful individuals. During our clinical practice, we found that the patients who had a strong desire for rhinoplasty were often accompanied by depression of the bilateral alar base, the concave of the columella base, and the protrusion of the upper lip. The simulation using 3D software indicates that the pyriform aperture augmentation can visually lower the protrusion of the lip, and increase the columella-labial angle and nasal tip protrusion at the same time. Therefore, pyriform aperture augmentation using a prosthesis should be an integral part of the surgical scheme for patients with mid-face concavity who desire to undergo comprehensive rhinoplasty.

INDICATIONS AND CONTRAINDICATIONS FOR PYRIFORM APERTURE AUGMENTATION

Comprehensive rhinoplasty with pyriform aperture augmentation is suitable for patients with mid-face concavity, deep nasolabial groove, protrusion of upper lip, short nose height, and insufficient

[a] Department of Plastic Surgery, Peking University Third Hospital, No.49 North Garden Road, Haidian District, Beijing 100191, China; [b] Department of Plastic and Burn Surgery, Peking University First Hospital, No.8 Xishiku Street, Xicheng District, Beijing 100034, China
* Corresponding authors.
E-mail addresses: anyangdoctor@163.com (A.Y.); lidong9@sina.com (L.D.)

Clin Plastic Surg 50 (2023) 133–140
https://doi.org/10.1016/j.cps.2022.08.003

external nose protrusion. In addition to the general contraindications of surgery, extremely long upper lip and wide alar are relative contraindications (**Fig. 1**). The reason is that the filling of the anterior nasal creston of the maxilla in the middle of the pyriform aperture will lower the upper lip; filling besides the pyriform aperture will widen the alar. Hence, if there is no combination of other restrictive surgery, these two symptoms are not suitable for pyriform aperture augmentation.

PREOPERATIVE EVALUATION AND SPECIAL CONSIDERATIONS

The 3D images of the patient's face are collected and analyzed using 3D surface imaging, and the degree of mid-face concavity is graded into five levels: grade I is severe depression; grade II is mild depression; grade III is normal; grade IV is mild protrusion; and grade V is a severe protrusion. Generally, the depth of the nasolabial groove is directly proportional to the severity of the mid-face concavity, accompanied by a small nasolabial angle. Therefore, pyriform aperture augmentation is required for grades I and II of mid-face concavity.

The length of the nose is also assessed and graded before operation: class I, nose length is equal to 1/3 of face height; class II, nose length is shorter than the 1/3 face height and the difference is less than 0.5 cm; class III, the length of the nose is shorter than the 1/3 face height and the difference is greater than 0.5 cm. Class II short nose only requires nose augmentation using prosthesis or nose tip augmentation using ear cartilage, whereas class III short nose needs nose extension surgery.

The various evaluation results of mid-face concavity and nose length determine the different surgical techniques that would be selected (**Table 1**).

SURGICAL PROCEDURES

Design three types of paired alar base prosthesis and columella base prosthesis according to the potential filling volume (**Fig. 2**). The size, shape, and thickness of the prosthesis are determined based on the severity and area of the facial depression. Normally, the thickness of the alar base and columella base prosthesis is between 0.5 and 0.8 mm.

Under general anesthesia with the patient in a supine position, the whole face is prepared and draped in a sterile fashion, local anesthetic solution for the incision and subcutaneous separation area is infiltrated (2% lidocaine 10 mL + 1:100,000 adrenalin). The alar base augmentation is performed using the incision at the inferolateral edges of both nostrils. The columella base augmentation is performed with an incision at the right infero-posterior edge of the nasal columella (**Fig. 3**), and the length of the incision is around 10 mm. The skin and subcutaneous tissue is incised, and the ophthalmic scissors and periosteal elevator are used to separate a cavity at the front of the periosteum. The lowest part of the cavity must be 5 mm above the upper gingival sulcus, and the separated space should be 2–3 mm broader than that of the prosthesis. The inner boundary of the alar base cavity is 2 mm outside the pyriform aperture, and the columella base cavity can be inserted into the nasal columella.

If the nasal septum needs to be extended, firstly it should be exposed following the classical method, and then the costal cartilage, nasal septal

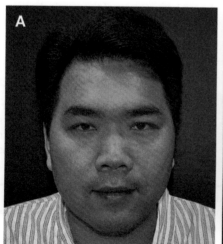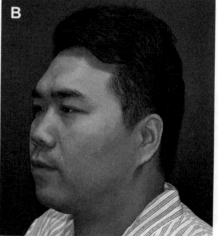

Fig. 1. Long upper lip and wide alar are relative contraindications of pyriform aperture augmentation. (A) front view. (B) lateral view.

Table 1
Surgical scheme selection according to the preoperative evaluation

Mid-face Concavity	Grade II	Grade II	Grate I
Nose length	Class I	Class II	Class III
Nasal dorsal height	Normal	Low	Low
Nasal alar base augmentation	√	√	√
Columella base augmentation		√	√
External nose augmentation		√	√
Nose extension			√
Surgical scheme	1	2	3

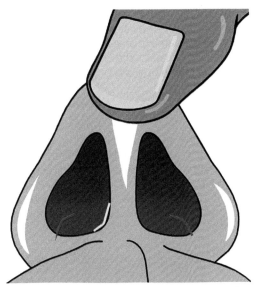

Fig. 3. Yellow line: an incision at the right infero-posterior edge of the nasal columella for the columella base augmentation. Red line: bilateral incision at the inferolateral edges of both nostrils for the alar base augmentation.

cartilage, or ear cartilage can be selected as the scaffold according to the extended length.

Expanded polytetrafluoroethylene (e-PTFE) nasal augmentation prosthesis and nasal base filling prosthesis are implanted into the separated cavity in the nasal dorsum, bilateral alar base, and anterior nasal crest of maxilla, respectively. The prosthesis can be fixed with 5-0 absorbable suture (**Fig. 4**).

The incision is closed with sutures and a thermoplastic splint is used for immobilization. A drain is placed in the separated cavity if nasal septum extension is performed.

POSTOPERATIVE CARE AND EXPECTED OUTCOME

The drainage tube should be removed when the drainage volume is less than 1 mL per day. The

fixing splint of the nasal dorsum is removed around 4 to 5 days. The upper lip fixing tape should be used for 4 to 5 days. The Incision suture is removed 5 to 7 days after the operation. Take antibiotics orally for 3 days after the operation to prevent infection. Limit laughter and excessive mouth

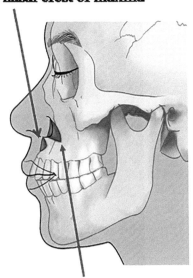

Anterior nasal crest of maxilla

Bilateral alar base

Fig. 4. Implant prostheses into the separated cavities at the bilateral alar base and the anterior nasal crest of maxilla.

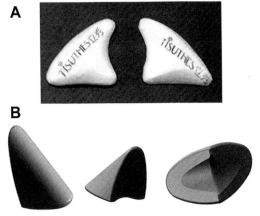

Fig. 2. Design prosthesis. (A) E-PTFE alar base implant for alar base augmentation. (B) Horseshoe implant for columellar base augmentation.

opening during tooth brushing to prevent the movement of the nasal base prosthesis. The edema of the surgical area usually partially subsides in about 2 weeks and completely dissipated 2 months after the operation.

MANAGEMENT OF COMPLICATIONS

Regular follow-up at 1 week, 1 month, 3 months, and 6 months after operation. If the prosthesis displacement occurs after operation, manual repositioning and external fixation should be done to revise the displacement. If there is an infection in the filling area, the prosthesis usually needs to be removed and implanted after 3 months.

REVISION OR SUBSEQUENT PROCEDURES

In case of prosthesis displacement, prosthesis reset is usually carried out 2 weeks after the surgery when the edema is completely dissipated. The replaced prosthesis should be fixed with 6-0 nylon thread through the skin or oral mucosa for 4 to 5 days.

CASE DEMONSTRATIONS

Case 1. A 25-year-old boy. Preoperative evaluation showed normal nose length, normal nasal dorsal height, grade II mid-face concavity, upper lip protrusion, and obvious nasolabial groove. Operation plan: medium e-PTFE nasal alar base

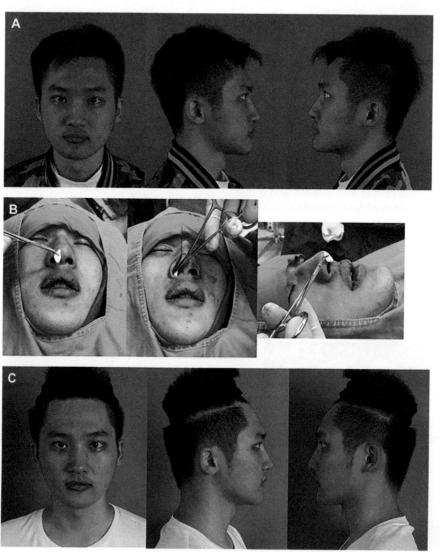

Fig. 5. A 25-year-old boy. Normal nose length, normal nasal dorsal height, grade II mid-face concavity. Operation plan: medium e-PTFE nasal alar base prosthesis and medium columella base prosthesis implantation. (*A*) Pre-operation. (*B*) Prostheses designed during operation. (*C*) 21 months post-operation.

prosthesis and medium columella base prosthesis were used to perform the pyriform aperture augmentation (**Fig. 5**).

Case 2. A 22-year-old girl. Preoperative evaluation showed normal nose length, relatively low nasal dorsum, grade II mid-face concavity, upper lip protrusion, and obvious nasolabial groove. Operation plan: medium e-PTFE nasal alar base prosthesis and medium columella base prosthesis were used for pyriform aperture augmentation, and e-PTFE prosthesis was used for rhinoplasty (**Fig. 6**).

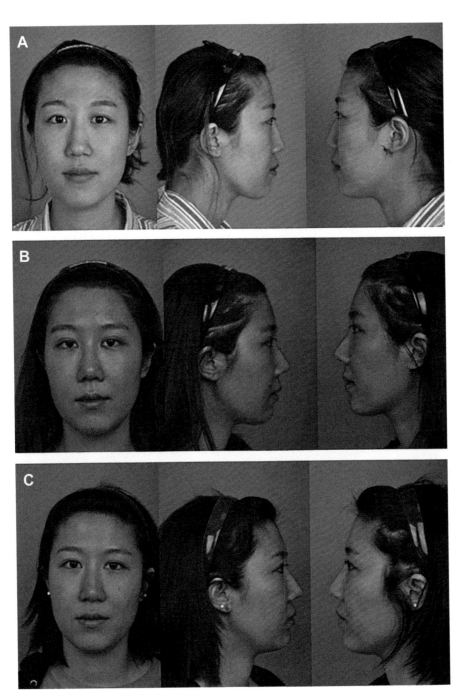

Fig. 6. A 22-year-old girl. Normal nose length, low nasal dorsum, grade II mid-face concavity. Operation plan: medium e-PTFE nasal alar base prosthesis and columella base prosthesis implantation, combined with nasal tip augmentation using ear cartilage. (*A*) Pre-operation. (*B*) 6 months post-operation. (*C*) 12 months post-operation.

Case 3. A 30-year-old man with Binder syndrome: Preoperative evaluation showed class II short nose, grade I mid-face concavity. Operation plan: large e-PTFE nasal alar base prosthesis and large columella base prosthesis were used for pyriform aperture augmentation. Costal cartilage was used for nasal septum extension and dorsal augmentation, and ear cartilage was used for tip reconstruction (**Fig. 7**).

DISCUSSION

A thorough and comprehensive preoperative morphological evaluation is crucial for plastic surgery. For rhinoplasty combined pyriform aperture augmentation, both the features of the external nose and the mid-face should be taken into consideration. In our surgery scheme, mid-face concavity and the length of the nose are measured

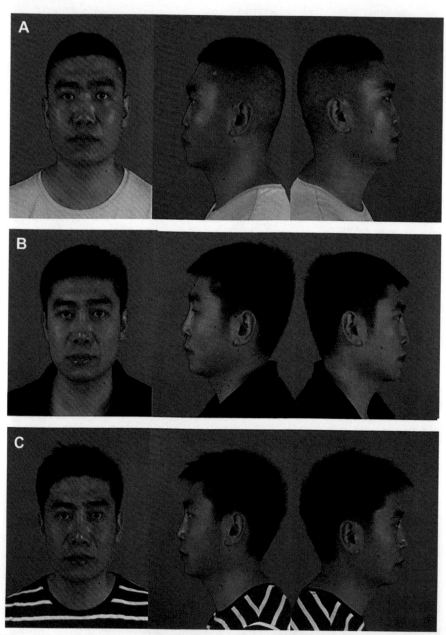

Fig. 7. A 30-year-old man with Binder syndrome. Class II short nose, grade I mid-face concavity. Operation plan: large e-PTFE nasal alar base prosthesis and columella base prosthesis implantation, combined with septal extension and dorsal augmentation using costicartilage. Nasal tip was also reconstructed. (*A*) Pre-operation. (*B*) 6 months post-operation. (*C*) 10 months post-operation.

and graded. The original data is collected using 3D imaging, which can ensure the objectivity and accuracy of the results. The degree of mid-face concavity and the level of the short nose helps us to determine the overall morphology of the patient's mid-face and assist the treatment selection.

Pyriform aperture augmentation not only improves the mid-face concavity, but also increases the columella-labial angle, nasofrontal angle, and the height of nasal sill.[1,2] More importantly, even a small amount of nose lengthening and nasal dorsum elevation can achieve a significant esthetic effect of external nose protrusion after the lifting of nasal base.[3] The key surgical areas are the periosteal surface region of inferolateral edge of the pyriform aperture and the anterior nasal crest of the maxilla. These areas are safe regions and can avoid nerve injury.[4]

From the perspective of minimally invasive, we performed alar base filling prosthesis and maxillary anterior nasal crest prosthesis with e-PTFE without using screw to fix it. Jiao Wei and colleagues used integral prostheses that covered the bilateral and below area of the pyriform aperture. The advantage of their prosthesis is stable implantation, but the disadvantages are extensively traumatic and the prosthesis shape is not easy to carve. Furthermore, once infected, it is easy to affect the whole implantation area.[5–7]

Anatomical studies showed that the maxillary anterior nasal crest of Chinese with mid-face concavity and short nose is obviously small. According to the shape of normal maxillary anterior nasal crest, we design three types of prosthesis with different sizes. The implantation of maxillary anterior nasal crest prosthesis can significantly reduce the protrusion of the upper lip and increase the nasolabial angle. It can also increase the nasal height and the visual protrusion of the external nose.

There are several key points of this operation. First, the cavity must be separated on the periosteum around the pyriform aperture of the maxilla. Second, the range of separated cavity for implantation should only be 2 mm larger than the size of prosthesis. Third, the inner boundary of the separated cavity should be 3 to 4 mm away from the edge of the pyriform aperture, the lower boundary should be 3-4 mm above the upper gingival sulcus, and the upper side of the cavity can be 2 mm wider than the prosthesis. In particular, the upper side of the separated cavity should not be too wide, which will lead to the displacement of the prosthesis. Besides, we also noticed that there are three patients who have alar width increase after surgery. This may have a relationship with the dissection of the muscle around the alar base.[8] The prosthesis can be sutured and fixed with an absorbable suture. In our unpublished study, (Li Dong, 2021) we performed pyriform aperture augmentation for 123 patients. The overall satisfaction rate was 92%. Prosthesis displacement occurred in 5 patients (4%), of which 2 cases occurred secondary infection. After removing the prosthesis for 3 months, the surgery was performed again and satisfactory results were achieved.

SUMMARY

Asians have a high proportion of mid-face concavity, and they also have a strong desire for rhinoplasty. Comprehensive rhinoplasty with pyriform aperture augmentation can significantly improve the esthetic relationship between the external nose and surrounding structures. The e-PTFE prosthesis has stable biocompatibility and the surgical method is also minimally invasive. The long-term effect of the surgery is stable and patients' satisfaction rate is high. This technique is especially suitable for composite rhinoplasty of Asian patients with mid-face concavity.

CLINICS CARE POINTS

- Some unpleasant facial profiles, such as a prominent mouth and short nose, may not occur solely. They may often combine with mid-face concavity or even be caused by it.
- Pyriform aperture augmentation includes nasal alar base augmentation and columella base augmentation.
- Thorough morphological evaluation should be performed before the operation. However, the esthetic definition and standard in the mid-face still need to be elucidated.

DISCLOSURE

This study has no conflicts of interest.

FUNDING

This work was supported by Key Clinical Projects of Peking University Third Hospital (No. BYSYFY2021005).

REFERENCES

1. Lee W, Park HJ, Choi HG, et al. Nostril base augmentation effect of alveolar bone graft. Arch Plast Surg 2013;40:542–5.

2. Jeon YT, Han SJ. Comparative study of the effect of paranasal augmentation with autologous bone in orthognathic surgery. J Oral Maxillofac Surg 2019; 77(10):2116–24.

3. Yaremchuk MJ, Vibhakar D. Pyriform aperture augmentation as an adjunct to rhinoplasty. Clin Plast Surg 2016;43(1):187–93.

4. Raschke R, Hazani R, Yaremchuk MJ. Identifying a safe zone for midface augmentation using anatomic landmarks for the infraorbital foramen. Aesthet Surg J 2013;33(1):13–8.

5. Lee TY, Chung HY, Dhong ES, et al. Paranasal Augmentation using multi-folded expanded polytetrafluorethylene (ePTFE) in the east asian nose. Aesthet Surg J 2019;39(12):1319–28.

6. Tang XJ, Zhang ZY, Shi L, et al. Accident entry of titanium screw into the sphenoid sinus during paranasal augmentation with porous polyethylene implant. J Craniofac Surg 2012;23(5):e394–6.

7. Wei J, Luo J, Herrler T, et al. A simple technique for the correction of maxillonasal dysplasia using customized expanded polytetrafluoroethylene (ePTFE) implants. J Plast Reconstr Aesthet Surg 2017;70(9):1292–7.

8. Kwon TG, Kang SM, Hwang HD. Three-dimensional soft tissue change after paranasal augmentation with porous polyethylene. Int J Oral Maxillofac Surg 2014;43(7):816–23.

Revision Rhinoplasty in Asians

Jiao Wei, MD, PhD, Chuanchang Dai, MD, PhD, Shengli Li, MD, PhD*

KEY WORDS

- Revision rhinoplasty • Complications • Asian • Implants • Autologous cartilage grafts

KEY POINTS

- Alloplast-related complications frequently seen in clinical practice are involved with implant deviation, extrusion, infection, and nasal contraction deformities after multiple surgeries or infection.
- Autologous cartilages are preferred in the cases of revision rhinoplasty.
- In revision rhinoplasty for Asian patients, costal cartilages play an important role as support grafts for nasal reconstruction.

INTRODUCTION

The demand on esthetic plastic surgery has been fueled by the achievements of economic development in the past several decades in Asian countries, social media coverageand the advances Internet communications also contribute to a spike in the number of people seeking the help of plastic surgery procedures, including rhinoplasty. The consequent cases for the purpose of the revision and enhancement in rhinoplasty, or secondary rhinoplasty, have been on the increase as well.

The alloplastic implants such as silicone and expanded polytetrafluoroethylene (ePTFE) and so on are still commonly applied in rhinoplasty mainly for nasal augmentation in Asian population, having proved to be safe and effective from a series of clinical studies.[1] However, inappropriate patient selection, in combination with poor surgical techniques using alloplasts by novices can bring about some complications. Revisional operations in rhinoplasty sometimes cannot be avoided even in the hands of an experienced surgeon. Alloplast-related complications frequently seen in clinical practice are involved with implant deviation, extrusion, infection, and nasal contraction deformities due to the postoperative infection or after multiple surgeries.

Another group of cases for revisional procedures in Asian rhinoplasty can be categorized as the complications or nasal deformities arising from the previous autogenous grafts including costal cartilage, auricular cartilage, septal cartilage, and the fascia from different areas of the body, which present with distinctive characteristics in a specified case. The case evaluation and its management would also be discussed in this article.

SPECIAL CONSIDERATIONS IN REVISION RHINOPLASTY IN ASIANS

Revision rhinoplasty usually requires a large quantity of materials for grafting and reconstruction of nasal structural supports. Autologous cartilages are preferred in the cases of revision rhinoplasty. Among the autologous cartilages, auricular, and septal cartilages are usually the first choice of grafts in the surgeons' mind in Asia for their easy harvest and low donor morbidities. Costal cartilage is often necessary when several graft pieces and strong support are needed in the recipient sites of nose. In cases with problems of the nasal skin envelope from the previous operations, the reconstruction of nasal skin and soft tissue loss

Conflicts of interest: There are no potential conflicts of interest regarding this article.
Department of Plastic & Reconstructive Surgery, Ninth People's Hospital of Shanghai Jiao-tong University School of Medicine, 639 Zhi Zao Ju Road, Shanghai 200011, P. R. China
* Corresponding author.
E-mail address: drlishengli@sina.com

Clin Plastic Surg 50 (2023) 141–149
https://doi.org/10.1016/j.cps.2022.08.004

should be considered accordingly, and nasal tip and columella are often affected in the cases of Asian revision rhinoplasty.

To compare with in the west, the procedure of filler injection in the Asian nose is not uncommon with the advantage of simplicity, relatively easy performance, short downtime, and to some extent, being the realistic simulation of the result of dorsal augmentation. Even so, it still can cause some problems involved with the filler material itself and nasal abnormalities following the filler injection, particularly for patients in pursuit of revision rhinoplasty following it.

IMPLANT-RELATED COMPLICATIONS

The silicone and ePTFE are the most commonly used alloplastic nasal implants in Asian rhinoplasty. They are used mainly for dorsal augmentation and, seldom for tip lengthening, even though ePTFE had been reported by some authors as a columellar strut or septal extension graft.[1,2] The main reasons for revision rhinoplasty in Asians are usually related to alloplast-related complications, such as implants visibility, deviation, extrusion, infection, and contracted nose.

Implant Visibility and Deviation

The implant visibility and deviation were common complications of the alloplastic implants in rhinoplasty. The contour and even deflection of the implants were manifested in the involved patients. In Asian population, the aesthetic criterion has some differences with that of Caucasian.[3] The natural appearance of height, width, length, and shape are widely accepted by Asian patients. The Asian female patients prefer a gentle slope from the supraorbital ridge to the tip, so is a lower nasion or nasal starting point which lies at the level between the mid-pupillary line and a bit above. It is not only necessary to consider the coordination between the nose and the forehead as well as cheeks but also the harmony between the nose and the whole face. Revision rhinoplasty is clearly warranted in the patients with obvious implant visibility and deviation. If the nasal dorsal height is too high because of the implant, or obviously deviated to either side, the implant removal and replacement should be carried out to obtain a gentle nasal profile (**Fig. 1**). Revision surgery should be performed to correct the deformities of implant displacement, deviation, and visibility after thorough clinical and psychological evaluation of the patient. Implant removal was the best choice for the patients with psychological disorders.

Extrusion

The excessive nasal skin tension, infection, or poorly healed incisions in primary rhinoplasty are the main reasons of implant extrusion. The most common sites of implant extrusion are located at the sites of the nasal tip and the previous incisions in Asian patients. To prevent pressure necrosis of the nasal tip skin, impending extrusion of any kind of implant material needs to be removed as early as possible. While removing the silicone implant, the capsule around it should be removed to allow the new graft fixation properly on the nasal dorsum. The ePTFE implant is often more difficult to dissect out due to their greater tissue adhesion, a wide dissection would be necessary to remove them during operation (**Fig. 2**).

Infection

Typical signs of infection include swelling, erythema, discharge, tenderness, or granulation tissue formation around the incision site (**Fig. 3**). If an obvious or diffusive signs of infection could not be fully controlled after the treatment by using antibiotics intravenously for 3 to 5 days, the surgeon should not hesitate to remove all implants. Early and prompt intervention could avoid or minimize soft tissue damage, postoperational scar, and contracture. The timing and surgical approaches in this kind of the revision rhinoplasty are controversial in the patients with a history of infection. Jang and colleagues[4] maintained that the revision rhinoplasty would be implemented at the time of implant removal without active infection or inflammation. Otherwise, revision rhinoplasty would be done for a few weeks later after the implant removal until the inflammation is completely controlled and before extensive skin contracture occurs. This is the rational decision the surgeon should be well aware of,furthermore,it should be added that, in some cases ,the signs of swollen and possible hypertrophic wound scar would be possibly reduced for 6 months or even longer after the emergency implant removal operation. Further revision surgery had better to be performed after the complete recovery of the soft tissue. The stretching massage of skin and mucosal tissue should be applied from early stage to decrease postoperative soft tissue contracture and scar formation. In the cases of severe infections, the costal cartilage grafts are recommended for later rebuilding the septal, nasal dorsum, and alar cartilage deformity instead of an alloplastic implant at least 6 months after the operation. The autologous

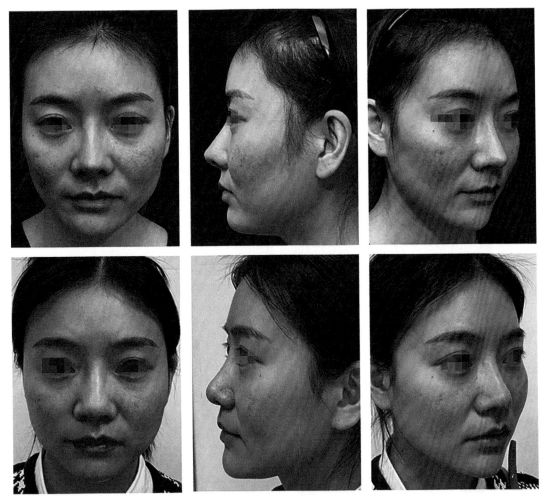

Fig. 1. A female patient with congenital short nose (above) previously underwent nasal elongation using silicone implant on the dorsum and auricular cartilage on the tip. The silicone implant was removed and an ePTFE implant reimplanted at the same time to correct the visibility and deviation of implants. Follow-up at 13 months postoperatively demonstrated a gentle nasal profile in aesthetics (below).

tissue could minimize the risks of reinfection and be conducive to rebuild a strong nasal framework.

SOFT TISSUES PROBLEMS
Contracture

Nasal contractures after rhinoplasty are usually caused by the alloplastic reaction, capsule, and fibrosis formation, infection, or inflammation. Its probability of occurrence is higher in Asian than Caucasian.[5] Before the surgery, it is necessary to evaluate nasal skin and lining extensibility, required extent of lengthening and elevation. If the nasal skin and lining are severely thickened and have lost its normal elasticity, the more robust support grafts or implants are recommended, mainly by the use of costal cartilage. The costal cartilage is

one of the most recommended autogenous materials in Asian patients. During the surgery, the nasal scar, the nasal mucosa of scroll area, and the soft tissue around the nose should be adequately released and mobilized to obtain the maximum amount of soft tissue coverage. The extended spreader grafts are placed in dorsal septum to reinforce septum support and support against the nasal contractures. The septal extension graft is fixed to the anterior nasal spine and caudal septum to adjust the position of nasal tip. According to the nasal height and length, the nasal grafts could be integrally designed in aesthetic standards (**Figs. 4 and 5**).[1,6] Hence, one of the most crucial factors in revision rhinoplasty is the extensibility of the nasal skin envelope and lining soft tissue. If there was a significant soft tissue defect, reconstruction of the soft tissue of the nose would be needed.[7]

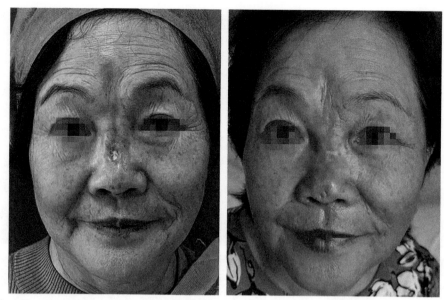

Fig. 2. A female patient with congenital saddle nose underwent a rhinoplasty using the ePTFE implant previously. The ePTFE implant was extruded from nasal skin at about 10 years later. The ePTFE implant was removed immediately after visiting us in clinic. The photos of preoperation (left) and 5 months (right) postoperatively demonstrated a well-healed wound.

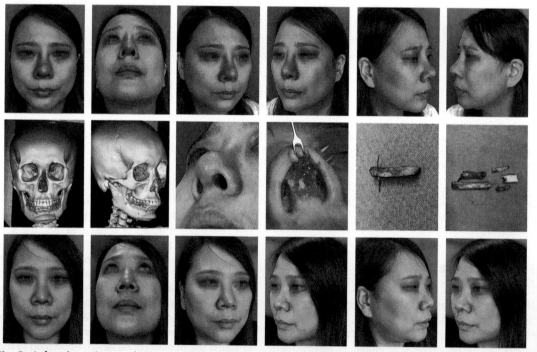

Fig. 3. A female patient underwent a rhinoplasty previously using the costal cartilage and ePTFE implants in other hospitals. The persistent and repeated infection occurred 6 months after operation with a swollen and red nose. The purulent exudation was found out in the incision of left nostril. Antibiotics were repeatedly administrated for a long time. The patient underwent an open rhinoplasty operation of debridement after being referred to us. The costal cartilage and ePTFE implants were removed and a drainage tube was placed in the nose for 2 days. The photos of preoperation (*above line*), 3D CT image reconstruction before the operation (*midline, left*), removed costal cartilage in operative (*midline, right*), follow-up at 6 months (*below line*) postoperatively demonstrated an entire recovery. The patient's psychologic condition improved significantly.

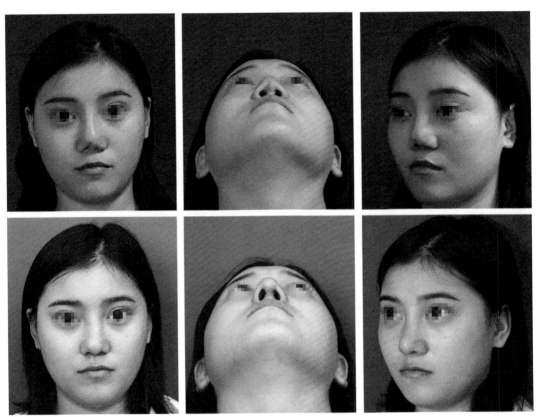

Fig. 4. A 29-year-old female patient with iatrogenic short nose (above) received nasal lengthening using costal cartilage framework. Nasal length was increased by 5 mm. Follow-up examination after 6 months showed satisfactory results (below).

Nasal Skin Defect and Necrosis

One of the most catastrophic complications of rhinoplasty is irreversible skin damage. In revision rhinoplasty in Asians, the cases with soft tissues defects are not rarely seen in clinical practice, especially occurring in nasal tip and columella. The defective nasal tip and columella were usually caused by the excessive skin tension after the placement of the oversized implants. The compromise in skin blood supply by excessive blood vessels destruction in operation is another factor of skin necrosis. To ensure a successful revision surgery of the soft tissue defects in Asian patients, the key point is to confirm the location, size, and depth of the soft tissue defect.

For the small size of nasal ala and columella defects, the local flap (eg, nasofacial groove flap, nasolabial flap) and an auricular cartilage composite graft would be indicated.[8] For the small size defects of nasal tip and columella, the local flap, for example, the nasal dorsal flap and the upper lip flap would be selected.[9,10] However, the facial scars are always encountered using the local flaps, which is usually difficult to accept

by the female patients seeking cosmetic surgery. In severe and large-area skin defects, a forehead flap, preauricular temporal artery flap, or a distant skin flap were reported for reconstruction.[11–13] The preauricular free flap could provide a perfectly texture and color-matched composite tissue with a stable blood supply. It is the best option for the repairment of large nasal tip and columella defects. The repaired size of defect would be up to 2 to 3 × 3 to 4 cm². The preauricular reversed superficial temporal artery flap was harvested and transferred to the nasal tip or columella defect as a free flap using supermicrosurgical techniques, which is a commonly used surgical approach in our department. The alar artery and angular vein were used as the recipient vessels for microsurgical anastomoses (**Fig. 6**).[11] The expanded forehead flap has been considered to be the best option for extensive nose reconstruction.[13] In this surgical procedure, the autologous costal cartilages were recommended for reconstruction of the nasal framework at the same time. It is worth noting that the skin repairment would be proposed at 6 months later of the primary rhinoplasty.

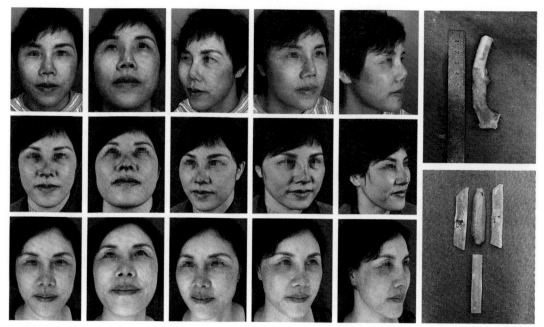

Fig. 5. A female patient with congenital short nose underwent nasal elongation using ePTFE implant. The skin nasal tip and columella had local necrosis after operation (*left, above line*). The soft tissue of the nose was contracted for 3 years. The scar of the nasal tip was not significantly improved after repeated laser treatment. The stretching massage of nasal skin and lining was instructed to implement for about 1 year. The costal cartilage graft was performed for nasal septum support by septal extension grafts and columellar strut. The photos of pre-operation (*left, above line*), intraoperative costal cartilage (right column), follow-up at 1 week (*left, middle line*), 12 months (*left, below line*) postoperatively demonstrated a significantly improvement of nasal appearance .

FILLER OR INJECTIONS-RELATED COMPLICATIONS

As a minimally invasive treatment, the number of injection rhinoplasty is rapidly increased in Asian these years. It has been proved to be effective in cosmetic rhinoplasty, yet some postoperative complication was also reported.[14–16] [17–20] The prognosis after injections in the nose mainly depends on the early detection of complications and the prompt managements.[18] Management strategies reported vary greatly.[19]

In Asian, the patients' complaints of the nasal unsightly nasal profile and transillumination are caused by overdose injection, thin nasal skin, and filler migration. Injections of hyaluronidase are the first choice for the removal of residual hyaluronic acid (HA) in the nose. The suction technique in closed approach or an operation in the open approach in rhinoplasty for removing fillers was performed to obtain a natural nasal shape (**Fig. 7**). At the same time of the filler removal, the augmentation rhinoplasty was always required by Asian patients. The revision operation should simultaneously implement in the cases without any signs of infection. The related deformities after the nasal injection need to be fully evaluated

before the revision procedure. The costal cartilage and the ePTFE, rather than silicone implants, were recommended by this kind of revision rhinoplasty to minimize the possibility of postoperative infection or the nasal transillumination.

DISCUSSION

The great advantages of autologous tissues are the low infection rate and low extrusion rates. Autologous cartilage grafts such as costal cartilage, auricular cartilage, septal cartilage, and fascia are reported in Asian rhinoplasty.

There still exist some problems about the applications of autologous tissues. The infection, warping, deviation, graft visibility, unnatural-looking appearance, even nasal tip, and columella skin necrosis are the involved complications needed to deal with, which had been reported in previous Asian rhinoplasty.[6,21] In Asians, autologous cartilage graft is widely used in revision rhinoplasty in the past decades. Based on our experience, the use of costal cartilage as an autologous graft is especially indicated in patients with severe short noses or following repeated revision surgery which is manifested in soft tissue contraction, poor septal cartilage, and tissue deficiency of nasal

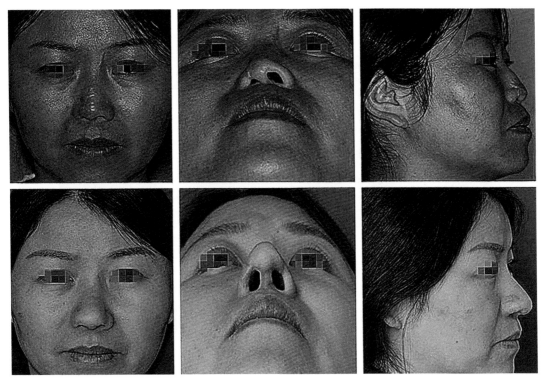

Fig. 6. A female patient underwent an HA injectant for rhinoplasty. The vascular embolization of the injected filler occurred. The skin defects of the nasal tip, dorsal, and alar necrosis were found 3 months postinjection (above). Taking the nasal alar artery and angular vein as the recipient vessels, the preauricular reversed superficial temporal artery flap was transferred by the supermicrosurgical method for reconstruction of the nasal defects. Seven months' postoperative view (below).

skin and lining. With an increasing incidence of revision rhinoplasty, costal cartilage has become one of the most popular choices of nasal grafts due to its robust strength and ample volume in Asian rhinoplasty.

The postoperative infection of the nose occurred not only in the early period but also in the scenario of delayed management of implant exposure. In the case of infection, the systematic antibiotics and local irrigation were administered for about 3 to 5 days. If there was no significant improvement in the symptoms of infections after this rigorous treatment, all implants should be removed to reduce further damage of the nasal tissues caused by the infection (see **Fig. 5**). In our experience, the further revision rhinoplasty in the unstable cases should be performed over 6 months later after achieving a full recovery of the nose.

The warping or deviation was a constant concern of the costal cartilage grafting. The main reasons of warping or deviation are the local calcification of the cartilage, local elastic differences of the costal cartilage after carving the cartilage into needed shape in operation, asymmetry of soft tissue elasticity or surgical sutures, and excessive

soft tissue tension. Attempts to avoid the above situation could reduce the occurrence of costal cartilage warping or deviation. Conventional measures to avoid warping include symmetric and concentric carving from the central portion of the cartilage, symmetric suture of bilateral nasal tissues, and adjustment of the length of the implanted cartilage to reduce excessive skin tension. The carved costal cartilage would be repeatedly immersed in warm saline.[22,23] The appropriate shortening of the costal cartilage length is necessary in the cases of excessive tip skin tension. To avoid implant deviation, deformation, and/or dislocation after the nasal elongation procedures, the supportive strength of the implants and the retraction force of the nasal skin and mucosa must be well-balanced (see **Figs. 4** and **5**).

The septal cartilage is often used to refine the nasal tip as a support structure in Caucasians. However, these approaches are not always suitable for Asians due to weakness and insufficiency in the nasal septum which is seldom applied in Asian revision rhinoplasty.[6,24] The auricular cartilage has an intrinsic curvature that could be used to provide an elastic support in the medial crura

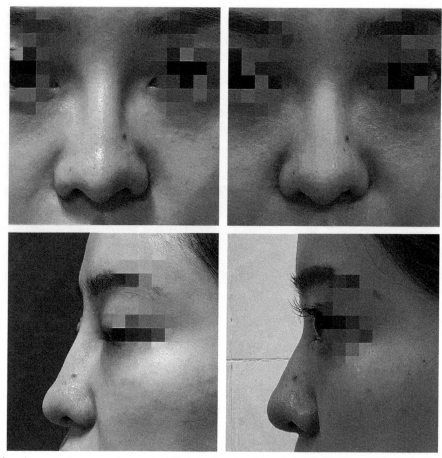

Fig. 7. A female patient once underwent a HA injection for rhinoplasty (*left*). The patient complained of the nasal transillumination and inaesthetic nasal profile. Filler removal was performed for a natural nasal shape with the photos of a follow-up 6 months late (*right*).

and cap grafting in the nasal tip. The autologous fascia grafting could be used to improve the skin thickness of nasal tip in selected cases.

SUMMARY

With the increasing demands of the rhinoplasty in Asian populations, there are mounting cases for the purpose of the revision or enhancement in rhinoplasty as well. To obtain a successful result of revision rhinoplasty in Asian, early detection, prompt management, and appropriate treatment of complications are essential for minimizing postoperative adverse consequences. There is no standard therapeutic technique for the various deformities and complications. The individual strategy needs to be comprehensive evaluation based on the anatomical and pathological features of patients, patients' demands, and the surgeon's experience. Psychological assessment of the patients before revision rhinoplasty, surgical risks, and the close observation during perioperative period is the great important factors to achieve the patient satisfactions.

Acknowledgements

This study was supported by Shanghai Clinical Medicine Research Center for the Plastic and Reconstructive Surgery, Shanghai Commission of Science and Technology (Grant ID: 22MC1940300)

CLINICAL CARE POINTS

- With an increasing incidence of revision rhinoplasty, costal cartilage has become one of the most popular choices of nasal grafts due to its robust strength and ample volume in Asian rhinoplasty.

- The early detection, prompt management, and appropriate treatment of complications are essential for minimizing postoperative adverse consequences.

- The balance of supportive strength of the implants and the retraction force of the nasal skin and lining was the critical element of stability after rhinoplasty.

REFERENCES

1. Wei J, Herrler T, Deng N, et al. The use of expanded polytetrafluoroethylene in short nose elongation: fourteen years of clinical experience. Ann Plast Surg 2018;81(1):7–11.
2. Yu BF, Qiu YQ, Du MX, et al. Contralateral hemi-fifth-lumbar nerve transfer for unilateral lower limb dysfunction due to incomplete traumatic spinal cord injury: a report of two cases. Microsurgery 2020;40(2):234–40.
3. Na HG, Jang YJ. Dorsal augmentation using alloplastic implants. Facial Plast Surg 2017;33(2): 189–94.
4. Jang YJ, Moon BJ. State of the art in augmentation rhinoplasty: implant or graft. Curr Opin Otolaryngol Head Neck Surg 2012;20(4):280–6.
5. Lan MY, Jang YJ. Revision rhinoplasty for short noses in the asian population. JAMA Facial Plast Surg 2015;17(5):325–32.
6. Wei J, Zhang J, Herrler T, et al. Correction of severe short nose using a costal cartilage extension framework. Ann Plast Surg 2020;85(5):472–5.
7. Jang YJ, Kim DY. Treatment strategy for revision rhinoplasty in asians. Facial Plast Surg 2016;32(6): 615–9.
8. Liu Y, Wei J, Dai C, et al. Supra Alar island flap and costal cartilage for "Arrow Tail" short nose deformity correction. J Plast Reconstr Aesthet Surg 2021; 74(7):1633–701.
9. Jung DH, Medikeri GS, Chang GU, et al. Surgical Techniques for the correction of postrhinoplasty depressed scars on the nasal tip. JAMA Facial Plast Surg 2015;17(6):405–12.
10. Weathers WM, Bhadkamkar M, Wolfswinkel EM, et al. Full-thickness skin grafting in nasal reconstruction. Semin Plast Surg 2013;27(2):90–5.
11. Wei J, Chen Q, Herrler T, et al. Supermicrosurgical reconstruction of nasal tip defects using the preauricular reversed superficial temporal artery flap. J Plast Reconstr Aesthet Surg 2020;73(1):58–64.
12. Li S, Cao W, Cheng K, et al. Microvascular reconstruction of nasal ala using a reversed superficial temporal artery auricular flap. J Plast Reconstr Aesthet Surg 2006;59(12):1300–4.
13. Weng R, Li Q, Gu B, et al. Extended forehead skin expansion and single-stage nasal subunit plasty for nasal reconstruction. Plast Reconstr Surg 2010; 125(4):1119–28.
14. Schuster B. Injection rhinoplasty with hyaluronic acid and calcium hydroxyapatite: a retrospective survey investigating outcome and complication rates. Facial Plast Surg 2015;31(3):301–7.
15. Fagien S, Bertucci V, von Grote E, et al. Rheologic and physicochemical properties used to differentiate injectable hyaluronic acid filler products. Plast Reconstr Surg 2019;143(4):707e–20e.
16. Kumar V, Jain A, Atre S, et al. Non-surgical rhinoplasty using hyaluronic acid dermal fillers: a systematic review. J Cosmet Dermatol 2021;20(8):2414–24.
17. Bouaoud J, Belloc JB. Use of injectables in rhinoplasty retouching: towards an evolution of surgical strategy? Literature review. J Stomatol Oral Maxillofac Surg 2020;121(5):550–5.
18. Kurkjian TJ, Ahmad J, Rohrich RJ. Soft-tissue fillers in rhinoplasty. Plast Reconstr Surg 2014;133(2): 121e–6e.
19. Beleznay K, Carruthers J, Humphrey S, et al. Update on avoiding and treating blindness from fillers: a recent review of the world literature. Aesthet Surg J 2019;39(6):662–74.
20. Bertossi D, Giampaoli G, Verner I, et al. Complications and management after a nonsurgical rhinoplasty: a literature review. Dermatol Ther 2019; 32(4):e12978.
21. Moon BJ, Lee HJ, Jang YJ. Outcomes following rhinoplasty using autologous costal cartilage. Arch Facial Plast Surg 2012;14(3):175–80.
22. Kim DW, Shah AR, Toriumi DM. Concentric and eccentric carved costal cartilage: a comparison of warping. Arch Facial Plast Surg 2006;8(1):42–6.
23. Park JH, Jin HR. Use of autologous costal cartilage in Asian rhinoplasty. Plast Reconstr Surg 2012; 130(6):1338–48.
24. Huang J, Liu Y. A modified technique of septal extension using a septal cartilage graft for short-nose rhinoplasty in Asians. Aesthetic Plast Surg 2012;36(5):1028–38.

Endoscopic-Assisted Transaxillary Breast Augmentation

Jie Luan, MD

KEYWORDS

• Breast augmentation • Transaxillary approach • Endoscope technique

KEY POINTS

- Endoscope technique is the best option for transaxillary breast augmentation. It greatly increases control over the process, avoids various drawbacks, reduces the incidence of complications, and improves the stability of clinical effects of transaxillary implant breast augmentation.
- Freestyle endoscopic technique may greatly improve the flexibility and efficiency of the endoscope operation through the axillary approach.
- In most Asian patients that need to lower the IMF, the high position dual-plane technique is helpful to keep the thickness of the inferior pole, avoid dynamic deformity and double-bubble deformity, and prevent long-term settling of the implant.

 Video content accompanies this article at http://www.plasticsurgery.theclinics.com.

INTRODUCTION

Breast augmentation with implants is becoming a more widely accepted and popular procedure in Asia. The axillary approach remains the preferred incision for Asian women. One of my findings suggested that the axillary approach was chosen up to 78% in Chinese women without any preaching.[1] The main reason for this is that Asian women are more concerned that the incision would expose that they had undergone previous mammoplasty surgery.

It is well known that among the three commonly used incision approaches, axillary incision augmentation mammaplasty with blind vision has the disadvantages of more trauma and pain, and longer recovery time with highest complication rate.[2]

In 1993, Eaves and colleagues[3] first used endoscope for breast augmentation through axillary approach, using a retractor-mounted endoscope system, which fixes the endoscope body on a U-shaped retractor. The endoscopic technique improved bleeding control and pocket dissection. However, the retractor-mounted endoscope has many disadvantages, such as: limited view field, inflexible operation, and hardship. Unlike the inframammary fold (IMF) incision, the type II and type III dual-plane cannot be achieved through the axillary approach. So the endoscope technique was not popularized for a long period of time.

To facilitate surgical operation through the axillary approach, I designed a special retractor and proposed a new technique called "freestyle endoscopic technique." This technology separates the endoscope from the retractor, so that the endoscope is moved and rotated independently, the field of view is fully exposed, and the electrosurgical knife is freely and conveniently moved in the pocket, which greatly improves the flexibility and efficiency of the endoscope operation.

In 2009 I proposed a technique to release the pectoralis major above the original IMF,[4] called high position dual-plane (high dual-plane). I found

Department of Breast Plastic Surgery, Plastic Surgery Hospital of Chinese Academy of Medical Sciences, 33 , Badachu Road, Shijingshan District, Beijing 100144, China
E-mail address: doctorluan@vip.163.com

Clin Plastic Surg 50 (2023) 151–162
https://doi.org/10.1016/j.cps.2022.08.010
0094-1298/23/© 2022 Elsevier Inc. All rights reserved.

that cutting the pectoralis major at a high position can release the connection between the proximal pectoralis major and the IMF, so that type II and III dual-plane is easily formed and effectively avoiding dynamic deformity and double-bubble deformity. The preserved distal pectoralis major muscle not only increases the thickness of the inferior pole of the breast, but also effectively prevents downward displacement of the smooth round implant to a certain extent.

In this article, I introduce the free-style endoscopic-assisted transaxillary breast augmentation with high dual-plane technique.

PREOPERATIVE EVALUATION AND SPECIAL CONSIDERATIONS
Patient Communication and Education

Issues that Asian women are usually concerned about include soft touch; hidden incision scars; narrow cleavage; and to solve such problems as nipple expansion, breast asymmetry, and breast ptosis. In fact, many patients' requirements cannot be achieved through a simple breast augmentation surgery, or they must incur higher costs and risks. Some deformities, such as breast asymmetry and separated nipples, are more obvious after breast augmentation. Therefore, adequate and effective communication before surgery is necessary. Through communication, patients should have reasonable expectations for the effect of surgery, have a clear understanding of their own limitations, and fully accept the risk of complications.

Preoperative Examination and Measurement

The primary purpose of preoperative examination is to understand the patient's physical condition, including systemic and local examinations, to make a correct and objective assessment of the patient's surgical conditions. Thin subcutaneous tissue, thoracic deformity, breast asymmetry, nipple asymmetry, excessive nipple spacing (nipple separation), constrictive IMF, and sagging breasts are the most common adverse conditions affecting postoperative outcomes. It is almost impossible for patients with the previously mentioned disadvantageous conditions to achieve satisfactory results. In some patients, fat grafting should be taken to mask these deformities and asymmetries as much as possible and reduce the poor postoperative appearance.

Linear measurements are the basis for evaluating basic conditions and symmetry, and for implant selection and preoperative design. The base width (BW) value is used to evaluate whether the breast bases are symmetric. For Asian women, patients with smaller breast width often require larger implants, so BW value is usually not an indicator for determining implant width. I suggest using the distance between parasternal line and anterior axillary line as the reference value for determine the width of the implant. The maximum width of the implant should be 1 cm less than the distance between parasternal line and anterior axillary line.

Digital technology that uses a three-dimensional scanner to record three-dimensional images of the breast is more and more commonly used in the measurement and evaluation of breast augmentation preoperation and postoperation. This digital technology can obtain more accurate measurement data than traditional methods, and can obtain data that cannot be measured using traditional methods. Three-dimensional scanning technology is an accurate, convenient, and repeatable measurement method for objective effect evaluation and research before and after breast surgery.[5,6]

Preoperative Marking

Because of the longer distance of the axillary approach, precise control of the boundary of the pocket is more difficult and requires careful preoperative design. The focus of preoperative design is to determine the boundaries of pocket dissection and important anatomic landmarks (**Fig. 1**).

No touch zone
For medium-sized Asian women, I generally recommend setting the width of the "no touch zone" at 2.5 cm.

Lateral border
The lateral dissection boundary is usually based on the medial boundary, plus 1 cm based on the width of the prosthesis and marked with a caliper. When the lateral border extends beyond the anterior axillary line, there is an increased risk of nipple areolar complex (NAC) sensory decrease and palpability of the implant.

New inframammary fold
IMF is one of the most important morphologic markers affecting the postoperative result of prosthetic breast augmentation. It is usually determined and marked by measuring the distance from the base of the nipple in the state of maximum retraction. There are many different formulas used to determine the new IMF. However, the formulas currently used ignore the influence of implant and breast projection.

Through years of aesthetic, morphologic, and clinical follow-up research,[7] I proposed a new

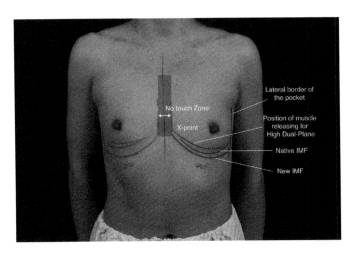

Fig. 1. Preoperative drawing.

IMF localization formula based on aesthetics, geometry, and tissue behavior (AGT):

New N-IMF (under max stretch) = 1/2(W + T) + 1/3(P + Pb),

where W is implant width; T is subcutaneous soft tissue thickness around the implant, simplified as STPTIMF measurement; P is implant projection; and Pb is breast projection.

When the original breast convexity is negligible, the formula is simplified as:

New N-IMF (under max stretch) = 1/2(W + P)

It should be noted that this formula is only suitable for dual-plane, subfascial plane, and submammary plane, not for the complete subpectoralis plane. It should also be emphasized that because the positioning of the new IMF is carried out with the nipple in the state of maximum upward stretch, the method of pulling the nipple greatly affects the accuracy of positioning. Pinch the tip of the ruler with thumb and forefinger, place the tip of thumb at the zero mark, and place this point at the base of the nipple. Use the middle finger to clamp the nipple from the opposite side of the thumb and pull it upward to the maximum extent. At the same time, place the soft ruler close to the skin surface of the lower pole of the breast, and make a mark according to the value calculated by the formula. Based on this marked point, draw a new IMF with the patient's upper arms raised (**Fig. 2**).

The location of pectoralis major muscle transection

This marking always starts from the intersection of the distal end of lower sternum and the parasternal line. I call this point the "X point." No matter what type of dual-plane is performed, the attachment of the pectoralis major on the sternum above this point must be preserved and cannot be severed. When forming a high dual-plane, mark 1 cm above the original IMF at the vertical line through the nipple, connect this point to the X point with a curve approximately parallel to the original IMF, and extend outward.

The original inframammary fold

The original IMF should be marked before surgery to show the relationship between the extent of dissection and the original IFM, especially when there is a tightening IMF that requires intraoperative release. It should be noted that the IMF moves up significantly when the upper arm is raised in some patients. Therefore, the moved position should be also marked as a reference for intraoperative release.

SURGICAL PROCEDURES
Axillary Incision and Approach

Please refer to Video 1 for details. The axillary incision is usually 4 cm long and is made on a hidden skinfold. The front end should not exceed the anterior axillary fold to avoid exposure. After making skin incision, dissect the subcutaneous tissue toward the lateral border of the pectoralis major muscle, on the surface of the superficial axillary fascia, and avoid entering the back of the superficial axillary fascia and injury to the axillary lymphoid tissue. In this layer, a superficial subcutaneous vessel that is perpendicular to the incision direction and runs across the anterior axillary fold is often seen (**Fig. 3**A), which should be detected and hemostasized in time. Dissect along the subcutaneous layer to the lateral edge of the pectoralis major muscle, and cut the pectoralis major

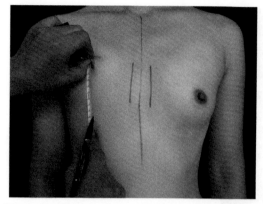

Fig. 2. Positioning of the new IMF. Place the zero mark of the soft ruler at the base of the nipple. Use the thumb and middle finger to clamp the nipple and the ruler. Pull them upward to the maximum extent. Mark at the new IMF position.

fascia in parallel. Enter the subpectoral space closely against the pectoralis major, which is a technique to avoid mistakenly entering the subpectoralis minor. After lifting the lateral edge of the pectoralis major, a bundle of lateral thoracic vessels and branches of the nerve is encountered between the pectoralis major and minor muscles (**Fig. 3**B), which are sentinel vessels that enter the subpectoral space. Coagulation and severing of this vessel allow unblocked access to the subpectoral space.

Principles of Endoscopic-Assisted Surgical Dissection

The endoscopic surgical dissection process should follow these basic principles:

1. Keep the surgical field of view clear by wiping the lens with a defogger, keeping the negative pressure suction system effective, and timely hemostasis. Do not perform any surgical dissection with unclear vision, otherwise there is a risk of serious complications.
2. Use electrosurgery or ultrasonic scalpel for dissection. The electrocautery should be set in spray or mixed coagulating mode. Do not use cutting mode during the whole process to avoid bleeding or deep tissue cutting. The use of ultrasonic knife clamping, cutting, sweeping, and other operations can more effectively complete hemostasis while separating, thereby ensuring a clean wound surface and a clear vision.
3. Prehemostasis: Under endoscopy, bleeding control is more difficult because of the long surgical approach. Once severe bleeding occurs, it greatly affects the clarity of the surgical field and makes hemostasis more difficult. The so-called prehemostasis means that the blood vessel is discovered in advance, and it is coagulated before it is cut off (**Fig. 4**). The ultrasonic scalpel itself has a good hemostatic effect, and generally there is little bleeding. Even if bleeding occurs, it is easy to control.

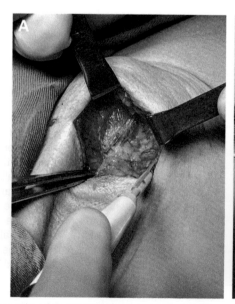
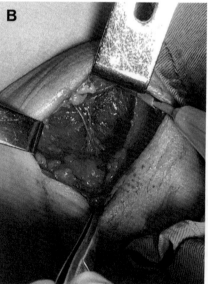

Fig. 3. Dissection of the transaxillary approach. (*A*) The superficial subcutaneous vessel across the anterior axillary fold. (*B*) The sentinel vessels between the pectoralis major and minor muscles.

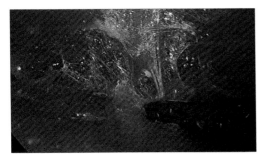

Fig. 4. Prehemostasis technique. Discover the perforating branch of the blood vessel and coagulate it before it is cut off.

4. Perform surgical dissections in the sequence of lateral superior to central-lateral, central-medial, and inferior pole.

Freestyle Endoscopic Technique

In 1998, I designed a retractor specially used for endoscopic breast augmentation and proposed a freestyle endoscopic breast augmentation technique (Fig. 5). The retractor is controlled by the assistant, while the surgeon holds the endoscope in one hand and the electric knife in the other. By coordinating the positional relationship between the endoscope and the electrosurgical knife, the surgeon can obtain the best viewing angle and the best operating space, while focusing on anatomic structure identification and accurate dissection performance under the endoscope. Through this technique, the surgeon's control of the endoscope and the electrosurgical knife becomes flexible, and the endoscope is placed on the side of the passage and the dissection cavity, which greatly expands the range of motion of the electrosurgical knife. In the freestyle endoscope operation mode, mastering the positional relationship of endoscope-electrosurgical knife-retractor is the key to ensure the success of the operation.

Key Points of Surgical Dissection in Each Region

Fig. 6 provides a typical placement for reference when separating different parts. The surgeon saves labor and can focus on the delicate and complex endoscopic operations.

Superior region
This is the area with the loosest tissue and the easiest surgical dissection, and a "sweep" technique is used. To ensure that the channel is wide enough, the lateral side needs to be dissected to the lateral edge of the pectoralis minor muscle.

Central-lateral region
Dissection was performed along the lateral border of the pectoralis minor muscle to the caudal end, and the lateral border was dissected by a combination of pressure and cutting (Fig. 7A). To the fourth and fifth intercostal space, the attachment of the pectoralis major muscle on each rib is cut from lateral to medial, and the central area below the nipple is dissected. It should be noted that large perforating vessels are often seen in the fourth and fifth intercostal spaces, and they should be cut off after prehemostasis. Turn the camera laterally to dissect at the surface of the serratus anterior along the lateral border of the pectoralis minor muscle. Care should be taken to observe and protect the lateral intercostal nerves (Fig. 7B), which usually run vertically upward and subcutaneously along with small blood vessels. If the nerve is too medial, more than 0.5 cm from the lateral border, it needs to be released. The sensibility of the nipple is affected. This should be adequately informed to the patient before surgery. Special attention should be paid to the level of surgical separation, neither too deep into the serratus anterior, nor too shallow to affect thickness of the tissue.

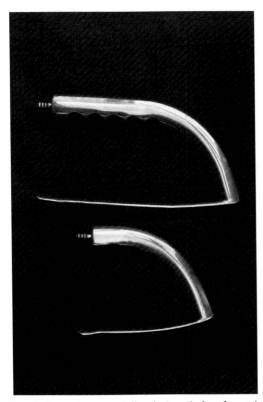

Fig. 5. Retractors specially designed for freestyle endoscopic breast augmentation technique.

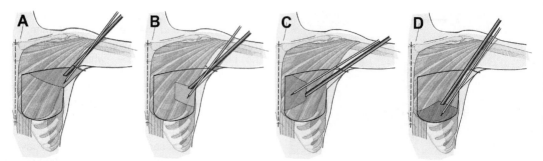

Fig. 6. Subregions of the pocket dissection. (*A*) The superior region. (*B*) The central-lateral region. (*C*) The central-medial region. (*D*) The inferior-inframammary fold region.

Central-medial region

The attachments of the pectoralis major muscle at the third to fifth ribs are cut off in sequence, and it should be noted that obvious intrathoracic perforators are often seen in the third intercostal space. When the perforators of the internal thoracic vessels are found in each intercostal space, it indicates that the distance from the medial border is close. After medial thoracic perforators are cut off, even with a puncture needle, the attachments of the pectoralis major muscle on ribs should be carefully identified and carefully cut off. Do not cut off the attachments of the pectoralis major to the sternum.

Inferior-inframammary fold region

This is also an area that requires careful separation. Cut off the muscle attachments on the sixth rib, and the upper edge of the external oblique muscle is seen on the lower lateral side. It is tightly adhered inward by the aponeurosis with the anterior sheath of the rectus abdominis and the lateral bundle of the pectoralis major. Dissect the superficial surface of the external oblique fascia from the deep surface of the pectoralis major muscle from the lateral side to the medial side, and avoid entering the deep surface of the external oblique muscle (**Fig. 7C**). The medial-inferior should be carefully dissected deep to the pectoralis major and superficial to the anterior sheath of the rectus abdominis. A considerable number of patients have low nipple positions, and the new IMF designed is correspondingly low. Under this circumstance, part of the medial-inferior attachments of the pectoralis major may be completely released, and only the lateral bundle of the lateral pectoralis major remains intact (**Fig. 7D**).

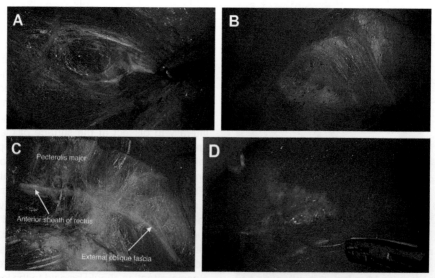

Fig. 7. Endoscopic-assisted surgical dissection. (*A*) Dissection in lateral side along lateral edge of the pectoralis minor muscle. (*B*) The lateral intercostal nerves should be protected if possible. (*C*) Avoid entering the deep surface of the external oblique muscle and anterior sheath of rectus. (*D*) Part of the medial-inferior attachments of the pectoralis major need to be completely released in some cases.

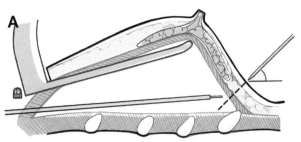
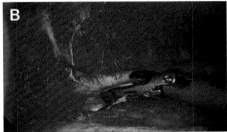

Fig. 8. Precise pocket boundary dissection. (*A*) Insert the needle according to the designed line on the body surface with an angle of 45°. Stop dissection after crossing the needle tip about 0.5 cm. (*B*) Dissect an accurate boundary of the pocket following the guidance of the needle.

Boundary Control of Surgical Dissection

To achieve precise control of the boundary of the pocket, the retractor is pointed in the direction of the boundary and the skin is stretched to simulate the tight state of the skin after the implant is placed. The assistant pierces the needle through the skin and subcutaneous tissue following the preoperative markers to provide guide to the operator. Usually, the implant causes traction on the surrounding skin, causing the skin to slide and shift toward the center. This shift is more pronounced on the lateral and lower parts of the breast. Therefore, for the medial, lower, and lateral boundaries, the methods of needle insertion and reference must be different. Dissection to the medial boundary and the IMF requires more caution. The needle insertion direction should be kept at a 45° angle to the body surface. When the surgeon sees the needle tip under the endoscope, it must continue to dissect a small distance forward. This distance is approximately equal to the thickness of the subcutaneous tissue there, typically about 0.5 cm (**Fig. 8**A, B). The lateral boundary is usually used to make final adjustments. The direction of the retractor should be outward, the direction of the needle is perpendicular to the skin, and the dissection is stopped when the needle tip is seen.

High Position Dual-Plane Creation

The concept of dual-plane was first proposed by Tebbetts,[7] which means that the pectoralis major muscle is cut off at 1 cm above the new IMF, and then the proximal end of the muscle is dissected upward to different levels to form type I, II, and III dual-plane.

In eastern women, most of the patients have breast dysplasia, and the designed new IMF position is usually lower than the original IMF, that is, the IMF must be lowered down. According to Tebbetts' method, the location of the transected muscle is usually below the native IMF in Asian women. Under the endoscopic-assisted axillary approach,

it is impossible to perform a reverse dissection from the broken end of the pectoralis major to create type II and III dual-plane, resulting in an insufficiently full lower pole shape and a series of problems in some patients, such as double-bubble and dynamic deformity (**Fig. 9**).

The high dual-plane technique is proposed for the previously mentioned problems. The pectoralis major muscle is released 1 cm above the original IMF to form a high dual-plane. The difference between this technique and traditional dual-plane technique is the position at which the muscle is transected.

The high dual-plane must be performed after the pocket is completely dissected. The operative space was fully exposed with a retractor, and the needle was punctured and positioned following the marked line on the body surface. Starting from the lateral edge of the pectoralis major, the muscle is released from the lateral side to the medial side with an electric knife or an ultrasonic knife to expose the posterior fat layer of the mammary gland. Manual pressure is applied to the outer skin surface to increase muscle tone for ease of cutting. It should be noted that the depth

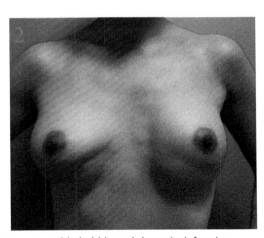

Fig. 9. Double-bubble and dynamic deformity.

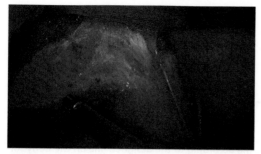

Fig. 10. Type II or III dual-plane creation. After releasing the muscle at a high position above the original IMF, create type II or III dual-plane by easily pulling the proximal end of the muscle upward using the retractor.

head under the skin or apply force forward, which may lead to severe complications of penetrating the subcutaneous tissue. When the muscle is completely severed above the original IMF, the retractor is placed on the proximal end of the muscle and pulled upward. Because the proximal end of the muscle is no longer bound by the original IMF, it is lifted to an appropriate height without stripping, forming a type II or type III dual-plane (Fig. 10).

Release of the Original Inframammary Fold

When the patient has signs of IMF tightening and the IMF has to be low, no matter what type of dual-plane is formed, the original IMF ligament must be released. Otherwise, the double-bubble deformity is caused by the tight fibrous strands at the IMF. The high dual-plane technique creates conditions for endoscopic-assisted IMF release through the axillary approach. Because the position of the severed muscle in the high dual-plane technique is located above the original IMF, the distal muscle retreats down to the IMF ligament and terminates, just exposing the fibrous connection between the IMF ligament and the subcutaneous tissue. It is easily released with either

of the electrocautery must be controlled to avoid damaging the subcutaneous fat as much as possible. In addition, the muscle is rich in blood supply, which should be electrocoagulated in advance and then cut off, so as to ensure reliable hemostasis. If the ultrasonic knife is used, the muscle and fascia should be sequentially clipped from the lateral edge of the pectoralis major. At the same time of clamping and cutting, apply force inward to lift up the muscle. Do not point the knife

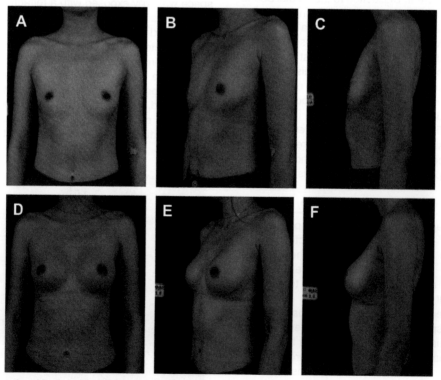

Fig. 11. Case 1, a 29-year-old woman. Primary breast augmentation with Mentor-CPG322-255cc implants. (A–C) Before operation. (D–F) Six months after operation.

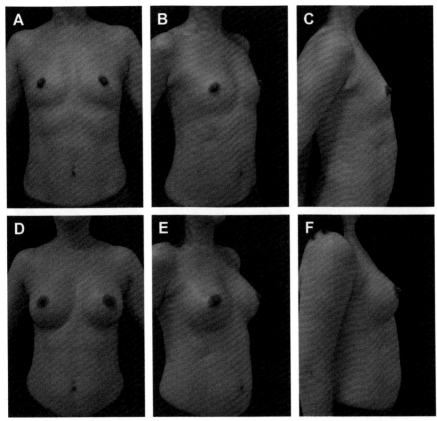

Fig. 12. Case 2, a 42-year-old woman. Primary breast augmentation with implants (Mentor-smooth round mp-250cc). (*A–C*) Before operation. (*D–F*) Two years after operation.

electrosurgery or ultrasonic scalpel. The operation is basically like that of muscle dissection, but the direction is different, and the layers are superficial. More attention should be paid to controlling the depth and preserving sufficient subcutaneous tissue thickness.

POSTOPERATIVE CARE AND EXPECTED OUTCOME

1. Use the elastic band on the upper pole of the breast at 1 month postoperation.
2. Remove drains when the daily volume of drainage is less than 40 mL.
3. Encourage patients to exercise their upper extremities early but avoid heavy loads and strenuous upper extremity exercises within 1 month.
4. For anatomic implant, it is recommended to ask the patient to lie on her stomach and place a hard pillow on the upper half of the breast, for at least 1 hour a day, starting 3 weeks after surgery. This helps to promote the capsule softening.

5. Keep in touch with the patient and review regularly.

CASE DEMONSTRATIONS

Figs. 11–14 provide case demonstrations.

MANAGEMENT OF COMPLICATIONS

The complications of endoscopic-assisted breast augmentation through the axillary approach are basically the same as those of other approaches. However, the axillary incision approach has a long operating distance, and even with the assistance of an endoscope, the risk of complications is greater than that of the areola approach or the IMF approach.

Pneumothorax

The main causes of pneumothorax are unfamiliarity with anatomy, misoperation of electrocautery, thoracic deformity, and so forth. During the operation of the electric knife, the electric coagulation

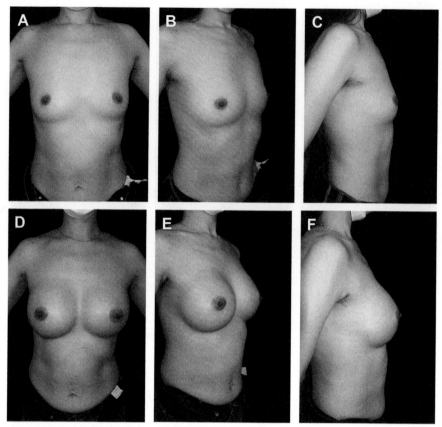

Fig. 13. Case 3, a 36-year-old woman. Primary breast augmentation with implants (Natrelle-STF1-SRF-295). (*A–C*) Before operation. (*D–F*) Two years after operation.

mode must be set in the whole process, and the pedal switch should be used to avoid accidently triggering the handle switch. When the patient has thoracic deformity or a rib is partially protruded, it is necessary to pay special attention to the direction of the electrocautery and the level of dissection to avoid accidental injury to the intercostal muscles. If a pneumothorax is inadvertently caused, the typical sign is that air bubbles emerge from the surface of the chest wall when the patient exhales. The incision should be sutured under the endoscope or through an additional areola incision. When the suture is ligated, it is necessary to cooperate with the anesthesiologist and inflate the lungs with a ventilator. Postoperative chest radiographs should be taken to check the compression of the lungs, and a thoracic drainage is used if necessary.

Hemorrhage

Hemostasis through the axillary approach is more difficult than other approaches. Mild bleeding under the endoscope is directly coagulated by electric knife, whereas hemorrhea needs to be compressed by small pieces of adrenaline saline gauze first, and then hemostasis with special bipolar electric coagulation forceps for endoscope when blood vessel constriction and bleeding is reduced. In case of uncontrolled hemorrhage, additional incision is made through the areola to stop the bleeding under direct vision if necessary.

Injury to Subcutaneous Tissue

Except for the release of IMF ligaments, electrosurgical or ultrasonic scalpel operations should not enter the subcutaneous adipose layer. Once the subcutaneous tissue is damaged, the local soft tissue will be too thin and the implant will be easily touched. In severe cases, the implant forms local wrinkles and sharp angles. Therefore, the level and depth of tissue dissection should be carefully controlled when stripping the lower polar boundary of the breast, severing the pectoral muscle and releasing the IMF ligament, especially in patients with thin subcutaneous tissue.

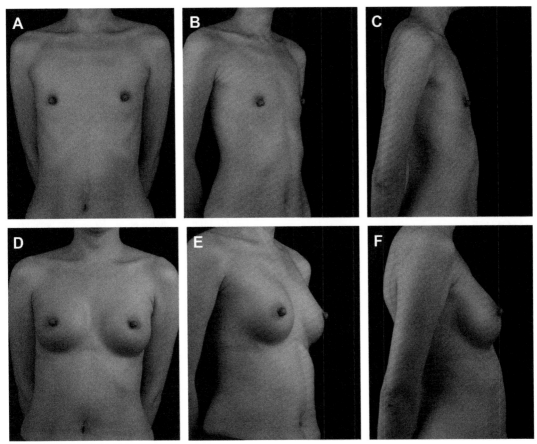

Fig. 14. Case 4, a 38-year-old woman. Primary breast augmentation with anatomic implants (Natrelle-ST-FF255). (*A–C*) Before operation. (*D–F*) Two years after operation.

Dynamic Deformity and Double-Bubble Deformity

The dynamic deformity is caused by the release of the muscle below the original IMF position, so that the proximal pectoralis major and the original IMF are not effectively released. In some cases, although the high dual-plane is performed above the original IMF, if the transection is not complete, there is still a bond between the muscle and the original IMF, which can also cause dynamic deformities. If there is constrictive IMF and the IMF ligaments are not released or partially released intraoperatively, a double-bubble deformity occurs. These two deformities are often associated.

Implant Malposition

The reasons for this complication include inaccurate preoperative design of IMF location, and insufficient or excessive dissection. Incompletely severed muscles during dual-plane formation can also cause upward displacement of the implant.

Therefore, it is necessary to precisely control the dissection boundary. If the dissection is insufficient, it is observed and adjusted after implantation of the implant or sizer. Once the dissection is excessive, sutures must be performed to reconstruct the IMF. IMF reconstruction can only be performed through other additional incisions (areola or inferior fold) if the surgeon has no experience with deep suturing through the endoscopic transaxillary approach. For slight malposition, adjustment is attempted by compression fixation for a long period after surgery.

SUMMARY

Current endoscope technique greatly increases control over the process, avoids various drawbacks, reduces the incidence of complications, and improves the stability of clinical effects of transaxillary implant breast augmentation. The freestyle endoscopic technique greatly improves the flexibility and efficiency of the endoscope operation through axillary approach. The high dual-plane technique makes it possible to create type II and III dual-plane, effectively avoids dynamic deformity and double-bubble deformity, increases the thickness of the inferior pole of the breast, and prevents the long-term settle down of the implant. The AGT formula for new IMF positioning and standard intraoperative navigation technique ensure a precise new IMF and improve predictability and controllability of the new IMF location. All these meet the requirements of Asian women for hiding the incision scar, while achieving safety and satisfactory surgical outcomes.

DISCLOSURE

The author has no financial interest to declare in relation to the drugs, devices, and products mentioned in this article.

SUPPLEMENTARY DATA

Supplementary data related to this article can be found online at https://doi.org/10.1016/j.cps.2022.08.010.

REFERENCES

1. Sun J, Liu C, Luan J, et al. Chinese women's preferences and concerns regarding incision location for breast augmentation surgery: a survey of 216 patients. Aesthet Plast Surg 2015;39(2):214–26.
2. Hidalgo DA, Spector JA. Breast augmentation. Plast Reconstr Surg 2014;133(4):567–83.
3. Eaves FF, Price CI, Bostwick J. Subcutaneous endoscopic plastic surgery using a retractor-mounted endoscope system. Perspect Plast Surg 1993;7:1–22.
4. Luan J, Mu D, Mu L. Transaxillary dual-plane augmentation mammaplasty: experience with 98 breasts. J Plast Reconstr Aesthet Surg 2009;62(11):1459–63.
5. Liu C, Luan J, Ji K, et al. Measuring volumetric change after augmentation mammaplasty using a three-dimensional scanning technique: an innovative method. J.Aesthetic Plast Surg 2012;36(5):1134–9.
6. Ji K, Luan J, Liu C, et al. A prospective study of breast dynamic morphological changes after dual-plane augmentation mammaplasty with 3D scanning technique. PLoS One 2014;9(3):e93010.
7. Tebbetts JB. Dual plane breast augmentation: optimizing implant-soft-tissue relationships in a wide range of breast types. Plast Reconstr Surg 2001; 107(5):1255–72.

Endoscopic-Assisted Abdominoplasty

Cheng-Jen Chang, MD, PhD, FACS, FICS[a,b,c,d,*]

KEYWORDS

• Endoscopy • Abdominoplasty • Diastasis recti • Fibrin sealants

KEY POINTS

- The major advantage of endoscopic-assisted abdominoplasty is the minimal scarring.
- A learning curve is required to achieve optimal technique and results.
- Certain patients with diastasis recti benefit from this surgery.
- Limitations of this technique must be acknowledged.
- The combination of the endoscopic technique with fibrin sealant can produce favorable results in an optimal surgical time frame.

INTRODUCTION

Regarding the treatment of postgestation abdominal wall deformities, studies continue to pursue optimal scar reduction that commonly results from the standard "dog ear technique."[1–8] Johnson developed endoscopically-assisted abdominoplasty in 1991. Evolving studies of endoscopic treatment of the abdominal wall have explored novel areas of application in pursuit of leaving minimal scarring and determining the precise patient base that would optimally benefit from such treatment.[9] In this review, the author introduces his preferred technique in endoscopic-assisted abdominoplasty. Indications of the procedure, preoperative evaluation and special consideration, surgical technique, postoperative care and expected outcome, management of complications, revision or subsequent procedures are described in detail. In addition, the pearls for the success are also discussed.

INDICATIONS AND CONTRAINDICATIONS

Patients that are (1) averse to postoperative abdominal scars, (2) require muscle fascia repair without panniculectomy, (3) have diastasis recti (Type A) and fascial laxity sufficiently serious as to benefit from repair, (4) have abdominal skin that would shrink without associated excision of excess skin in conjunction with liposuction in a preoperative evaluation, and (5) have a body mass index between 24 and 35 can attain optimal results. Patients with ventral or umbilical hernia must be ruled out preoperatively. Open procedure is an option for patients with a large pannus and poor skin elasticity.

PREOPERATIVE EVALUATIONS AND SPECIAL CONSIDERATIONS

Each patient should undergo routine laboratory work, an electrocardiogram, chest X-ray, human

[a] Department of Plastic and Reconstructive Surgery, Chang Gung Memorial Hospital, Chang Gung University, No. 5, Fuxing Street, Guishan District, Taoyuan City 333423, Taiwan; [b] Department of Plastic Surgery, Taipei Medical University Hospital, Taipei Medical University, No. 252, Wuxing Street, Xinyi District, Taipei City 110301, Taiwan; [c] Department of Surgery, School of Medicine, College of Medicine, Taipei Medical University, No. 252, Wuxing Street, Xinyi District, Taipei City 110301, Taiwan; [d] Graduate Institute of Biomedical Optomechatronics, College of Biomedical Engineering, Taipei Medical University, No. 252, Wuxing Street, Xinyi District, Taipei City 110301, Taiwan
* Department of Plastic Surgery, Taipei Medical University Hospital, Taipei Medical University, No.252, Wu Hsing Street, Taipei City 110, Taiwan.
E-mail address: chengjen@h.tmu.edu.tw

Clin Plastic Surg 50 (2023) 163–170
https://doi.org/10.1016/j.cps.2022.08.008
0094-1298/23/© 2022 Elsevier Inc. All rights reserved.

immunodeficiency virus test, and thorough consultation with an anesthesiologist. Visual documentation is conducted pre- and postoperatively. Patients who've had previous abdominal surgery are fully examined to evaluate the optimal endoscope approach, whereas patients who have abdominal lipodystrophies, umbilical widening, or protrusion must show optimal skin elasticity and no excess skin for correction.

There are four types of diastasis recti with stretched muscle or skin tissue patients: (Type A), over-stretched rectus sheath at abdominal center; (Type B), laxity of the central and lateral abdominal area, along with the infraumbilical aponeurotic layer at either lateral side; (Type C), spreading of muscle tissue involving the congenital lateral insertion of the recti muscles; and (Type D), advanced spreading of muscle tissue with minimal support of tissue along patient's waistline has occurred. Preoperative type classification is determined using ultrasonography (**Fig. 1**).

SURGICAL PROCEDURES

The abdominal perimeter should first be marked during assessment from the costal margin (lower ribcage) on the right and left to the top of the xiphoid process of the sternum; then bilaterally along the anterior axillary lines, down to the supra-inguinal areas and the bottom of the suprapubic lines (**Fig. 2**). Internal elliptical markings are also made on the protruded lines of the bilateral rectus abdominis muscle. Both external rectal sheaths are marked with methylene blue on the midline and lateral borders. Markings are also made on the midsection to lift the pocket and apply plication (folding) of external layers of rectal sheaths of the bilateral rectus abdominis muscle. Areas of excessive fat are marked and designated

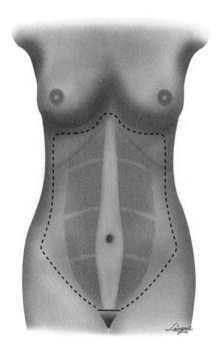

Fig. 2. Abdominal perimeter markings during preoperative assessment. (*Courtesy of* Ya-lin Lai, NTUA, New Taipei City, TW.)

for subsequent liposuction with outlined depressive areas to avoid over-liposuction.

Dissection is performed simultaneously as video endoscopic imaging relays the procedure to a connected monitor (Snowden-Pencer, Tucker, GA, USA). Once the patient receives general anesthesia and an endotracheal tube is inserted, the patient is placed in the supine position with arms extended at 80° to 90° on cushioned arm boards with the monitor in the surgeon's direct line of vision (**Fig. 3**). An indwelling Foley catheter is inserted following hair removal. To avoid visible scarring, a suprapubic incision is made below the hairline just above the rectal sheath of no more than 5 cm. During dissection at the periumbilical area, finger insertion in the umbilical fossa for prevention of umbilical injury is used if indicated. A 10mm-diameter endoscope with an angle of either 0° or 30°extends the pocket dissection from the xiphoid and subcostal margin to the side walls of the anterior axillary lines and down to reach the lower abdomen. This dissection creates a skin pocket using 1-0 Prolene transcutaneous sutures to lift for tenting and thorough passage of the scope (**Fig. 4**).

The lower abdominal dissection may be conducted using an endoscopic retractor to improve visualization of the dissected field. Regarding internal stitching for plication of the external rectal

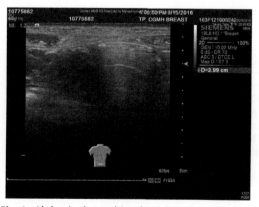

Fig. 1. Abdominal stretching (area between two focal markings) in the junction of the central rectus sheath.

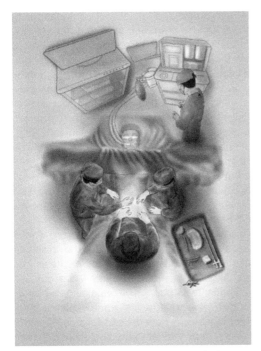

Fig. 3. Assigned stations for a right-handed surgeon according to lithotomy or operative positions (Clockwise: from top: anesthesiologist, nurse, surgeon, and assistant doctor). (*Courtesy of* Ya-lin Lai, NTUA, New Taipei City, TW.)

sheath, 2-0 Prolene sutures are double enforced by first running the sutures from the distal section of the suprapubic area to the proximal section of the infraumbilical area and then back down to the distal section where a closure tie is made at the suprapubic area. For the same procedure, a 2-0 Prolen was used for double enforcement by first running sutures from the distal of supraumbilical area to the proximal section of lower sternal area, and then back down to the distal for a closure tie to be made at the supraumbilical area (**Fig. 5**). Before wound closure, a final endoscopic hemostasis in the pocket is confirmed and repositioning of the umbilicus skin flap is set while avoiding tension to prevent poor circulation.

POSTOPERATIVE CARE AND EXPECTED OUTCOME

Although some outpatients can be discharged the same day, most patients, especially those undergoing multiple procedures or with additional medical concerns, should receive overnight care and observation. Abdominal pressure belts/garments are recommended for 3 to 6 weeks for external support. Patients are closely observed and documented at 3, 12, and 24 weeks after surgery to assess optimal correction of the abdominal protrusion from suture plication of the external rectal sheath.

All 88 patients (100%) in our study reported numbness with local paresthesia at the first 3-month assessment, which subsided gradually in all patients at the 6-month follow-up. In total, nine patients (10.2%) experienced ecchymosis, and seromas affected 3 patients (3.4%). These minor concerns were treated by syringe aspiration for 2 to 4 days and patients were guided on self-care for the prevention of seroma formation. One patient (1.1%) had dyspnea immediately after surgery but recovered after oxygen (O_2) administration. One patient (1.1%) showed minimal skin loss, but this patient recovered within 3 months following surgery and reported no further complications. No patients showed signs of hematoma nor any perioperative complications, such as prolonged seroma formation or substantial subdermal irregularities. Hypertrophic scars were apparent in three patients (3.4%) without any signs after scar revision.

MANAGEMENT OF COMPLICATIONS

Intraoperatively, numerous vessels must be transected and cauterized to create a pocket. The preservation of perforator vessels and nerves reduces

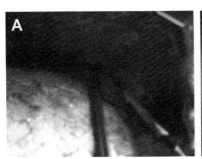
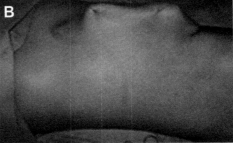

Fig. 4. Internal dissection displayed with video endoscope (A). Skin pocket using 1-0 Prolene sutures for tenting to facilitate scope passage (B).

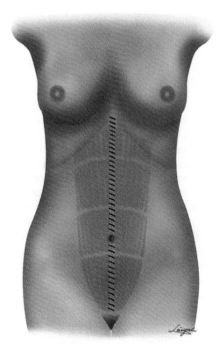

Fig. 5. Image of internal stitching using 2-0 Prolene sutures for plication of external rectus sheath. (*Courtesy of* Ya-lin Lai, NTUA, New Taipei City, TW.)

postoperative complications such as seromas, hematomas, numbness, and paresthesia. All complications were resolved and subsided within 6 months postoperatively. At the final follow-up visit, no patients showed treatment-related complications.[10]

REVISION OR SUBSEQUENT PROCEDURES

Minor hypertrophic scars, if evident, can be addressed by scar revision. Subsequent "dog ear" revision for abdominal wall contouring is not required unless the patient seeks complete body contouring and optimal reshaping.[11–13] For patients that undergo liposuction, a tumescent solution with 500 g of lidocaine, 0.5 mg of epinephrine, and 10 mEq of $NaHCO_3$ in 1000 mL normal saline is injected into the fatty layer of the abdominal wall following endoscopic surgery after the completion of the plication of the external rectal sheath. If liposuction were performed before subverting the flap of the abdominal wall, the work on the right anatomical layers would be challenging. During liposuction, removal of fat above the Scarpa fascia may enhance skin contraction; however, may result in surface layer irregularities.

To seal the tissue before wound closure, 4 mL of fibrin sealant was sprayed into the dissected pockets[14,15] In our study of 52 diastasis recti (Type A) patients, fibrin sealants were not used for 26 patients (Group I). The remaining 26 patients (Group II) were treated with fibrin sealants before wound closure. A paired *t* test for comparison of the two groups indicated no significant difference in reactions between the groups ($P > 0.05$). However, inpatient care was significantly less for those that received with fibrin sealants before endoscopic-assisted abdominoplasty wound closure than those that weren't assessed (**Table 1**).

CASE DEMONSTRATIONS
Case 1

A 40-year-old female patient with diastasis recti underwent endoscope-assisted abdominoplasty (**Fig. 6A-E**). Internal endoscopic dissection created a skin pocket for the plication of the external rectal sheath. Postoperative assessment demonstrated that these procedures were

Table 1
Results and observed side effects of 52 endoscopy-assisted abdominoplasty patients with and without fibrin sealant

Side Effects	Early (%) (3 weeks)		Late (%) (6 months)		Final (%) (≥6 months)	
Group[a]	I	II	I	II	I	II
Numbness and paresthesia	26(50)	26(50)	0	0	0	0
Ecchymosis	8 (15.4)	1(1.9)	0	0	0	0
Hypertrophic scar	2 (3.8)	1(1.9)	0	0	0	0
Seroma	3 (5.8)	0	0	0	0	0
Skin loss	1(1.9)	0	0	0	0	0
Hematoma	0	0	0	0	0	0

($P > 0.05$).
 [a] Group I: without fibrin sealant Group II: with fibrin sealant.

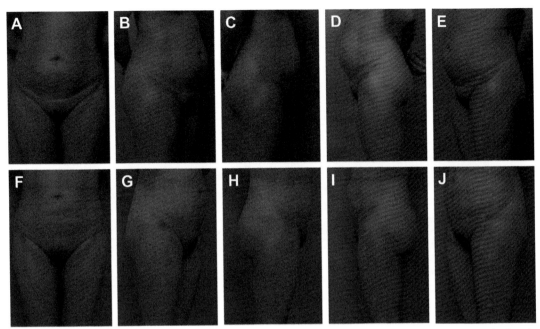

Fig. 6. Frontal, oblique, and lateral images of a 40-year-old female patient with abdominal protrusion before (A–E), and at 26-month follow-up after endoscope-assisted abdominoplasty (F–J).

effective in correcting the abdominal protrusion (Fig. 6F-J).

Case 2

A 50-year-old patient with diastasis recti deformity received combined endoscope-liposuction reconstructive surgery (Fig. 7A–C). Endoscope-assisted abdominoplasty was performed by means of a periumbilical incision with a 4-cm suprapubic incision. Plication of the external sheath of the rectus fascia was completed using 2-0 Prolene running sutures from below and above the umbilicus. A 300 mL tumescent solution was injected into the subcutaneous fatty layer of the abdominal wall.

Liposuction followed, removing 100 mL of fat and yielded favorable results (Fig. 7D–F).

Case 3

A 35-year-old female patient with diastasis recti underwent endoscope-assisted abdominoplasty through her previous scar of appendectomy (Fig. 8A, B). Internal endoscopic dissection

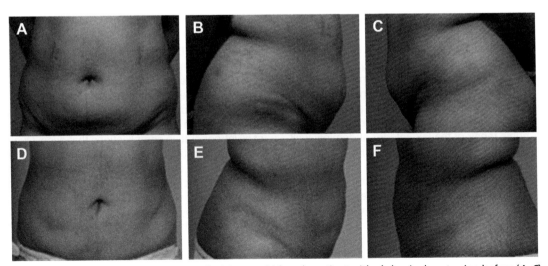

Fig. 7. Frontal and lateral images mages of a 50-year-old female patient with abdominal protrusion before (A–C), and at 21-month follow-up (D–F) after endoscope-assisted abdominoplasty.

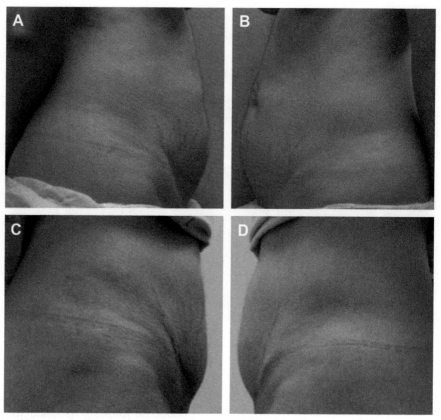

Fig. 8. Bilateral images of a 35-year-old female with postgestation diastasis recti deformity (*A, B*) before, and at 11-month result following plication of the external rectus sheath by endoscope-assisted abdominoplasty through previously incised scar of appendectomy (*C, D*).

created a skin pocket for plication of the external rectal sheath with 4 mL fibrin sealant application and produced favorable results (**Fig. 8**C, D).

DISCUSSION

In 1996, plastic surgeons began to use endoscopic techniques for forehead lifting, hyperactive muscle ablation, midface lifting, soft tissue removal, and augmentation mammoplasty.[16,17] From an aesthetic perspective, the endoscopic approach for abdominoplasty is advantageous. Endoscopic procedures for performing xiphoid-to-pubis repair of the lax anterior abdominal wall, fascia, and muscle through the limited incision are indicated for patients who require effective repair of the muscle and fascia without the excision of excess skin. Patients that meet the postoperative evaluation to undergo treatment are categorized as follows: Type A, stretching in the junction of the rectus sheath at the center of the abdominal area that central plication of the rectus sheath (PRS) is performed; Type B, laxity of the central and lateral abdominal area and the infraumbilical aponeurotic layer at either lateral side which a central PRS and L-shaped plication of the external oblique aponeurosis is performed; Type C, requiring congenital lateral insertion of the recti muscles due to the outward spreading of muscle tissue that requires moving the muscles to the center of the patient's body for the procedure; and Type D, advanced spreading of muscle tissue with minimal support along the patient's waistline where PRS and advancement of the external oblique muscles are indicated and thus, endoscopic abdominoplasty is not recommended.

Surgeons are responsible to fully inform patients of all intraoperative complications that arise. Quality standards that serve as procedural goals for treatment are required for both the open and endoscopic techniques so that, the endoscopic abdominoplasty techniques are successfully administered by surgeons who perform conventional open abdominoplasty. Furthermore, the quality of muscle and fascia repair must be at least equal to that obtained using the open technique. An endoscope can be used to enter previously incised scars following procedures such as appendectomies, cesarean sections, and laparotomies. Umbilical incisions can also be made in Y- or Z-shaped forms, where the skin flap is subverted for dissection with the creation of an umbilical incision.

Endoscopic dissection requires careful attention to hand-eye coordination by both surgeons and assistants to obtain adequate exposure by lifting the abdominal wall. Only when thorough knowledge of hemostasis, smoke filtering, fluid removal, scope care, and steady positioning of the electrode tip can the procedure run efficiently. Another challenging aspect of endoscopic abdominoplasty is repairing the fascia. A patient's tissue can be redirected with a cervical tenaculum or autosuture disposable fascia stapler. If arterial or active bleeding occurs it must be ligated intraoperatively. Previous studies have noted tissue ischemia or even skin necrosis may result once perforator vessels are cauterized or cut during dissection.[18,19] However in our study, these complications can be prevented when ligation or bleeder coagulation was conducted properly.

Essential sealant procedural steps to ensure the ultimate safety of the patient have been reported and should therefore be applied meticulously, such as awareness of the tissue samples that are exchanged or transferred among patients to prevent infection or present risk for hypersensitivity, allergic, and/or anaphylactic reactions.[20] Although no significant difference in complications was observed in our study, the use of fibrin sealants in conjunction with endoscope-assisted abdominoplasty demonstrated a positive effect against the formation of seromas and helped reduce hospitalization length.

Advantages observed in our endoscopic abdominoplasty study include a decreased incidence of scarring, bleeding, numbness, edema, and, primarily, the minimization of scarring. Painful discomfort and numbness were not observed. Noted disadvantages were observed after large vessel ligation, rather than cutting, was employed. For future studies, when large vessels are handled, steps to avoid intensified bleeding should be taken with a suitable product and endoscope use. A learning curve representing the observation and administration of these treatments by experts in the field of abdominoplasty can be referenced for mastering relevant techniques. We must focus on the aforementioned points to achieve the most favorable outcome and results for both surgeon and patient.

SUMMARY

Endoscopic-assisted abdominoplasty can be used for diastasis recti deformities with minimal excess skin. Advantages of endoscopic surgery include diminished incidence of scarring, pain sensation, numbness, bleeding, seroma, and edema. New training, a learning curve, and proper instrumentation are required, and the limitations of this technique must be acknowledged. The techniques and outcomes can be extended to support the use of robotic surgery for abdominoplasty.

CLINICS CARE POINTS

- Preoperative knowledge of anatomical landmarks and neurovascular bundles in the abdominal wall is essential.
- Existing comorbidities must be identified preoperatively.
- The quality of fascia repair must be at least equal to conventional abdominoplasty.
- A learning curve for mastering the technique is required and should only be performed by surgeons who presently conduct conventional open abdominoplasty treatment.

FUNDING

Research grants were awarded by Taipei Medical University Hospital (TMU106-AE1-B06), National Science and Technology Council (MOST 111-2221-E-038-012-), Taiwan.

DISCLOSURE

The author has no financial interests to declare in relation to the drugs, devices, or products mentioned in this article.

ACKNOWLEDGMENTS

Recognition and appreciation to the TMU Office of Research and Development, Yae-Lin Lai from the National Taiwan University of Arts, and Wallace Academic Editing, for their illustration and editorial contribution.

REFERENCES

1. Carson WG. Arthrosocopy of the shoulder, anatomy and technique. A review paper. Orth Rev 1992;XXI: 143.
2. Grimes D. Frontiers of the operative laparoscopy: a review and critique of the evidence. Am J Obstet Gynecol 1992;166:1062.
3. Gadacz TRUS. Experience with laparoscopic cholecystectomy. Am J Surg 1993;165:450.

4. Chow JC. Endoscopic release of the carpal ligament: a new technique for carpal tunnel syndrome. Arthroscopy 1989;5:19.

5. Sasaki GH. Endoscopic aesthetic, and reconstructive surgery. Philadelphia: Lippincott-Raven; 1996. p. 120–47.

6. Core GB, Vasconez LO, Askren C, et al. Coronal face-lift with endoscopic techniques. Plast Surg Forum 1992;XV:227.

7. Ramirez OM. The subperiosteal rhytidectomy: the third generation face lift. Ann Plast Surg 1992;28: 218–32.

8. Ho LYC. Endoscopic assisted transaxillary augmentation mammoplasty. Br J Plast Surg 1993;46:332–6.

9. Johnson GW. The Johnson endoscopic abdominoplasty. Presented at the endoscopic Plastic Surgery Educational Seminar (in cooperation with the Lipoplasty Society of north America) September, 1994;21.

10. Chang CJ. Assessment of videoendoscopy-assisted abdominoplasty for diastasis recti patients. Chang Gung Med J 2013;36(5):252–6.

11. Bronestedt S, Olson S, Rank F. Wound healing and formation of granulation tissue in normal and defibrinogenerated rabbits. Eur Surg Res 1978;10(suppl 10):104.

12. Marchac D, Sandor G. Face lifts and sprayed fibrin glue: an outcome analysis of 200 patients. Br J Plast Surg 1994;47:306–9.

13. Mandel MA. Closure of blephaloplasty incisions with autulogous fibrin glue. Arch Ophthalmol 1990;108:842–4.

14. Marchac D, Ascherman J, Arnaud A. Fibrin glue fixation in forehead endoscopy:evaluation of our experience with 206 cases. Plast Reconstr Surg 1997; 100:704–12.

15. Bozola AR, Psillakis JN. Abdominoplasty: new concept and classification for treatment. Plast Reconstr Surg 1988;82:983–93.

16. Chang CJ. Combining the CO2 laser and the endoscope to remove soft tissue masses from the forehead area. Photomed Laser Surg 2005;23:509–12.

17. Chang CJ, Yu DY, Chang SY, et al. Comparing the effectiveness of for laser vs. Conventional endoforehead lifting. J Cosmet Laser Ther 2018;20(2):91–5.

18. Ousterhout KD. Combined suction assisted lipectomy, surgical lipectomy and surgical abdominoplasty. Ann Plast Surg 1990;24:126–32.

19. Stewart KJ, Stewart DA, Coghlan B, et al. Complications of 278 consecutive abdominoplasties. J Plast Reconstr Aesthet Surg 2006;59:1152–5.

20. Grossman JA, Capraro PA. Long-term experience with the use of fibrin sealant in aesthetic surgery. Aesthet Surg J 2007;27:558–62.

Buttock Augmentation with Fat Grafting

Weigang Cao, MD, PhD*, Lingling Sheng, MD, PhD

KEYWORDS

• Fat grafting • Buttock augmentation • Gluteoplasty • Gluteal reshaping • Liposuction

KEY POINTS

- Accurate patient evaluation, proper preoperative planning are keys to obtaining aesthetically body silhouette and buttock contour.
- Gluteal fat graft should be transferred into the subcutaneous layers evenly with small aliquots from the deep supramuscular fascia layer to the superficial subdermal layer.
- Deep musculature fat injection is highly not recommended to avoid the risks of fatal fat embolism resulting from possible inadvertent intravascular penetration.
- A pleasing buttock and S-shaped body curvature is achieved not only by volume augmentation of buttock proper but also by volume reduction of its surrounding areas through liposuction.
- An efficient and cost-effective fat harvesting method is introduced.

INTRODUCTION

According to the latest data from the American Society for Aesthetic Plastic Surgery (ASAPS) and the International Society of Aesthetic Plastic Surgery (ISAPS), buttock augmentation (BA) continues to gain popularity in the US and around the world despite of spread of COVID-19 pandemic in recent 2 years. It is one of the most significant increases in the number of procedures performed over the course of a 5-year period up 95% and 19.3% in 2020 compared with 2016 in the US and worldwide, respectively. The growth is even much higher if observed over a longer period of time. Buttock augmentation procedure performed in 2020 is 40,320 in the US and has increased by more than 7 times over the past decade.[1,2] Moreover, the percentage of fat grafting is continuous increasing from 89% in 2015 up to 95% in 2019 among the buttock augmentation procedures performed.[1] However, despite these dramatic trends, there are still few data available about BA with fat grafting for Chinese patients. Here we introduce our experiences in BA with fat grafting in Chinese women over the past decade. Ethnic preference for buttock aesthetics in Asians especially in Chinese is evaluated and a pertinent strategy for buttock contouring is proposed.

AESTHETIC CONSIDERATIONS OF BUTTOCK AUGMENTATION FOR CHINESE PATIENTS

There are significant differences in preferences for buttock size and lateral thigh fullness in different ethnicities, cultures, and nationalities. In contrast to the expectation of being a voluminous hip and narrower waist which meant waist-to-hip ratio (WHR) to be less than 0.65 in Hispanic Americans, in African Americans, a relative smaller well-shaped round buttock with a WHR of 0.7 is usually

This work was supported by Shanghai Municipal Key Clinical Specialty (shslczdzk00901).

Department of Plastic & Reconstructive Surgery, Ninth People's Hospital, Shanghai Jiao Tong University School of Medicine, 639 Zhi-Zao-Ju Road, Huangpu District, Shanghai 200011, P.R.China

* Corresponding author.

E-mail address: drcaoweigang@icloud.com

Clin Plastic Surg 50 (2023) 171–179
https://doi.org/10.1016/j.cps.2022.08.005

expected in Caucasian and Asian patients. Nevertheless, controversies and even confusion regarding the preferences of an ideal buttock WHR still remain due to strong media influence and new fashion trends in the modern age. Wong and colleagues[3] performed a population analysis of the characteristics of the ideal buttocks through digitally created images of buttocks with varying proportions on posterior and lateral views. They demonstrated that the most attractive buttocks WHR are 0.65 (44.2% of respondents) and 0.60(25% of respondents) from the posterior view. Interestingly, most of those respondents are white/Caucasian (56.4%). Moreover, a slim figure with elongated thighs is thought to be more attractive in Asians, especially in the Chinese population, this is probably due to relatively shorter height in Eastern Asian women, whereas a slim figure with long straight lower limbs without lateral thigh prominence usually looks taller. Visually elongated appearance of the lower limbs can be achieved by reducing the lateral thigh prominence through liposuction on the outer thighs, which makes the buttocks more prominent, but not voluptuous if the middle-lateral buttock depression is fully corrected with fat grafting. In general, Eastern Asians are usually more conservative, they expect their buttocks to prominence at the mid-buttocks but less prominent (with a lateral WHR of 0.75 in contrast to a ratio of 0.70–0.725 in other ethnicities) on a lateral view,[3] thus a harmonious combination of shaped buttocks and elongated slim lower limbs with smooth transitions between the buttocks and its surrounding areas was then created, this kind of figure is highly favored by the Chinese population. This ethnic preference has also been confirmed by Wong's study with regard to vertical ratios of the lateral buttock prominence on the posterior view, in which they demonstrated that Pacific Islander, Chinese, Japanese, and other Southeast Asian preferred the placement of the lateral prominence at the lower 70% of the buttocks (70:30 vertical ratio) as the most attractive, whereas white/Caucasian, black/African, and Native American preferred the buttocks with an inferior gluteal convexity (with the lateral prominence positioned at the inferior gluteal fold) as the most attractive.[3]

SURGICAL TECHNIQUES
Anesthesia and Wetting Solution Infiltration

General anesthesia with tracheal intubation or deep sedation was usually applied. In most instances, the patient is placed in the prone position, prepared, and draped. The fat grafts were usually aspirated from peri-gluteal areas such as hips,

flanks, sacrum, the lumbar regions, the lateral and medial thighs. Otherwise, the patient is placed in the supine position first if the fat grafts are harvested from the abdomen or the anterior thighs, then turned over on the stomach after fat harvesting for facilitating fat injection. Modified wetting solution[4] (500 mg lidocaine, 5 mg 1:1000 epinephrine, and 60 mL 5% sodium bicarbonate are added to 3 L saline solution) is infiltrated into the subcutaneous plane of the donor sites 30 minutes before aspiration. The wetting solution was heated to 37 degree Celsius during large volume liposuction to reduce possible hypothermia and postoperative shivering.

Preoperative Marking

Marking is performed with the patient in the standing position, different color markers are used to distinguish the donor sites for liposuction and the recipient sites for fat grafting as well as incision sites. The black indicates the liposuction areas around the buttocks, which include the lower back, flanks, hips, sacrum, and both thighs; the blue indicates the grafted areas, which include the midlateral buttock depressions and buttock proper; the green indicates the subgluteal "pillar" in the posterior thigh immediately below the buttock whereby the subcutaneous fat tissues especially the deep layer of fats should not be suctioned to prevent buttocks from ptosis, while the red indicates incisions placed at the top end of intergluteal fold and the middle of the inferior gluteal fold (**Fig. 1**).

Fat Aspiration and Processing

Syringe liposuction can be used if a small amount of fat grafts is needed during the correction of small areas of gluteal depression. Otherwise, a suction machine is preferred to aspirate fat in relatively large volume gluteal augmentation and body contouring procedures for faster and more efficacious aspiration, especially in lean patients. A blunt tip Mercedes cannula 3 to 5 mm (**Fig. 2**) in diameter is used and the aspirated fat is collected in a sterile canister and condensed by gravitation simultaneously (**Fig. 3**).

The canister contains a special metal grating filter for removing the fibrous tissues from aspiration, the filtered fat grafts can easily pass through an injection cannula 2 mm in diameter without clog during fat injection. The negative pressure is controlled under 50 KPa during the aspiration for decreasing possible injuries to adipocytes. Once upper limit of 700 mL fat tissues is reached in the canister, the fat tissues are then transferred to 60 mL syringes and decanted for

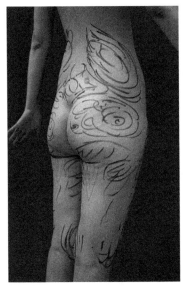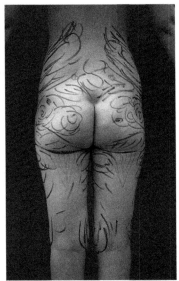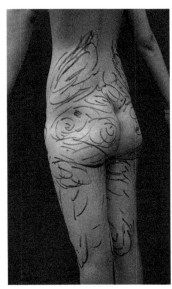

Fig. 1. Areas for liposuction, fat grafting, incision sites, and subgluteal supporting "pillar" are marked with different color markers during preoperative design.

10 minutes. Finally, the fat is transferred to 5 mL or 10 mL syringes ready for injection.

Fat Injection

The liposuction entry incisions can also be used to inject fat grafts into buttocks. Occasionally, small stab incisions located in the hip region are used for facilitating injection. Fat grafts are only injected into the subcutaneous layer from deeper plane of gluteal fascia toward superficial subdermal plane. Deep intramuscular and submuscular injection is not recommended to avoid risks of inadvertent intravascular penetration of gluteal vessels and subsequent fatal fat embolism. Small aliquots of fat grafts are evenly distributed in a fanning motion into both the deeper and superficial layers of the subcutaneous tissues with multiple-tunnel, multiple-plane, and multiple-point techniques (**Fig. 4**). For areas with severe depressed deformities or fibrotic adhering between the derma and the deep musculature, 3-dimensional percutaneous releasing of fibrotic adhesion with a 16G needle or a V-dissector is necessary, the resulting small spaces are then filled with fat grafts.

Postoperative Care and Expected Outcome

The sanguineous fluids and tumescent fluids residing in the subcutaneous tissue spaces are thoroughly evacuated before the incisions are closed with layered sutures. Drains are

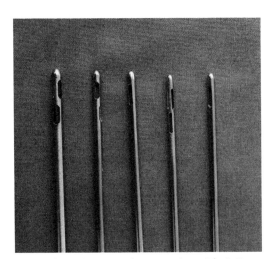

Fig. 2. Blunt tip Mercedes cannulas with 3–5 mm diameter for fat harvesting.

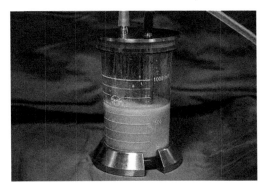

Fig. 3. The aspirated fat is filtered and condensed by gravitation in a sterilized canister.

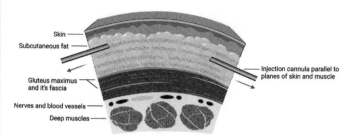

Fig. 4. Fat grafts are only injected into the subcutaneous layer with the injecting cannula parallel to the planes of the skin surface and underlying gluteus maximus muscle when the cannula is withdrawn (figure was created with Biorender.com).

unnecessary. After the skin closure, compression elastic garments are applied immediately before the patient is sent to the recovery room. Intravenous antibiotics for the prevention of infection are usually prescribed for 3 days following 2 days of oral antibiotics if large volume of fat grafting is performed, otherwise, only oral antibiotics for 3 to 5 days are given if small amounts of fat grafts are transferred in touchups.

The patient is asked to lie in the prone position when fully awakened and avoid sitting or lying on the buttocks for the first 2 weeks. The patient is also instructed to sit on the thighs with buttocks off the edge of a sitting stool or chair with no back to avoid buttocks being compressed. Early ambulation is encouraged but exercises are prohibited in the first 2 weeks, normal ambulation or light exercises is usually resumed 1 month after the operation but vigorous movement and strenuous exercises are not recommended in the first 6 months.

Mild edema and ecchymosis in the operated areas might be encountered and subsided in 2 weeks. The size of buttocks remains stable in 1 to 3 months and the ideal buttock contouring outcome and figure silhouette with smooth transition between convexities and concavities are expected through fat grafting to the buttocks combined with liposuction procedures on the surrounding areas of the buttocks as well as on the other body parts.

Management of Complications

Complications are rare if principles for fat grafting are adhered to. No major complications were observed in our series. The senior author (C.W.) had one case of suspicious infection in one buttock and the patient had an uneventful recovery after antibiotics treatment.[4] Another case reported buttock paresthesia which resolved in 3 months. One case complained of a small subcutaneous nodule in her right buttock and the lump was excised through a small incision and confirmed as an oily cyst. No other liponecrosis such as sclerotic induration, calcified solid lumps,

hematoma, seroma, and other complications were developed.

Revision or Subsequent Procedures

Most of the patients were satisfied with the outcomes after one session of contouring. Some patients wanted to improve overall body contour through staged liposuction procedures and achieve prominent buttock projection with further fat grafting procedures. Touchup was performed in 3 to 6 months if the concave deformity was not fully corrected. Otherwise, secondary large volume fat grafting was usually arranged at least in a 6-month interval from the last operation.

Case Demonstration

Case 1, A 35-year-old female with BMI of 20 kg/m² (weight 52 Kg, height 161 cm), who presented for improving her body contour. She had a square buttock framework with severe point-C depressions without significant fat accumulation on the outer thighs. Circumferential abdominal liposuction was performed and total 460 cc (240 cc for right buttock, 220 cc for left buttock) fat grafts were transplanted into both buttocks and lateral depressed areas. Thirty-nine months later, she came back for further improvement. Liposuction on her back, sacrum, hips, and flanks was carried out and additional 275 cc fat grafts were injected into each buttock (**Fig. 5**).

Case 2 A 25-year-old young lady with BMI 20.8 kg/m² (weight 58 Kg, height 167 cm) wanted to improve her silhouettes through breast and buttock augmentation with fat grafts. She had 2 operations in 9 months, liposuction on her lateral and medial thighs and 250 cc fat grafts to the breasts were carried out first, 9 months later, second operation was performed, buttock and breast augmentations with fat grafting (260 cc to each breast, and 250 cc to each buttock) were performed, The donor sites of fat grafts include abdomen, flanks, and hips. Eight years later, she came back for her last body contouring surgery to correct her anterior thigh protruding and add more volume to her buttocks. 200 cc fat grafts

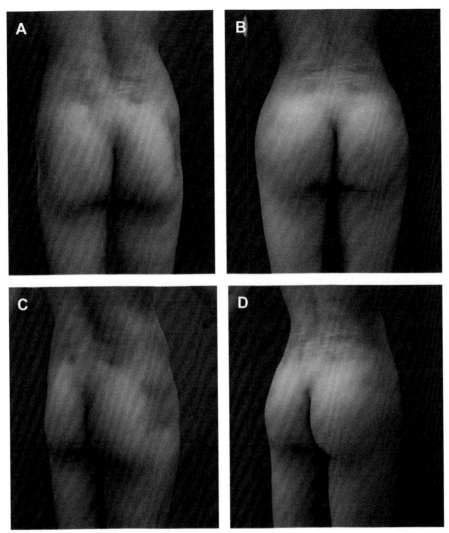

Fig. 5. Two sessions of buttock augmentation with fat grafting (right 515 cc, left 495 cc) combined with liposuctions on abdomen, back, sacrum, hips, and flanks. Preoperatively (*A*, *C*); Postoperative images 33 months after 2nd procedure (*B*, *D*).

were injected into each buttock. **Fig. 6** demonstrated the pleasing S-shaped curvature with a smooth back-hip-buttock-thigh transition 8 years after the first operation.

Case 3. A 29-year-old young lady with a BMI of 21.5 kg/m^2 (weight 60 Kg, height 167 cm) suffered from the congenital dislocation of her right hip joint and had a right hip replacement 7 years ago. She was unpleased with her depressed deformities on both buttocks, especially with her ugly scar on her right buttock and right thigh. After liposuction on her abdomen, waist, and hips, 180 cc and 230 cc fat grafts were injected into the left buttock, right buttock, and thigh, respectively. The deformities have been largely corrected and asymmetry has been greatly reduced. **Fig.7** shows the results 19 months after the operation.

Case 4. A 23-year-old young girl with a BMI of 19.7 kg/m^2 (weight 55 kg, height 167 cm), had buttock augmentation with hydrophilic polyacrylamide gel (PAAG) injection in a private clinic in South Korea but unfortunately got infected with persistent lower fever. She got severely depressed deformities on her buttocks and groin regions after serial debridement and clearing of fillers. She presented for correcting deformities and improving body curvature. 720 cc (right 350 cc, left 370 cc) fat grafts during the first operation were transplanted. Five months later, she had a second procedure, 220 cc fat grafts were injected into each buttock. **Fig. 8** shows the comparison of preoperative and 10 months later after 2 sessions of fat grafting and liposuction on her upper back, hips, flanks, abdomen, and anterior thighs.

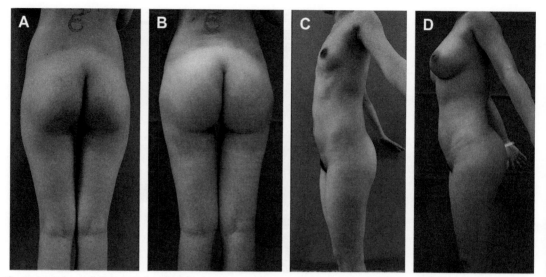

Fig. 6. Long-term follow-up of total body contouring procedures with 2 sessions of augmentation mammoplasty (510 cc to each breast in total) and one session of gluteoplasty (250 cc to each buttock) with fat grafting. Preoperatively (A, C); and 8 years after the first operation before the correction of anterior thigh protruding (B, D).

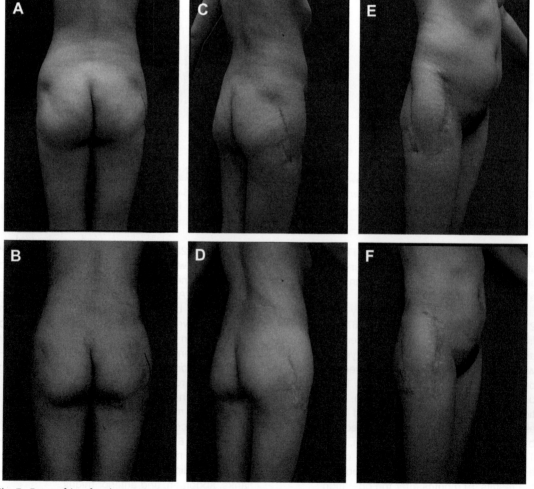

Fig. 7. Fat grafting for the correction of gluteal and thigh depressed deformities resulted from right hip replacement surgery. Before the operation (A, C, E); 19 months after the fat injection (B, D, F).

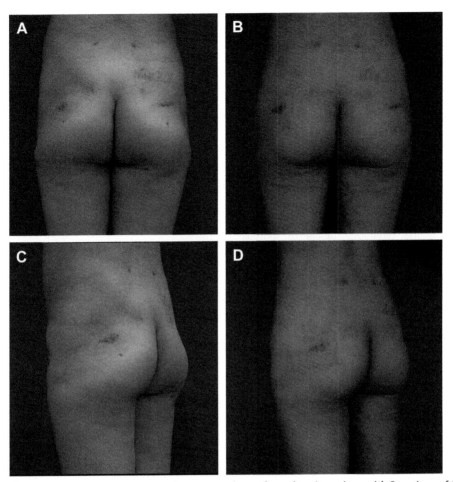

Fig. 8. Correction of iatrogenic depressed deformities on buttocks and groin regions with 2 sessions of fat grafting (right 570 cc, left 590 cc) after clearing of PAAG. Before fat grafting (*A*, *C*); 10 months after the second procedure (*B*, *D*).

DISCUSSION

Almost every physically healthy patient with realistic expectations is eligible to undergo BA with fat grafting, but excellent results largely depend on the presence of proper patient characteristics in addition to meticulous manipulations by skillful surgeons.

Each patient' s buttock frame type should be judged and defined as Square, Round, A-shape, or V-shape according to Mendieta's classification system,[5] fat depositions around the buttocks such as lateral thighs, lower back, flanks, and hips as well as other possible fat grafts donor sites should also be carefully evaluated. Much of cases in our series have Square shape or A-shape frame but with moderate to severe mid-lateral C depression deformity, which makes the body silhouette irregular and has an unsmooth transition between the buttocks and the thighs as well as waist. The biggest appeal of Eastern

Asian patients is usually reshaping the buttocks to obtain a smooth transitional S-shaped curvature from lower back, buttocks to thighs rather than enlarging buttocks alone. This can be accomplished by not only adding volume to the buttocks and enhancing buttock projection through fat grafting, but also reducing widths of waist and thigh circumferences through liposuction on the sacral-lumbar region, the lower back, flanks, and hips as well as the protruding lateral thighs. In contrast, the posterior thighs under the inferior gluteal fold should only be suctioned conservatively or not be suctioned, otherwise, buttocks ptosis will inevitably occur due to loss of support from underlying "pillar-like" subcutaneous tissues.

Various authors have reported their successful experiences worldwide in terms of fat grafting to buttocks subcutaneously and intramuscularly.[4,6–11] However, greater concerns for gluteal fat injection are raised in recent years due to fatal complications related to buttock augmentation with fat grafting.[12–14] Most of deaths were resulted from cardiovascular pulmonary fat embolism because of gluteal veins penetration or laceration during deep intramuscular or submuscular fat injection.[12–16] In addition, recent studies about gluteal vein anatomy showed that both superior and inferior gluteal veins are immediately deep to gluteus maximus approximately 6 cm deep with a ≥6 mm caliber. The distribution of those veins suggests that there is no "safe zone" in the intramuscular or submuscular planes.[17,18] Nevertheless, buttock augmentation with fat grafting would be a very safe procedure if the fat grafts were injected only in the subcutaneous tissue layers above the tenacious fascia of gluteus maximus.[4,13,15,16]

The other recommended safe techniques for buttock augmentation with fat grafting include placing the patient in the jackknife position, avoidance of downward injection, the use of cannulas larger than 4.1 mm in diameter, continual motion during injection and so on.[13,14,18] Recent reports have demonstrated that there was a significant decrease in recent pulmonary fat embolism and mortality rate and an improvement in the safety of the procedure after the application of those recommended techniques.[19,20] However, the senior author (C.W.) preferred to use a smaller caliber blunt tip cannula (2.0 mm to 2.4 mm in diameter) for fat injection,[4,6–9] because this cannula provides more accurate and even distribution of small fat particles in a relative thinner subcutaneous layer in Eastern Asian patients. In addition, the blood vessels in the subcutaneous layer have a relative smaller caliber than that in muscles and below the gluteus maximus,[17,18] thus risks of penetration into blood vessels are greatly reduced.

The drawback of subcutaneous injection alone is limited volume of fat grafts injected due to relative limited subcutaneous space. Staged sessions would be recommended rather than large volume injection in one session for those patients who want their buttocks more projecting, otherwise, overloaded fat grafts would be necrotic and subsequent complications would be resulted. Sometimes, a few cases have moderate to severe depression deformities and scar contractures due to the injection of penicillin in childhood and other factors such as surgery, trauma and infection (see **Figs. 7** and **8**), scar contracture released with a 16G needle or a V-dissector is necessary for the correction of these deformities and subsequent small spaces after releasing should be filled with fat parcels to prevent scar adhesion recurrence.[4]

SUMMARY

Buttock augmentation with fat grafting has become one of the fasted growing procedures in plastic surgery society in the past decade. Patient characteristics and expectations should be carefully evaluated and individualized plan should be discussed with the patient during preoperative consultation. Excellent buttock contouring result depends not only on fat grafting for the enlargement of buttock volume but also on the removal of fat by liposuction on areas around the buttocks.

Strict following proper principles and careful maneuvers perioperatively, the procedure can be performed safely and create an S-shaped body curvature from back-buttock-thigh with a smooth transition between concavities and convexities.

CLINICS CARE POINTS

- Proper preoperative patient evaluation and combined techniques of fat grafting and liposuction are keys to obtaining successful contouring outcomes
- Adherence to principles of fat grafting to the buttocks and avoiding intramuscular and submuscular injection is the top priority of patient safety
- Individualized planning for each patient is paramount important for high patient satisfaction

DISCLOSURE

The authors have nothing to disclose.

REFERENCES

1. American Society for Aesthetic Plastic Surgery. Available at: https://www.surgery.org/sites/default/files/ASAPS-Stats.2020.pdf. Accessed May 24, 2021.
2. Number of worldwide procedures performed by plastic surgeons in 2020. Available at: https://www.isaps.org/wp-content/uploads/2022/01/ISAPS-Global-Survey_2020.pdf. Accessed February 15, 2022.
3. Wong WW, Motakef S, Lin Y, et al. Redifing the ideal buttocks: a population analysis. Plast Reconstr Surg 2016;137:1739–47.
4. Wang G, Ren Y, Cao W, et al. Liposculpture and fat grafting for aesthetic correction of the gluteal

concave deformity associated with multiple intraglu-teal injection of penicillin in childhood. Aesth Plast Surg 2013;37:39–45.

5. Mendieta CG, Sood A. Classification system for gluteal evaluation Revisited. Clin Plast Surg 2018; 45:159–77.

6. Mendieta CG. Gluteal reshaping. Aesthet Surg J 2007;27:641–55.

7. Toledo LS. Gluteal augmentation with fat grafting the Brazilian buttock technique: 30 Years' experience. Clin Plast Surg 2015;42:253–61.

8. Rosique RG, Rosique MJF, De Moraes CG. Gluteo-plasty with autoulogous fat tissue:Experience with 106 consecutive cases. Plast Reconstr Surg 2015; 135:1381–9.

9. Rosique RG, Rosique MJF. Gluteoplasty: a Brazilian perspective. Plast Reconstr Surg 2018;142:910–9.

10. Ghavami A, Villanueva NL. Gluteal augmentation and contouring with autologous fat transfer: Part I. Clin Plast Surg 2018;45:249–59.

11. Cárdenas-Camarena L, Durán H. Improvement of the gluteal contour modern concepts with systema-tized lipoinjection. Clin Plast Surg 2018;45:237–47.

12. Cárdenas-Camarena L, Bayter JE, Aguirre-Serrano H, et al. Deaths caused by gluteal lipoinjec-tion: what are we doing wrong? Plast Reconstr Surg 2015;136:58–66.

13. Mofid MM, Teitelbaum S, Suissa D, et al. Report on mortality from gluteal fat grafting: recommendations from the ASERF task force. Aesthet Surg J 2017; 37(7):796–806.

14. Villanueva NL, Del Velcchio DA, Afrooz PN, et al. Staying safe during gluteal fat transplantation. Plast Reconstr Surg 2018;141:79–86.

15. Del Vecchio DA, Villanueva NL, Mohan R, et al. Clin-ical implications of gluteal fat graft migration: a dy-namic anatomical study. Plast Reconstr Surg 2018; 142:1180–92.

16. Wall S Jr, Delcecchio D, Teitelbaum S, et al. Subcu-taneous migration: a dynamic anatomical study of gluteal fat grafting. Plast Reconstr Surg 2019;143: 1343–51.

17. Ordenana C, DallaPozza E, Said S, et al. Objec-tifying the risk of vascular complications in gluteal augmentation with fat grafting; A latex casted cadaveric study. Aesth Surg J 2020;40: 402–9.

18. Turin SY, Fracol M, Keller E, et al. Gluteal vein anat-omy: Location, caliber, impact of patient positioning, and implications for fat grafting. Aesthet Surg J 2020;40:642–9.

19. Rios L, Gupta V. Improvement in Brazilian Butt Lift(BBL) safety with the current recommendations from ASERF,ASPS and ISAPS. Aesthet Surg J 2020;40:864–70.

20. O'Neill RC, Hanson SE, Reece E, et al. Safety considerations of fat grafting in buttock augmen-tation. Aesthet Surg J 2021;41(Suppl 1):S25–30.

Vaginal Rejuvenation with Acellular Dermal Matrix

Yunzhu Li, MD[a], Ruijia Dong, MD[b], Jiuzuo Huang, MD[a], Yiding Xiao, MD[a], Jie Chen, BSN[a], Hailin Zhang, MD[a], Xiao Long, MD[a,*], Xiaojun Wang, MD[a,*]

KEYWORDS

- Female genital cosmetic surgery • Vaginal rejuvenation • Labiaplasty • Labia majora augmentation
- Vaginoplasty

KEY POINTS

- Vaginal laxity, usually secondary to normal aging and childbirth, affects women's sexual satisfaction and results in psychological disorders.
- Vaginoplasty and perineoplasty with acellular dermal matrix (ADM) can be considered for patients with mild to moderate vaginal laxity.
- The combination of multiple female genital cosmetic surgeries based on the individual demand of every patient magnifies the surgical effect.

 Video content accompanies this article at http://www.plasticsurgery.theclinics.com.

INTRODUCTION

Hormone change related to normal aging and pregnancy and pelvic injury because of childbirth and previous pelvic surgery interferes with the normal function of genital skin, mucosa, and pelvic muscle, leading to aesthetic and functional genital problems.[1–3] Aesthetically, the altered appearance of the vulva is characterized by enlarged labia minora, flatted labia majora, and widened vagina orifice. Functionally, patients may suffer from vulva friction, hygiene difficulty, chronic irritation, stress urinary incontinence (SUI), decreased sexual satisfaction, and secondary psychological disorders.[2,4,5] Owing to the increasing requirements that women have for the quality of life and widespread propaganda, the demand for female genital cosmetic surgery has steadily increased in recent years.[6]

Female genital cosmetic surgery is a relatively new concept that consists of multiple procedures, usually including labiaplasty, clitoral prepuce reduction, labia majora augmentation, and vaginoplasty.[7] In this article, we introduce the modified vaginoplasty with acellular dermal matrix (ADM) and briefly reviewed our experience in the combination of multiple procedures to achieve the optimal effect.

INDICATIONS AND CONTRAINDICATIONS OF YOUR PREFERRED RECONSTRUCTION

Vaginal laxity can be described as "widening" or "looseness" of the vagina. Symptoms included dysfunction of the muscles around the vagina and the vaginal urethral sphincter, accompanied by prolapse or ptosis caused by the reduced strength of the vaginal mucosa and the fascia around the vaginal lumen.[4] As a result, the symptoms of vaginal laxity are complex, usually including symptoms of SUI, reduced vaginal sensation during intercourse, and worse general

[a] Department of Plastic and Reconstructive Surgery, Peking Union Medical College Hospital, Peking Union Medical College and Chinese Academy of Medical Sciences, No.1 Shuaifuyuan Road, Dongcheng District, Beijing 100730, China; [b] Department of Plastic and Reconstructive Surgery, Beijing Tsinghua Changgung Hospital, School of Clinical Medicine, Tsinghua University, No.168 Litang Road, Changping District, Beijing 102218, China
* Corresponding author.
E-mail addresses: pumclongxiao@126.com (X.L.); pumchwxj@163.com (X.W.)

Clin Plastic Surg 50 (2023) 181–187
https://doi.org/10.1016/j.cps.2022.07.007
0094-1298/23/© 2022 Elsevier Inc. All rights reserved.

sex life.[8] Women complaining of any of the above symptoms are candidates for vaginal rejuvenation. Widened vaginal orifice and reduced vaginal contraction found upon digital palpation are surgical indications as well (Fig. 1).

Active vulva infection is an absolute contraindication. Besides, as the procedure is minimally invasive and does not involve any incision of the vaginal mucosa and surrounding muscles, previous damage to the anal sphincter muscles during childbirth will not be corrected, and these patients should be excluded. Moreover, to prevent injury to the uterine during the process of blind dissection, patients with uterine prolapse should also be excluded.

Preoperative Evaluation and Special Considerations

Before surgery, trimanual examination and vaginal wet mount should be conducted to exclude patients with uterine prolapse, previous damage to the anal sphincter muscles during childbirth, and active vulva infection.

The vulva is a three-dimensional structure; thus, its proper evaluation should involve lithotomy position, standing position, and overlooking position images (Fig. 2).

The application of questionnaires including the Vaginal Laxity Questionnaire (VLQ) and Female Sexual Function Index (FSFI) and objective evaluation, including vaginal tactile imaging and perineal ultrasound, is encouraged.[9–11] On the one hand, it creates scales allowing clinical involvement and the patient's degree of concern to be scored. On the other hand, it provides values to

be tracked, and quantitative improvements may be evaluated.

Surgical Procedures

All operations were performed with the patients under sufficient local tumescence anesthesia (0.5% lidocaine with 1:400,000 epinephrine).

The first step is vaginoplasty. Two incisions are made at the 3 and 9 o'clock positions on the mucocutaneous junction of the vaginal orifice. A retriever is used to create four U-shaped tunnels in the submucosal muscular layer in the posterior vaginal wall through these 2 incisions, each one being 1 cm apart from the other. The first tunnel is about 4 cm away from the vaginal orifice, while the last tunnel is almost at the vaginal orifice. Then, a 15 × 1 cm piece of ADM (Beijing Jayyalife Biological Technology Co., Ltd., Beijing, China) is introduced into the tunnels. By pulling both ends of the implanted ADM, the mucosa folds of the posterior vaginal wall are increased, and the vaginal orifice is narrowed.

The second step is perineoplasty. Three incisions are made on the central perineal tendon and bilateral ischial tubercles. A retriever is used to create a " ∞ " -shaped tunnel in the submucosal muscular layer on the perineum. A piece of ADM is introduced into the tunnel, tightened, and sutured to the deep tissue. This way, the superficial transverse perineal muscle is reinforced and fixed to the perineal body (Fig. 3, Video 1).

For good wound healing and implant integration, the mucosal layer and skin layer should be closed with 3-0 absorbable sutures separately.

Postoperative Care and Expected Outcome

Once the procedures are completed, the digital rectal examination (DRE) should be performed, and blood present on the glove may indicate the vaginal-rectal fistula. A 3-day course of postoperative antibiotics is recommended. The use of analgesics is not required either during or after the operation. Intercourse should be prohibited for one month.

Management of Complications (Revise this part and add management of actual complications in your case series, if any).

So far, we have had a few cases with implant visibility around the incision site as a result of poor wound healing. We believe it was because we closed the incisions in one layer and did not close the mucosal layer and skin layer separately. After we closed the two layers separately, the complication did not happen again. (We do not think it is worth mentioning and as long as the readers stick to the instructions we introduced in

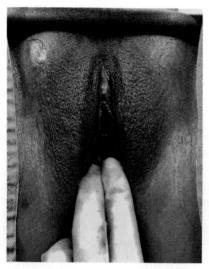

Fig. 1. Photograph of a 39-year-old parturient woman with a widened vaginal orifice.

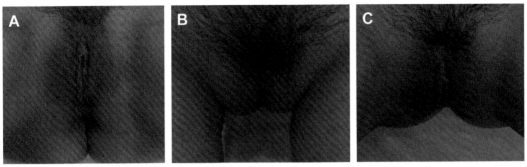

Fig. 2. Standard photographic assessment of the vulva of a 33-year-old female; (*A*) lithotomy position; (*B*) standing position; (*C*) overlooking position.

the *Surgical Procedures* part, such complications could be avoided.)

SUBSEQUENT PROCEDURES

The female genitalia includes the mons pubis, labia majora, labia minora, clitoris, urethral opening, and vaginal opening. Any pathogenic factor resulting in vaginal laxity is likely to create problems in other organs, such as labia minora hypertrophy and labia majora atrophy. To achieve the optimal effect, vaginal rejuvenation with ADM

should be accompanied by other procedures in patients with indications. Labiaplasty is the most frequently performed female genital cosmetic surgery.[12] The edge resection usually is the first choice if the patients would like to abdicate the natural pigmentated transition of the labial edge, which they consider an aging look (**Fig. 4**A–C). If patients have enlarged clitoral prepuce, which comes in the horizontal or vertical direction, clitoral prepuce reduction should be performed simultaneously to avoid large overhanging clitoral prepuce after simple labiaplasty.[13]

The injection of hyaluronic acid (HA) into the labia majora improves the pathological changes associated with labia majora atrophy.[14] A critical anatomical structure of the labia majora is the adipose sac lying underneath the dartos, containing fat tissue. It is a fibrous connective tissue that divides the fat into individual chambers, creating cylinder-like lobes. To achieve a natural filling result and prevent the formation of nodules, the needle is inserted from different sites in the pubis or the labia majora to create multiple tunnels for injection, and the filler is administrated while removing the needle to assure the full coverage of the adipose sacs (see **Fig. 4**D).

Case Demonstrations (up to 4 Cases)

Case 1 A 42-year-old female underwent vaginal rejuvenation with ADM. An immediate tightening effect was achieved in the vaginal orifice (**Fig. 5**). The 3-month-postoperative transvaginal ultrasound confirms the successful neo-vascularization of ADM (**Fig. 6**).

Case 2 A 46-year-old female patient complained of an unaesthetic vulva and decreased sexual experience, whose preoperative exam indicated enlarged labia minora, deflated labia majora, and loose vagina. She underwent a combination of labiaplasty, labia majora augmentation of HA, and vaginoplasty (**Fig. 7**).

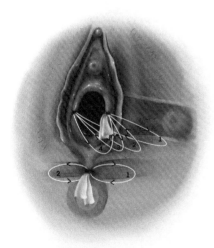

Fig. 3. The operation is performed in 2 steps. The first step is to implant ADM into the posterior vaginal wall. As indicated by the arrowheads, four U-shaped tunnels are created; the second step is to implant ADM into the perineal body. (*From* Li Y, Xia Z, Bai M, et al. New Method for Genital Aesthetic Surgery: An Easy-To-Learn Two-Step Approach With Acellular Dermal Matrix (ADM) [published online ahead of print, 2022 Mar 30]. Aesthet Surg J. 2022;sjac071; with permission.)

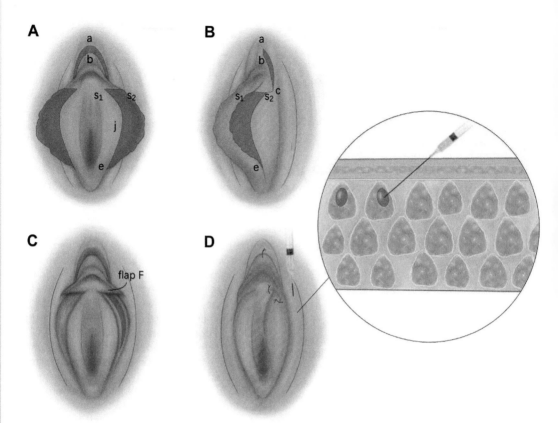

Figure 4. (*A–C*) Surgical procedures of edge resection of hypertrophic labia minora and clitoral hood: Linear incision s_1e (s_2e) is designed on bilateral labia minora. A minimum residual labial width of 1.0 cm should be retained. The widest point j of labia minora is approximately located at the level of the urethral orifice. A U-shaped resection within the boundary of points abc is designed on the clitoral hood. It helps to treat vertical excess and horizontal excess at the same time. The flap F is obtained by extending the incision along s_1, and s_2 and preserving an adequate amount of soft tissue underneath. Followed by 5-0 Vicryl continuous intradermal suture along the entire course of labia minora and clitoral prepuce, the bilateral flaps F are approximated into the lines of labia minora closure; (*D*) labia majora augmentation should fully cover the adipose sacs to avoid nodule formation.

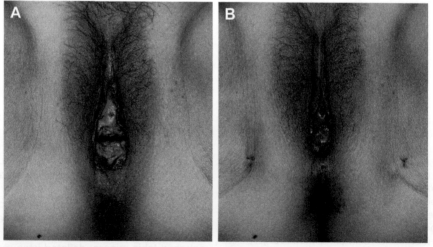

Fig. 5. Photograph of a 42-year-old woman who underwent vaginal rejuvenation with ADM. (*A*) Preoperative view; (*B*) immediate postoperative view. (*From* Li Y, Xia Z, Bai M, et al. New Method for Genital Aesthetic Surgery: An Easy-To-Learn Two-Step Approach With Acellular Dermal Matrix (ADM) [published online ahead of print, 2022 Mar 30]. Aesthet Surg J. 2022;sjac071; with permission.)

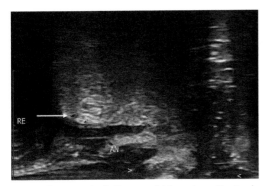

Fig. 6. Ultrasound of 42-year-old female patient who underwent vaginal rejuvenation three months ago. Blood flow signal detected around the implanted ADM (*arrowhead*), indicating successful vascularization of ADM.

Case 3 A 62-year-old woman who underwent the surgery four years ago. Three-dimensional transvaginal ultrasound detected blood flow signals around the implanted ADM and thickened the lower posterior vaginal wall (**Fig. 8**).

DISCUSSION

Traditional vaginal tightening surgery involves incision of the posterior vaginal wall, exposure of the vaginal mucosa and levator ani muscle, reapproximating of the vaginal sphincter muscle, and resection of the loose vaginal mucosa. It solves the problem of vaginal laxity while repairing uterine prolapse and rectocele at the same time.[15] However, the procedures are aggressive, and the excision of vaginal mucosa might lead to fibrosis and scar tissue and eventually result in vaginal dryness and dyspareunia.[16] A new trend is the nonsurgical vaginal rejuvenation with radiofrequency and laser devices. But there are still disputes regarding its efficacy and safety.[17]

ADM is taken from human allograft skin, with all cells in the dermis removed by means of tissue engineering. The remaining three-dimensional scaffold structure comprises collagen and elastic fibers, allowing for rapid vascularization and infiltration by regenerating host cells.[18] Another worth mentioning feature is that ADM possesses high resilience and tensile strength; the maximum load at ADM break was between 181.92 N and 492.11 N and the tensile strength was between 14.34 MPa and 26.12 MPa, with an elongation ratio between 104% and 126%.[19] Its good performance in both elasticity and flexibility enables it to stretch over forces and to return to its original shape later, which is highly compatible with the nature of the vagina.

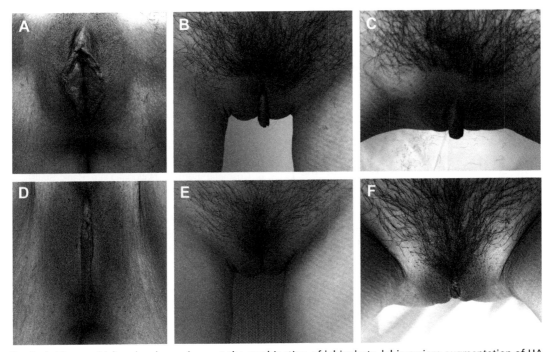

Fig. 7. A 46-year-old female who underwent the combination of labiaplasty, labia majora augmentation of HA, and vaginoplasty; (A) preoperative view in lithotomy position; (B) preoperative view in the standing position; (C) preoperative view in overlooking position; (D) 1-month postoperative view in lithotomy position; (E) 1-month postoperative view in standing position; (F) 1-month postoperative view in overlooking position.

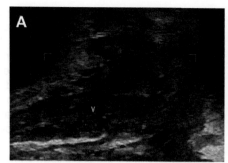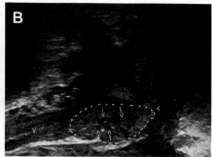

Fig. 8. Ultrasound of a 62-year-old woman who underwent vaginal rejuvenation with ADM four years ago. (*A*) Blood flow signal detected around the implanted ADM (*arrowhead*); (*B*) ADM (*dotted line*) thickens the lower posterior vaginal wall. (*From* Li Y, Xia Z, Bai M, et al. New Method for Genital Aesthetic Surgery: An Easy-To-Learn Two-Step Approach With Acellular Dermal Matrix (ADM) [published online ahead of print, 2022 Mar 30]. Aesthet Surg J. 2022;sjac071; with permission.)

The vaginal artery, originating from the internal iliac artery, runs along the anterior and lateral walls of the vagina. In addition, vaginal venous plexuses are located at the sides of the vagina.[20] The distribution of arteries and veins allows the posterior vaginal wall to be a safe zone for operation. In addition, the surgery is minimally invasive, preserving intact vaginal mucosa. Hence, its risk of wound dehiscence and scar formation is low, and it enables a quick recovery for patients.

SUMMARY

Vaginal rejuvenation with ADM is a minimally invasive procedure with low complication risk and high efficacy for patients with vaginal laxity. Combined with other female genital cosmetic surgeries based on the individual demand of every patient will magnify the surgical effect.

CLINICS CARE POINTS

- Standard photographic assessment of the vulva should include lithotomy position, standing position, and overlooking position images.
- Preoperative exams should include a trimanual examination and vaginal wet mount.
- Sufficient local tumescence fluid, restricting the operations to the lower third of the vagina, and putting a finger in the rectum during the procedure helps protect the rectum.

CONFLICT OF INTEREST

All authors declare that they have no conflicts of interest.

SUPPLEMENTARY DATA

Supplementary data related to this article can be found online at https://doi.org/10.1016/j.cps.2022.07.007.

REFERENCES

1. Sturdee DW, Panay N. Recommendations for the management of postmenopausal vaginal atrophy. Climacteric 2010;13:509–22.
2. Palacios S. Vaginal hyperlaxity syndrome: a new concept and challenge. Gynecol Endocrinol 2018; 34:360–2.
3. Gulia C, Zangari A, Briganti V, et al. Labia minora hypertrophy: causes, impact on women's health, and treatment options. Int Urogynecol J 2017;28(10): 1453–61.
4. Lukacz ES, Lawrence JM, Contreras R, et al. Parity, mode of delivery, and pelvic floor disorders. Obstet Gynecol 2006;107(6):1253–60.
5. Miklos JR, Moore RD. Labiaplasty of the labia minora: patients' indications for pursuing surgery. J Sex Med 2008;5:1492–5.
6. Cosmetic Surgery National Data Bank Statistics. Aesthet Surg J 2018;38:1–24.
7. Elective female genital cosmetic surgery: ACOG committee opinion summary, number 795. Obstet Gynecol 2020;135:249–50.
8. Campbell P, Krychman M, Gray T, et al. Self-reported vaginal laxity- prevalence, impact, and associated symptoms in women attending a urogynecology clinic. J Sex Med 2018;15(11):1515–7.
9. Qureshi AA, Sharma K, Thornton M, et al. Vaginal laxity, sexual distress, and sexual dysfunction: a cross-sectional study in a plastic surgery practice. Aesthet Surg J 2018;38(8):873–80.
10. Egorov V, Murphy M, Lucente V, et al. Quantitative assessment and interpretation of vaginal conditions. Sex Med 2018;6(1):39–48.

11. Manzini C, Friedman T, Turel F, et al. Vaginal laxity: which measure of levator ani distensibility is most predictive? Ultrasound Obstet Gynecol 2020;55(5): 683–7.

12. Plastic surgery statistics report, Available at: https://www.plasticsurgery.org/documents/News/Statistics/2020/plastic-surgery-statistics-full-report-2020.pdf,2020. Accessed Feburary 15, 2021.

13. Hunter JG. Labia minora, labia majora, and clitoral hood alteration: experience-based recommendations. Aesthet Surg J 2016;36:71–9.

14. Turlier V, Delalleau A, Casas C, et al. Association between collagen production and mechanical stretching in dermal extracellular matrix: in vivo effect of cross- linked hyaluronic acid filler. A randomized, placebo-controlled study. J Dermatol Sci 2013;69: 187–94.

15. Pardo JS, Solà VD, Ricci PA, et al. Colpoperineoplasty in women with a sensation of a wide vagina. Acta Obstet Gynecol Scand 2006;85(9):1125–7.

16. Abedi P, Jamali S, Tadayon M, et al. Effectiveness of selective vaginal tightening on sexual function among reproductive aged women in Iran with vaginal laxity: a quasi-experimental study. J Obstet Gynaecol Res 2014;40(2):526–31.

17. U.S. Food and Drug Administration, UPDATE on serious complications associated with transvaginal placement of surgical mesh for pelvic organ prolapse: FDA safety communication. Available at: https://www.fda.gov/files/medical%20devices/published/Urogynecologic Surgical-Mesh–Update-on-the-Safety-and-Effectiveness-of-Transvaginal-Placement-for-Pelvic-Organ-Prolapse-%28July-2011%29.pdf, 2011. Accessed Feburary 15, 2021.

18. Capito AE, Tholpady SS, Agrawal H, et al. Evaluation of host tissue integration, revascularization, and cellular infiltration within various dermal substrates. Ann Plast Surg 2012;68(5):495–500.

19. Nam SY, Youn D, Kim GH, et al. In Vitro characterization of a novel human acellular dermal matrix (BellaCell HD) for breast reconstruction. Bioengineering (Basel) 2020;7(2):39.

20. Gray H. Female reproductive system. In: Standring S, editor. Gray's anatomy: the anatomical basis of clinical practice. 42nd edition. Amsterdam: ELSEVIER; 2020. p. 1309–13.

Primary Breast Augmentation with Fat Grafting

Jeng-Yee Lin, MD, PhD[a], Lee L.Q. Pu, MD, PhD[b],*

KEYWORDS

- Breast augmentation • Fat grafting • Autologous fat transplantation • Fat injection • Fat transfer
- Adipose-derived stem cells

KEY POINTS

- Fat grafting to breasts is a good choice for breast augmentation.
- Autologous fat transfer avoids foreign body reaction or capsular contracture, which potentially complicates the implant-based breast augmentation.
- Meticulous fat graft harvesting, processing, and injection is the key to a successful result in the mega-volume fat grafting.
- Pregrafting skin expansion is necessary for patients with tight breast skin tissue.
- Postoperative care with immobilization of the graft is imperative for a satisfactory outcome.

INTRODUCTION

There has been a renewal of interest in the fat grafting to breasts recently. Reasons for revisiting of these techniques are its advantages over implant-based breast augmentation, including avoidance of foreign body with implants and its associated complications such as capsular contracture and malposition deformity. Initially, the safety and efficacy of fat grafting to the breasts had been questioned mainly due to the issues of low graft survival percentage and its associated complications. The statement from the American Society of Plastic Surgery Fat Grafting Task Force in 2009 suggested that fat grafting may be indicated for breast augmentation and reconstruction.[1] Emerging reports in the literature have also echoed the safety and efficacy of fat grafting to breasts because the postoperative incidence of malignancy is not increased[2,3] and the limited

data regarding the radiologic impact of fat grafting to breasts suggest that there is little interference with breast cancer screening.[4]

The technique for fat grafting should be performed in 3 stages: harvesting of adipose tissue from proper donor sites, processing of lipoaspirate to remove impure nonfat tissues, and meticulous reinjection of the purified fat grafts to ensure an even distribution of the grafts in the breasts. Proper patient selection is the key to achieving a superior outcome of primary fat grafting for breast augmentation, specifically referring to the need for a special consideration to the skin pliability and stretching ability of the patient's chest skin. In this article, the authors share their established and rationalized techniques of fat grafting for primary breast augmentation and propose an algorithmic approach to fat necrosis after fat grafting for breast augmentation as a way of managing complications.

[a] Freya Aesthetic Institute, 5F, No. 300, Song Long Road, Taipei 100, Taiwan; [b] Division of Plastic Surgery, Department of Surgery, University of California Davis Medical Center, 2335 Stockton Blvd., Room 6008, Sacramento, California 95817, USA
* Corresponding author.
E-mail address: llpu@ucdavis.edu

Clin Plastic Surg 50 (2023) 189–200
https://doi.org/10.1016/j.cps.2022.07.002

INDICATIONS AND CONTRAINDICATIONS

Patients who have abundant adipose tissues as the donor site for harvest and pliable skin pocket and sufficient tissue dimension that serves as a good recipient base for injection of adequate volume of graft will be well indicated for breast augmentation with fat grafting. The patient who expects a volume of 120 to 150 cc increase is also a good candidate because this procedure has limitation in the increment of breast size in one session of fat grafting. There is no absolute contraindication for this procedure. However, patients who do not have sufficient adipose tissues to be harvested and those who have deficient breast skin envelopes and disagree to undergo either internal or external tissue expansion when necessary are not good candidates for this procedure.

PREOPERATIVE EVALUATION AND SPECIAL CONSIDERATIONS

Patients with a higher risk of breast cancer should be well informed that long-term safety issue of fat grafting to breasts in patients of this category has not been fully investigated. Therefore, it is suggested that patients with a higher risk of breast malignancy not have fat grafting to breasts unless they are willing to pay an additional attention and effort in breast cancer surveillance after the operation. Fat necrosis can develop in the form of solid tumors and calcification that potentially complicates breast cancer screening.

The volume of available fat is important for preliminary assessment of the volume to be harvested for single or multiple sessions of fat grafting depending upon patient's expectation. Estimation of the volume of body fat is conveniently achieved by palm measurement in which one palm size is about 180 to 200 cm^2 depending on the surgeon's palm size.[5] The thickness of fat tissue is tested by a pinch test. The volume of fat to be collected is calculated by the product of the estimated surface area and thickness of fat to be suctioned (volume = palm size 200 cm^2 × thickness of fat to be suctioned). In general, a total of 700 to 800 mL of lipoaspirates (not including the infranatant) can be harvested from both thighs and is enough for most patients.

A special attention should be paid to the breast skin tightness or constricted breast. The skin tightness can be tested by stretching and pulling breast skin off the body with how much effort and strength. Patients with a short nipple to inframammary fold distance may serve as a sign of tight lower pole skin. Note especially that

expansion of the skin dimension in the lower pole is an indispensable part for achieving an esthetic breast contour in tight breast skin envelope. In addition to the ideal contour of breast shape, patients who desire an increment of more than 2 breast cup size should be informed of the necessity of multiple sessions of grafting.

SURGICAL PROCEDURES

Favorable donor sites include areas that uniformly have abundant or excess adipose tissues to be harvested such as abdomen, flanks, buttocks, medial and lateral thighs, or knees. Generally, donor sites are selected where body contouring with liposuction is easily accessible in the supine position. Although viability of adipocytes within the fat grafts from different donor sites has been reported to be equal, higher cell concentration of lipoaspirates is found in the lower abdomen and inner thigh[6] in the young (21–37 years old) female group (**Fig. 1**). They are also better donor sites of adult mesenchymal stem cells and therefore should be chosen as the "preferred" donor sites for fat transplantation.[7]

Fat Graft Harvesting

The surgical procedure is normally performed under general anesthesia, or intravenous sedation. The tumescent solution used for donor site analgesia or hemostasis should contain lidocaine that synergizes with general anesthesia. However, we suggest that lidocaine concentration be kept to a minimum because lidocaine toxicity is detrimental to adipocyte function and viability.[8] Generally, we use 0.01% lidocaine in Ringer's lactate if performed under general anesthesia. The tumescent solution contains epinephrine with a concentration of 1:200,000. Vasoconstriction effect from

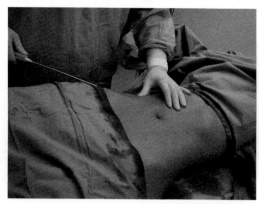

Fig. 1. Liposuction for harvest of fat graft from lower abdomen and inner thighs as the preferred donor sites.

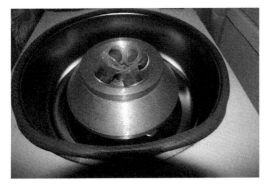

Fig. 2. Centrifugation of the lipoaspirate in the 50 mL syringes with 3000 rpm (1200g) for 3 minutes.

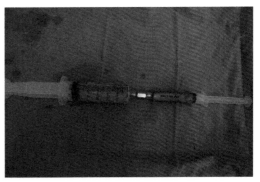

Fig. 4. Transfer of centrifuged fat graft from 50 mL syringe to 10 mL syringe for better control of injection.

epinephrine promotes hemostasis and reduces the risk of intra-arterial injection of the fat graft.

A 4-mm incision is made for infiltration of tumescent solution and for graft harvest with a No. 11 blade in the locations where the scar can be hidden in the groin crease with clothing. The tumescent solution is then infiltrated evenly to the donor site 10 to 15 minutes before fat extraction, which makes harvesting of fat graft easier and less traumatic. The ratio of aspirated fat to tumescent solution volume is about 1:1. The suction power for suction-assisted lipectomy using the machine was set to a negative pressure as low as 70 mm Hg. Lipoaspirates are collected into a 2 L or 3 L canister, which has a draining hose attached to its bottom. The watery part at the bottom of the canister is drained out after lipoaspirate is set standstill for a while by gravity. The fat portion in the lipoaspirates is then collected through the hose connection into syringes of the volume size of the surgeon's preference for convenience of centrifugation.

Fat Graft Processing

The authors choose a 50 mL Luer-Lok syringe for more efficient fat graft processing in mega-

volume fat grafting. The fat portion of the lipoaspirates can be easily transferred to a 50 mL Luer-Lok syringe, which is snugly attached to the flexible hose that drains out the lipoaspirates. The Luer-Lok aperture of the syringe is then locked with a plug. After careful removal of the plunger, all lipoaspirate-filled syringes are then centrifuged with 3000 rpm (about 1200g) for 3 minutes as advocated by Coleman (**Fig. 2**). Centrifugation with a greater g force or longer duration may be harmful to adipocytes and is therefore not recommended.[9]

In authors' experience, centrifuged lipoaspirates can be concentrated into 60% of its original

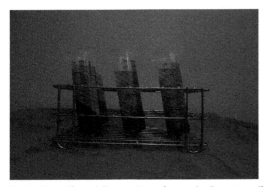

Fig. 3. Centrifuged lipoaspirate layers in 3 parts: oil (*top*), centrifuged fat (*middle*), and water part (*bottom*).

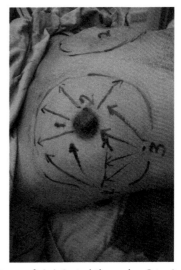

Fig. 5. Far graft is injected through a 3 to 4 mm incision in the inferior or lateral inframammary fold or around the areola border. Fat graft is injected into all layers (subcutaneous tissue, breast parenchyma, and above, inside, and under pectoralis muscle) of breast tissue and fanned out in a radial fashion to achieve an even distribution of graft in the breast tissue.

volume. Therefore, an estimated 700 to 900 cc lipoaspirate is needed for conversion into 400 to 600 mL of concentrated fat for injection after centrifugation. Every effort should be made to stick to the "no touch" principle in which fat graft exposure to air should be kept to a minimum to avoid graft contamination. After centrifugation, lipoaspirates in the syringe are divided into 3 layers: the oil content in the upper layer, fatty tissue in the middle layer, and the watery portion at the bottom (**Fig. 3**). The oil can be decanted from the syringe. The residual oil is wicked with a cotton strip or swab. The fluid at the bottom can be easily drained out once the plug at the Luer-Lok aperture is removed. The concentrated fat in the 50 mL syringe can then be transferred to a 10 mL syringe (our preferred size of syringe for fat injection in primary fat grafting to breasts; **Fig. 4**). Pay attention to the air bubbles inside the syringe and they should be removed and thus quantification of the volume injected can be precise.

Placement of Fat Grafts

Injection of fat graft to the breast requires an understanding the relevant anatomy in this area for safety and efficacy of this operation. The key to a successful fat graft injection is to achieve an even distribution of fat grafts in the recipient site. A 15-cm 12-gauge cannula is attached to a 10 mL syringe containing the fat graft, which is then slowly injected into the breast and fanned out in a radial fashion through a 3 to 4 mm incision. Fat graft is injected in small amounts as the cannula is withdrawn; we use multiple passes, with multiple tunnels, and within multiple tissue planes. Specifically, small aliquot of graft (0.5 mL) should be injected while withdrawing the cannula for a distance of at least 12 to 15 cm. One practical

way to avoid repeated injection at the same spot is that the resistance is always felt during the advancement of the cannula into the virgin tissue before graft injected. Topographically, fat graft is injected into the subcutaneous layer, inside or behind the breast parenchyma, inside the pectoralis muscle (the proximal part of muscle), and behind the muscle as if the graft is totally infiltrated into the breast tissue. The choices of incision location include the inferior and lateral positions near the inframammary fold and around the border of nipple areolar complex where scars can be easily hidden (**Fig. 5**). Injection should be as gentle as possible to avoid a possible injury to vessel or nerve. Advancement of the cannula with too much force would compromise vascularity of the recipient tissue that is important to nourish the graft and increases the chance of complications. The end point of fat injection is based on the tension across the skin pocket due to filling of the fat graft as judged by the operating surgeon. In general, the injection volume of concentrated fat is between 150 and 250 mL for each side of breast depending on the patient's original breast tissue volume. Deeper to the subpectoral level lies the rib cages and intercostal muscles and thus injection should not point downward toward the thorax once the cannula is deep to subpectoral level because pneumothorax may occur once cannula penetrates the pleura.

Preexpansion of tight breast skin pocket

Tissue expansion can be external vacuum expansion (EVE) or internal expansion with implant placement. EVE such as Brava system is to create a continued negative pressure on the breast skin mounted by a dome-shaped device. Successful application of EVE requires attentive education to

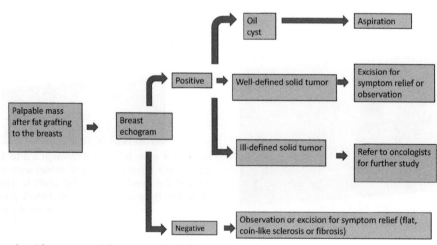

Fig. 6. The algorithm proposed for approach of fat necrosis following fat grafting to the breasts.

the patients and strict patients' compliance. Therefore, the authors preferred implant or tissue expander for internal expansion, which provides a stable and reliable expansion of the breast skin pocket especially at the lower pole of the breast. The implant/tissue expander is placed subpectorally to achieve an esthetically larger breast mound, and this procedure is no different from implant-based breast augmentation surgery. The implant/tissue expander expansion can be effective in as short as 1 to 2 months after implantation. Surgeons should avoid injection into the capsule cavity left after implant explantation because fat grafts in the cavity will not survive and fat necrosis will develop eventually. Fat graft should be injected to the areas anterior to the anterior wall of the capsule. If unfortunately capsular contracture develops, then capsulotomy or capsulectomy should be done to release the contracture holding skin from expanding to a good contour. Capsulotomy was performed for Grade 1-2 capsular contracture and partial capsulectomy on the anterior wall for Grade 3-4 capsular contracture to ensure an adequate expansion of subcutaneous skin pocket for maximum lipofilling, especially in the lower pole of the breast.

POSTOPERATIVE CARE AND EXPECTED OUTCOME

Patients are instructed not to exercise strenuously using pectoralis major muscles in the first 3 months

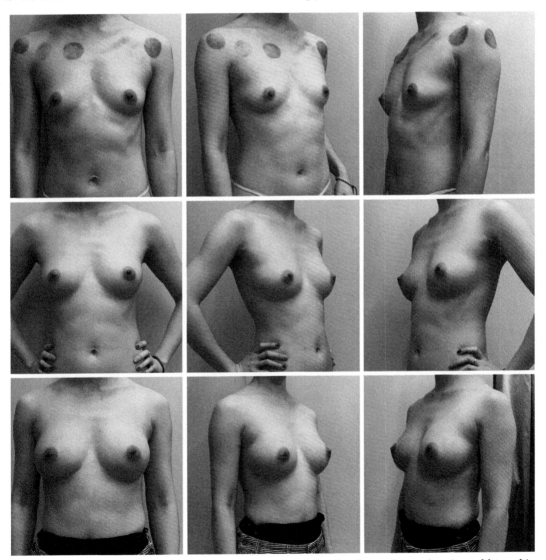

Fig. 7. Comparison of the preoperative original photos, 12 months after first and second sessions of fat grafting to the breasts. The first and second sessions of fat grafting are 12 months apart. The volume of first session grafting is 210 cc on each side breast. The volume of second session is 190 cc on each side.

following the surgery. It is also imperative that patients not have hard compression or tight clothing on the breasts for the same period postoperatively. The rationale is that mobility and tight compression on the graft recipient site may violate neovascularization to the fat grafts. Swelling in the recipient site is expected for 1 or 2 weeks. The long-term fat graft retention rate has been reported with variable success in the literature.[10,11] Based on our experience, about 60% (or about 110–130 mL) of the long-term graft volume retention rate can be achieved.[12]

MANAGEMENT OF COMPLICATIONS

Serious complications such as pneumothorax at graft injection or breast tissue infection is very rare. Meticulous injection and awareness of the direction of the cannula tip can avoid inadvertent pulmonary puncturing. Aggressive antibiotic treatment pending bacteria culture is necessary and serial debridement and adequate drainage are imperative for salvage if infection develops.

The most commonly seen complication of fat grafting to the breasts is fat necrosis.

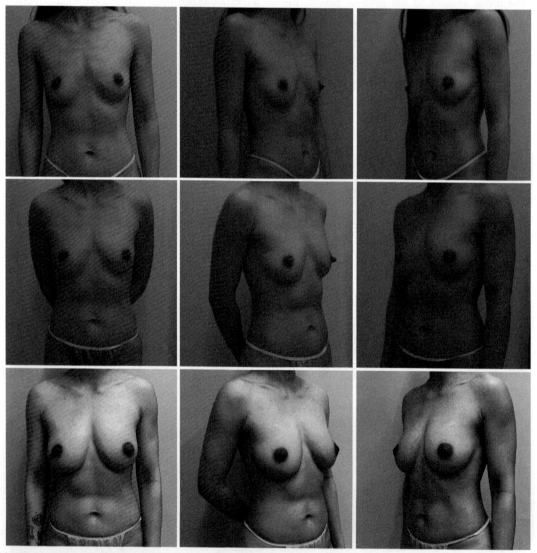

Fig. 8. Comparisons of original preoperative photos and the first and second postoperative photos are done and demonstrate the satisfactory outcomes both at 5 years of follow-up. The first and second sessions of fat grafting to the breast are 5 years apart. The first and second session of fat grafting volume for both side breasts were 220 and 200 cc, respectively.

Nonabsorbed necrotic fat in the form of oily cyst, sclerotic induration, and calcified solid tumor may cause palpability, pain on palpation, skin retraction, dermatitis, and postinflammatory hyperpigmentation. Although there has been no scientific data showing that fat necrosis-related tumors and calcifications can interfere with breast cancer screening, they may potentially complicate breast health check-up. Therefore, complications from fat necrosis in the breast should be managed promptly and properly. We suggest that any palpable mass noticed postoperatively should have breast imaging study such as breast echogram, which is noninvasive and relatively quick to perform as a screening tool.[12] Oily cyst located superficially can simply aspirated using syringe with an 18-gauge needle. Hard fibrotic or calcified nodules can be excised through a stab incision directly above the lesion site or mammotome that is used for core needle breast biopsy. In the author's practice, we manage fat necrosis through an algorithm using a mammotome (**Fig. 6**).

REVISION OR SUBSEQUENT PROCEDURES

Once the final result (with a waiting period of 4–6 months) has achieved, the need for subsequent

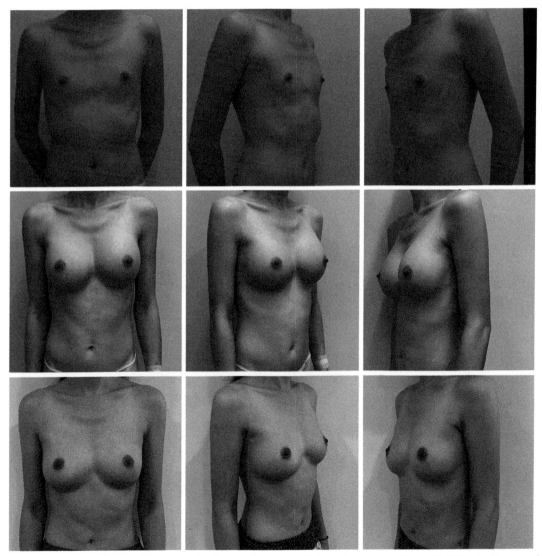

Fig. 9. Comparison photos of preoperative breasts (*upper row*), breast augmentation with 300 mL silicone gel implants (*middle*), and implant explantation with simultaneous fat grafting to the breasts (*bottom*). Skin expansion with breast implant augmentation lasts for 1 year before explantation and immediate injection with 230 mL of fat graft to the breasts.

revision to improve the breast contour is rare. However, patient may need a repeated injection for further augmentation. There is no scientific study, which has addressed the timing of subsequent fat grafting. It is difficult to assess the surgical outcome at the initial stage following the operation. In general, we have observed the transplanted fat gradually loses its volume with time and usually becomes stabilized at 4 to 6 months postoperatively. Therefore, the timing of a subsequent fat grafting procedure should be deferred to at least 3 to 4 months after the previous transplantation. In addition, patients should be informed that the result of the breast volume is still subject to change in accordance with the body weight change even when the outcome is finalized.

CASE DEMONSTRATION
Case 1

A 30-year-old woman had undergone 2 times of fat grafting to her bilateral breasts for augmentation. Her breast skin tissue is soft, and pliable when stretched. The volume of first session grafting is 210 cc on each side breast. The volume of second session is 190 cc on each side. Comparison photos of original and the first and second grafting to the breasts are shown (**Fig. 7**). The patient is satisfied with the surgical results with no complications.

Case 2

This 35-year-old woman received fat grafting for bilateral breast augmentation twice. Her breast

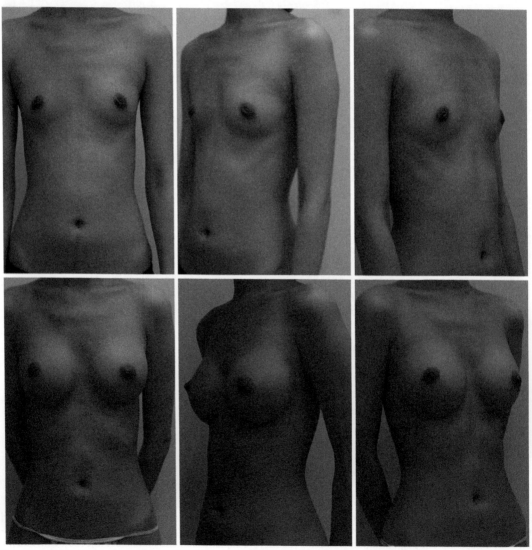

Fig. 10. Preoperative and postoperative photos of breast augmentation with 330 mL gel implants are shown.

skin envelope is elastic and pliable during stretching. Comparisons of original preoperative photos and the first and second postoperative photos are done and demonstrate the satisfactory outcomes in long-term follow-up (**Fig. 8**).

Case 3

This 25-year-old woman requests fat grafting for breast augmentation and wishes to have 2 to 3 breast cup size increase. Her original breast skin tissue is tight and therefore pregrafting tissue expansion is planned. Breast augmentation with 300 cc silicone gel implants was done. Explantation was done 1 year later and immediate fat grafting was performed with injection volume of 230 cc to the bilateral side breasts. A satisfactory result is shown 6 months after breast implant explantation and simultaneous fat grafting (**Fig. 9**).

Case 4

Breast augmentation with the implant of 330 mL (**Fig. 10**) through transaxillary approach was planned in this 22-year-old woman as the method of preexpansion of breast skin before fat grafting to the breasts. Two sessions of fat grafting to the breasts were done after explantation. The first session of fat grafting of 200 mL was done immediately in each side breast after explantation. The second session of fat grafting of 210 mL in each breast was done 4 years following the first grafting. Comparison of postoperative photos of first and second session of fat grafting are shown

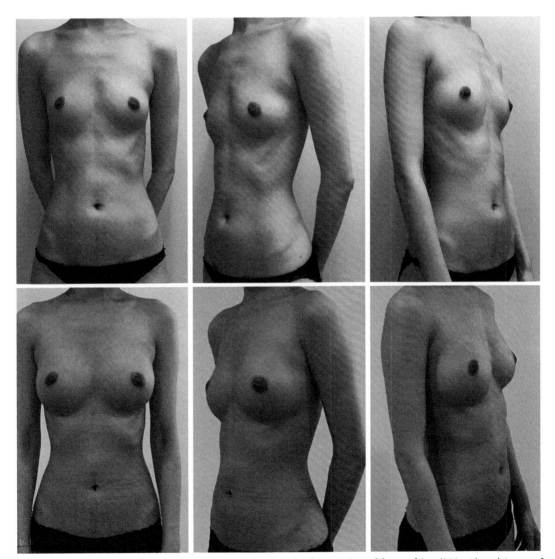

Fig. 11. Comparison of postoperative photos 4 years after the first session of fat grafting (200 mL) and 1 year after the second session of fat grafting (210 mL) are shown.

(Fig. 11). Comparing photos of the original breasts and after the second session of fat grafting are also shown (Fig. 12).

DISCUSSION

Surgical techniques are important to a successful result in primary breast augmentation with fat grafting. Delicate graft harvesting, refinement of graft processing to provide pure parcels of adipose tissue with integrity and meticulous reinjection of adipose tissue to the recipient sites are all equally essential for the long-term fat graft retention. We prefer to use 4 mm cannula for harvesting. Harvesting cannulas with a larger caliber are managed to collect larger adipose parcels and

have been shown to improve adipocyte viability and long-term graft survival.[13] This can be accounted for by the fact that larger caliber cannulas lead to less shearing force and less traumatic to adipocytes during procurement. Higher viability of adipocytes with 4 mm cannulas was demonstrated compared with 2 and 3 mm cannulas in a randomized prospective study reported by Ozsoy and colleagues.[14]

Despite the literature has thus far failed to reveal a single superior method for fat graft processing, centrifugation is perhaps the most recognized technique for processing and has been considered the standard. In order to effectively remove the impure materials, including the excess infiltration solution, hematogenous cells, free oil, and the

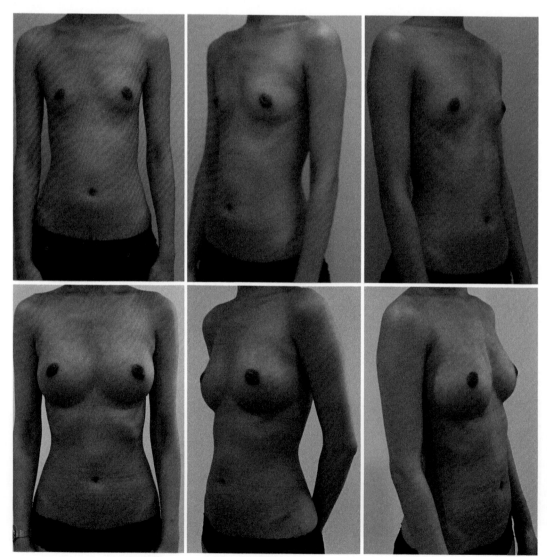

Fig. 12. Preoperative and postoperative photos comparing the original breasts and the final outcome (1 year after the second session of fat grafting) are also shown.

nonfat elements within the lipoaspirates and to obtain more concentrated fat grafts. Not only do these nonfat elements cause inflammation that can be harmful to the fat graft but also injection of debris gives an illusion of adequate volume correction. Moreover, centrifugation separates adipocytes from the substances that may degrade them such as blood cells, proteases, and lipases. In addition, recent studies have shown that proper centrifugation can concentrate not only adipocytes and adipose-derived stem cells (ADSCs) but also several angiogenic growth factors such as fibroblast growth factor and vascular endothelial growth factor within the processed fat grafts.[15] Maximizing the number ratio of ADSCs to the graft promotes the graft survival have been reported by many authors in the literature.[16] However, the exact benefits of ADSC for graft survival and the optimum ratio of ADSC to adipocyte have been elusive and contradictory results of ADSC-assisted lipotransfer have been reported[4] and thus a larger scale of clinical trials is needed.

The principle of reimplantation of fat grafts is based on optimizing recipient site vascularity for increased graft survival.[17] Graft through nutrition by tissue fluid absorption can survive up to 48 hours, whereas the neovascularization proceeds with the rate of 1 mm per day. Therefore, ideally, the diameter of graft parcel should not exceed the diameter of 2 mm to avoid central necrosis.[5,18] Following this science rationale, 1 mL of fat graft should spread across a path of at least 25 to 30 cm in length when injected as a microcylinder with a diameter of 2 mm or 0.5 mL of graft over a path at least 12 to 15 cm in length.

Overcorrection for "better" graft survival in the recipient site seems to be lack of scientific support. Excessive overcorrection, which increases the complications of fat necrosis and infection especially for breast augmentation that proceeds with mega-quantity fat injection, is not recommended.

SUMMARY

Breast augmentation with primary fat grafting offers an option for breast augmentation and is a procedure that requires a comprehensive understanding of the science of autologous fat transplantation. The surgeon should master the techniques of liposuction and fat injection using the appropriate instruments. Moreover, proper patient selection is also important for a successful outcome. The surgeon should stick to all the principles that have been described here to ensure a satisfactory result.

CLINICS CARE POINTS

- Evaluation of the appropriate candidate for fat grafting to the breasts is a critical step for an optimal result, including the availability of fat graft harvest, and pliability of breast skin envelope.

- Meticulous graft injection following the principle of multiple planes and multiple tunnel and avoidance of over grafting is the key to a successful result and reduction of complications.

- Preexpansion of breast skin and tissue is an important step for achieving an esthetic breast shape and larger volume of graft retention before fat grafting to the breasts in patients with constricted breasts or tight breast skin envelopes.

DISCLOSURE

The authors have nothing to declare regarding the products, drugs, or devices mentioned in this article.

REFERENCES

1. Gutowski KA. Current applications and safety of autologous fat grafts: a report of the ASPS fat graft task force. Plast Reconstr Surg 2009;124(1):272–80.
2. Coleman S, Saboeiro AP. Fat grafting to the breast revisited: safety and efficacy. Plast Reconstr Surg 2007;119(3):775–85.
3. Zheng DN, Li QF, Lei H, et al. Autologous fat grafting to the breast for cosmetic enhancement: experience in 66 patients with long-term follow up. J Plast Reconstr Aesth Surg 2008;61:792–8.
4. Parikh R, Doren P, Mooney B, et al. Differentiating fat necrosis from recurrent malignancy in fat-grafted breasts. Plast Reconstr Surg 2012;130(4):761–72.
5. Khouri RK, Rigotti G, Cardoso E, et al. Megavolum autologous fat transfer: part II. Practice and techniques. Plats Reconstr Surg 2014;133(6):1369–77.
6. Padoin AV, Braga-Silva J, Martins P, et al. Sources of processed lipoaspirate cells: influence of donor site on cell concentration. Plast Reconstr Surg 2008; 122(2):614–8.
7. Yoshimura K, Suga H, Eto H. Adipose-derived stem/progenitor cells: roles in adipose tissue remodeling and potential use for soft tissue augmentation. Regen Med 2009;4(2):265–73.
8. Keck M, Zeyda M, Gollinger K, et al. Local anesthetics have a major impact on viability of

preadipocytes and their differentiation into adipo-cytes. Plast Reconstr Surg 2010;123(5):1500–5.

9. Kurita M, Matsumoto D, Shigeura T, et al. Influences of centrifugation on cells and tissues in liposuction aspirates: optimized centrifugation for lipotransfer and cell isolation. Plast Reconstr Surg 2008;121(3):1033–41.

10. Hyakusoku H, Ogawa R, Ono S, et al. Complications after autologous fat injection to the breast. Plast Reconstr Surg 2009;123(1):360–70.

11. Petit JY, Lohsiriwat V, Clough KB, et al. The onco-logic outcome and immediate surgical complica-tions of lipofilling in breast cancer patients: a multicenter study—milan-Paris-Lyon experience of 646. Plast Reconstr Surg 2011;128(2):341–6.

12. Lin JY, Song P, Pu LLQ. Management of fat necrosis after autologous fat transplantation for breast augmentation. Plast Reconstr Surg 2018;142(5):665–73.

13. Kirkman JC, Lee JH, Medina MA III, et al. The impact of liposuction cannula size on adipocyte viability. Ann Plast Surg 2012;69(4):479–81.

14. Ozsoy Z, Kul Z, Bilir A. The role of cannula diameter in improved adipocyte viability: a quantitative anal-ysis. Aesthet J Surg 2006;26(3):287–9.

15. Pallua N, Pulsfort AK, Suschek C, et al. Content of the growth factors bFGF, IGF-1, VEGF, and PDGF-BB in freshly harvested lipoaspirate after centrifuga-tion and incubation. Plast Reconstr Surg 2009;123(3):826–33.

16. Coleman SR. Structural fat grafting: more than a per-manent filler. Plast Reconstr Surg 2006;118(3S):108S–20S.

17. Kakagia D, Pallua N. Autologous fat grafting: in search of the optimal technique. Surg Innov 2014;21(3):327–36.

18. Khouri RK, Rigotti G, Cardoso E, et al. Megavolume autologous fat transfer: part I. Theory and principles. Plast Reconstr Surg 2014;133(3):550–7.

Moving?

Make sure your subscription moves with you!

To notify us of your new address, find your **Clinics Account Number** (located on your mailing label above your name), and contact customer service at:

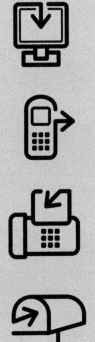

Email: journalscustomerservice-usa@elsevier.com

800-654-2452 (subscribers in the U.S. & Canada)
314-447-8871 (subscribers outside of the U.S. & Canada)

Fax number: 314-447-8029

Elsevier Health Sciences Division
Subscription Customer Service
3251 Riverport Lane
Maryland Heights, MO 63043

*To ensure uninterrupted delivery of your subscription, please notify us at least 4 weeks in advance of move.

Printed and bound by CPI Group (UK) Ltd, Croydon, CR0 4YY

08/05/2025

01864715-0016